CURRENT ANTIBIOTIC THERAPY

CURRENT ANTIBIOTIC THERAPY

EDITORS

A. M. GEDDES, F.R.C.P.E.
Consultant Physician, East Birmingham Hospital, Birmingham

J. D. WILLIAMS, M.D., M.R.C.Path.
Consultant Microbiologist, Dudley Road Hospital, Birmingham

1973
CHURCHILL LIVINGSTONE
EDINBURGH AND LONDON

First published 1973

International Standard Book Number
0 443 00975 9

Any correspondence relating to this volume should be directed to the publishers at 15 Teviot Place, Edinburgh EH1 2XX

Printed in Great Britain by
William Clowes & Sons Limited
London, Colchester and Beccles

PREFACE

Although penicillin was discovered by Alexander Fleming in 1929, it did not become generally available for the treatment of patients until thirty years ago. Since then there has been an almost constant flow of new antibiotics. Unfortunately, the microbiological Utopia which was envisaged in the 1940's has not materialized and infection remains a significant cause of morbidity and mortality. Viral and fungal infections, bacterial resistance to chemotherapeutic agents and adverse reactions to antibiotics are problems which concern all who are interested in the treatment of patients suffering from infective disease.

Under the joint sponsorship of the Midland Medical Society and the Board of Graduate Studies of the University of Birmingham, and with financial support from Beecham Research Laboratories, a Symposium entitled 'Antibiotics After Thirty Years' was held in Birmingham in February 1972. The meeting was designed as a dialogue between clinicians and bacteriologists and many important aspects of antimicrobial chemotherapy were discussed by a distinguished group of speakers. The proceedings of the symposium are published in this volume.

It is with deep regret that we record the death of one of the contributors, Sister M. E. Harris, who died as the result of an accident some weeks after the meeting.

We are grateful to Dr. R. B. Hunter for giving the Opening Address of the meeting and to the session Chairmen. We are especially indebted to Mr. D. Goodchild and Professor A. P. D. Thomson for their help with the organization of the symposium and to Professor Francis O'Grady for his advice and support.

We wish to acknowledge the invaluable assistance of Miss P. M. Kirby, Mrs. G. Jeffries, Mrs. D. Hammond, Mrs. A. Smith and Dr. J. Kosmidis in the preparation of this book.

CONTRIBUTORS

P. ACRED, B.Sc., Chemotherapeutic Research Centre, Beecham Research Laboratories, Brockham Park.

SIR MELVILLE ARNOTT, M.D., F.R.C.P., Professor of Cardiology, University of Birmingham.

A. W. ASSCHER, M.D., F.R.C.P., Reader in Medicine, Welsh National School of Medicine, Cardiff.

G. A. J. AYLIFFE, M.D., M.R.C.Path., Consultant Microbiologist, Hospital Infection Research Laboratory, Birmingham.

D. J. BAUER, Ph.D., F.R.C.Path., Wellcome Laboratories of Tropical Medicine, Beckenham.

M. V. BAIMBRIDGE, F.R.C.S., Consultant Surgeon, St. Thomas's Hospital, London.

G. C. BRANDER, B.Sc., M.R.C.V.S., Nutritional Research Centre, Beecham Research Laboratories, Tadworth.

W. BRUMFITT, M.D., F.R.C.Path., Professor of Microbiology, Royal Free Hospital, London.

A. B. CHRISTIE, M.D., F.R.C.P., Consultant Physician, Fazakerley Hospital, Liverpool.

N. DATTA, M.D., M.R.C.Path., Senior Lecturer in Microbiology, Royal Postgraduate Medical School, London.

S. EYKYN, M.B., Ch.B., Lecturer in Microbiology, St. Thomas's Hospital, London.

A. M. GEDDES, F.R.C.P.E., Consultant Physician, East Birmingham Hospital, Birmingham.

R. R. GILLIES, M.D., F.R.C.Path., Senior Lecturer in Bacteriology, University of Edinburgh.

J. C. GOULD, M.D., F.R.C.Path., Director, Central Microbiological Laboratories, Edinburgh.

M. E. HARRIS, R.G.N., Nursing Officer, Regional Renal Unit, East Birmingham Hospital, Birmingham.

R. B. HUNTER, M.B.E., M.D., F.R.C.P., Vice-Chancellor, University of Birmingham.

J. C. KOSMIDIS, M.D., Research Fellow, East Birmingham & Dudley Road Hospitals, Birmingham.

H. P. LAMBERT, M.D., F.R.C.P., Consultant Physician, St. George's Hospital, London.

D. J. LANE, M.D., M.R.C.P., Consultant Physician, The Churchill Hospital, Oxford.

E. J. L. Lowbury, M.D., F.R.C.Path., Consultant Bacteriologist, Burns Research Unit, Accident Hospital, Birmingham.

J. F. Munro, F.R.C.P.E., Consultant Physician, Eastern General Hospital, Edinburgh.

F. W. O'Grady, M.D., F.R.C.Path., Professor of Bacteriology, St. Bartholomew's Hospital, London.

M. T. Parker, M.D., F.R.C.Path., Director, Staphylococcal Reference Laboratory, Central Public Health Laboratory, Colindale.

A. Percival, M.R.C.Path., Senior Lecturer in Microbiology, University of Liverpool.

R. G. Petersdorf, M.D., F.A.C.P., Chairman, Department of Medicine, University of Washington, Seattle, U.S.A.

I. Phillips, M.D., M.R.C.Path., Reader in Microbiology, St. Thomas's Hospital, London.

M. H. Richmond, Ph.D., Professor of Microbiology, University of Bristol.

M. Ridley, M.R.C.Path., Consultant Microbiologist, St. Thomas's Hospital, London.

K. B. Rogers, M.D., F.R.C.Path., Consultant Microbiologist, Children's Hospital, Birmingham.

G. N. Rolinson, D.Sc., Chemotherapeutic Research Centre, Beecham Research Laboratories, Brockham Park.

E. K. Smith, M.R.C.O.G., Senior Registrar in Obstetrics, Walsgrave Hospital, Coventry.

R. Sutherland, B.Sc., Chemotherapeutic Research Centre, Beecham Research Laboratories, Brockham Park.

O. L. Wade, M.D., F.R.C.P., Professor of Clinical Pharmacology, University of Birmingham.

H. J. O. White, M.Chir., F.R.C.S., Consultant Surgeon, United Bristol Hospitals, Bristol.

A. G. W. Whitfield, M.D., F.R.C.P., Professor of Post-Graduate Studies, University of Birmingham.

R. R. Willcox, M.D., M.R.C.P., Consultant Venereologist, St. Mary's Hospital, London.

J. A. Williams, Ch.M., F.R.C.S., Consultant Surgeon, United Birmingham Hospitals, Birmingham.

J. D. Williams, M.D., M.R.C.Path., Consultant Microbiologist, Dudley Road Hospital, Birmingham.

R. E. O. Williams, M.D., F.R.C.Path., Professor of Bacteriology, St. Mary's Hospital, London.

H. I. Winner, M.D., F.R.C.Path., Professor of Bacteriology, Charing Cross Hospital, London.

ADDITIONAL PARTICIPANTS IN DISCUSSIONS

Dr. S. Campbell, *Kent*; Dr. E. A. P. Croydon, *Beecham Research Laboratories, London*; Dr. L. Goldman, *Leo Laboratories, London*; Dr. W. Griffel, *Oxfordshire*; Mr. D. M. Hancock, *Sunderland Group Hospitals, Sunderland*; Professor G. R. F. Hilson, *St. George's Hospital, London*; Dr. J. L. Honigman, *I.C.I. Ltd., Macclesfield*; Dr. I. Lennox-Smith, *Roche Laboratories, London*; Mr. R. L. Lamming, *Nobles Hospital, Douglas, Isle of Man*; Dr. J. G. Lewis, *Edgware General Hospital, Edgware, Middx*; Dr. D. Shanson, *University College Hospital, London*; Dr. N. A. Simmons, *Guy's Hospital, London*; Dr. Hillas Smith, *Royal Free Hospital, London*; Dr. J. S. Stevenson, *Stobhill General Hospital, Glasgow*; Dr. Joan Stokes, *University College Hospital, London*; Dr. J. Vahrman, *Westminster Hospital, London*; Miss P. M. Waterworth, *University College Hospital, London*; Dr. G. M. Williamson, *Pfizer Ltd., London.*

FOREWORD

In the symposium on which this book is based many facets of antibiotic therapy were discussed. I do not wish to detail these discussions but would like to mention a few of the historical events in antibiotic development.

Because of the toxicity of antiseptic compounds most people in the 1930's considered that cure of infections with systemic agents was not a profitable exercise. It was only when Domagk and Beauvais published their work on sulphonamides that attitudes began to change. Fleming's pioneer work on penicillin had been largely ignored but the sulphonamides stimulated further efforts and with the support of the Rockefeller Foundation the major advances of Florey, Chain and their colleagues were possible.

One would have thought that this discovery of penicillin and its introduction in the 1940's for clinical use would have been sufficient for a generation but before long chloramphenicol was being widely used in South East Asia for the treatment of mite typhus, and is now crucial in the treatment of typhoid fever. Then in 1944 Waksman and his colleagues described the isolation of streptomycin, an antibiotic much less toxic than actinomycin, which had a broader spectrum than penicillin; it was active against gram-negative organisms and subsequently was shown to be effective treatment in a variety of forms of tuberculosis. Now it is an essential, indispensable part of that treatment.

The research and development of the pharmaceutical industry has given rise to hundreds of new anti-bacterial substances. Many of these are only of biochemical interest; only a few of clinical importance, such as the tetracyclines, kanamycin, lincomycin, the polymyxins and the anti-fungal antibiotic amphotericin B. All these, no mean achievement, were discovered in industrial laboratories. The last of the vitally important groups, cephalosporin-C, was isolated in a small Public Health Laboratory in Sardinia by an Italian Public Health Officer, Dr. Brotzu, who noted its striking action against salmonellae. The structure of cephalosporin was determined at Oxford by Abraham and Newton and, with x-ray crystallography studies by Dorothy Hodgkin, its structure was proved to be similar to that of penicillin. It contains the four-membered beta-lactam ring but this is fused with the six-membered thiazine ring instead of with the five-membered thiazolidine ring. Penicillin and cephalosporins, as you know, can be interconverted by chemical methods.

The massive screening programme of the pharmaceutical industry began to peter out in the late nineteen-fifties. It became evident that conventional screening was not getting anywhere and it was not a profitable line to pursue. Therefore attention was directed to the efforts by Sir Ernest Chain to try and modify the penicillin molecule. He started in 1955 and a number of Beecham's research workers came and worked with him. In 1956 they went back to their own laboratory, where they managed to identify by simple chromatographic means a substance formed in the culture fluid in the absence of the precursor acid which behaved chemically like penicillin but had little or no biological activity. They showed that after phenacetylation of the culture fluid benzylpenicillin was formed. This substance proved to be the nucleus of the penicillin molecule, 6-aminopenicillanic acid.

Three groups of semi-synthetic penicillins have resulted from this work. First, the acid stable penicillins—not very different from benzylpenicillin but with improved chemical and physical properties. Secondly, penicillins resistant to penicillinase and therefore active against the penicillin-resistant staphylococci and thirdly, broader spectrum penicillins, the prime example of which is ampicillin: much less toxic than chloramphenicol or the tetracyclines.

I would like to congratulate the Board of Graduate Studies of the University of Birmingham, the Midland Medical Society and Beecham Research Laboratories for their initiative in arranging this Symposium. I do not know whether a steady state will ever be reached in the antibiotic field but it is undoubtedly an opportune moment to examine the situation and I congratulate them for calling together such a distinguished group of people. A much wider audience will benefit from this publication.

R. B. HUNTER

CONTENTS

1

ANTIBIOTICS IN PERSPECTIVE

Dialogue between

FRANCIS O'GRADY AND H. P. LAMBERT

Dr. Lambert

Francis O'Grady and I have taken as our task in this opening session on 'Antibiotics in perspective' the drawing up of a profit and loss account of antibiotic experience and the delineation of the principal requirements which we think are still unmet. We thought that two separate talks, each of us taking our assigned role as bacteriologist and clinician might lead to the danger seen in medical symposia as often as in Pinter's plays, of two approaches which run parallel but by the same token never meet. We decided therefore that we would make our presentation in the form of a dialogue. The wide scope of our brief means that we shall raise many points that we will be unable to answer, and I hope some of these will serve as foci for later discussion.

Professor O'Grady

I suppose the best way of trying to get the antibiotic situation into perspective is to begin at the beginning and remind ourselves what the infectious diseases situation looked like thirty or more years ago when effective chemotherapy first became available. Would you like to show us what the situation was?

ANTIBIOTICS AND MORTALITY FROM INFECTIOUS DISEASES

Dr. Lambert

One fairly familiar way of trying to start a profit and loss account is to look at the incidence of mortality of certain infectious diseases before and after the antibiotic era. As you know, this tends to give rather surprising results. It is often difficult to discern the effect of antimicrobial drugs amid the remarkable changes, so easy to show, but so recalcitrant to precise analysis, which were wrought by social changes in the rich countries in the last century. One example in which the effect of antimicrobial agents can be seen is that of scarlet fever with the effects of sulphonamides and penicillin probably discernible in the curve of declining mortality. In tuberculosis also the chart shows a considerable steepening of the graph, with declining mortality after the introduction of antituberculous chemotherapy. These effects, however, are small compared with those not directly attributable to antibiotics and you can construct similar curves, for example of the decline of mortality in, say, enteric fever before the introduction of chloramphenicol.

These familiar statistics have often led to two quite opposing misconceptions. On the one hand people have doubted whether any real effect of antimicrobial agents on infectious disease is discernible but of course you only have to consider meningococcal meningitis, pneumococcal pneumonia, or subacute bacterial endocarditis to refute this fallacy—rather like Dr. Johnson discussing with Boswell Bishop Berkeley's theory of the unreality of physical objects. Boswell said the theory could not possibly be refuted and Dr. Johnson hit his foot against a stone with such force that he rebounded from it and said 'Sir, I refute it thus' and I think that if we look at meningococcal meningitis we can refute it thus.

TABLE 1

MORTALITY FROM MEASLES

	Age	
	Under 1 year (%)	*Under 5 years* (%)
Glasgow 1908	12	6
London fever hospitals 1911–14	23	14
Nigeria 1958–61	20	26
England and Wales 1960	0·104	0·030

The opposite fallacy is much more important as an influence which underlies much inappropriate use of antibiotics. This is to suppose that the change of pattern we now see such as the rarity of mastoiditis and other suppurative complications of upper respiratory tract infection and the low mortality of measles and of pertussis are the direct result of antibiotic treatment in the individual patient. These changes clearly cannot be much to do with antibiotics in any very direct way but the expectation of danger which rightly concerned the pre-antibiotic doctor is often still present when the natural history of infectious disease has changed beyond all recognition. Even now you can see simultaneous but quite different patterns of infectious disease in rich as compared with developing countries, differences which cannot be attributed either to variations of the causal agent or to patterns of treatment. Table 1 summarizes Morley's analysis of measles mortality in Nigeria today which looks identical to the list of measles complications in Glasgow or London in 1910. I think this type of fallacy, based on misinterpretation of changing patterns of infection, has dogged antibiotic usage for many years, for example, in gastro-enteritis and in the acute infections of childhood.

AVAILABILITY OF ANTIMICROBIAL AGENTS

Professor O'Grady

It seems pretty clear from what you say that the outstanding successes have generally been associated with the introduction of agents highly effective against the specific pathogen. A dramatic example is penicillin treatment for haemolytic streptococcal infection. One of the things we must look at therefore is the extent to which we have available at the present time agents which are effective against the major pathogens. If we construct a list (Table 2) of the

TABLE 2

AGENTS IN CURRENT THERAPEUTIC USE ACTIVE AGAINST MAJOR PATHOGENS

Haemolytic streptococcus Pneumococcus	Penicillin	Erythromycin	Lincomycin
Staphylococcus	Cloxacillin	Cephalosporins	Fucidin
Enterobacteria	Tetracyclines	Chloramphenicol	Aminoglycosides
Pseudomonas	Polymyxins	Carbenicillin	Gentamicin
Fungi	Polyenes	5-Fluorocytosine	Griseofulvin
Viruses	Idoxuridine	Methisazone	Amantadine

major pathogens: the haemolytic streptococcus, the pneumococcus, the staphylococcus, various kinds of enterobacteria, the pseudomonas and fungi and those extremely important and generally resistant organisms, the viruses, we can match them all with agents. I have included by no means all those which are available in current therapeutic use and which are effective in the laboratory against each of these major organisms. So that from the point of view of availability of effective agents we obviously have the problem licked. We have the agents; the only difficulty is the inability of you chaps to make proper use of them!

RESULTS OF ANTIBIOTIC THERAPY

Dr. Lambert

We started with the idea of a profit and loss account and I think we can draw this up under three general headings. One is success, and the second is modified success and the third is total failure. The successes we don't really have to talk about much but we can point to streptococcal sepsis as a most striking example, not only in the declining mortality figures which we mentioned at the beginning, but in the virtual disappearance of death from puerperal sepsis and indeed of the *Streptococcus pyogenes* as an important cause of puerperal sepsis. It would be hard to think of a more dramatic example than this.

What I think is much more important is to consider the reasons why antimicrobial drugs fail when, as Francis O'Grady has shown, there is nearly always an antibiotic for most of the organisms we have to contend with. These sort of difficulties where success is modified in practice come about for a number of totally different reasons. One main reason is that we are often in deep difficulties about achieving causal diagnoses. There are certain situations in which the clinical diagnosis not only implies a specific organism but also implies a drug sensitivity pattern and classical examples again would be scarlet fever and enteric fever. The difficulty is that on most occasions this is not so, and we either know roughly the organism but not the antibiotic resistance pattern, or even more confusing, we do not know which organism we are dealing with. Now, why are bacteriologists so little help to us in these common situations?

SOME SOURCES OF MISLEADING LABORATORY REPORTS

Professor O'Grady

I am unhappily forced to accept that the microbiologist often fails to help, and may even actually deceive his clinical colleagues—and that for a number of different reasons (Table 3). He may examine the wrong germs, or test their sensitivities to the wrong agents, or even when he tests the right germs and the right agents he not infrequently comes up with the wrong answer. In the first place, instead of discarding those organisms which are contaminants or commensals and plainly have nothing whatever to do with the patient's infection, he laboriously examines and reports them and gives their sensitivities, thereby creating the impression that they play some important pathogenic role. Moreover, from time to time he reports completely inappropriate agents. An outstanding example is the report that organisms recovered from the respiratory tract are sensitive to nitrofurantoin. No doubt they are, but since nitrofurantoin does not reach the lungs it is quite useless in the treatment of pulmonary infection. Now, either the clinician knows that, in which case he thinks the microbiologist is daft—which is probably what he thinks anyway—or he does not, in which case he treats the patient with nitrofurantoin and not surprisingly the patient is not benefited at all!

TABLE 3

CONTRIBUTION OF MICROBIOLOGIST TO UNHELPFUL OR MISLEADING RESULTS

Wrong germs
  commensals, contaminants
Wrong agents
  e.g. respiratory bacteria
    'sensitive nitrofurantoin'
Wrong answers
  e.g. *Escherichia coli*
    'resistant sulphonamide'
    staphylococci
    'sensitive penicillin'

Finally, although microbiologists would hotly have denied this at one time, some of the sensitivity reports are wrong. Several surveys conducted in various parts of the world have shown just how frequently antibiotic sensitivities reported by laboratories have been erroneous, almost all the mistakes being caused by some very well-known catches such as reporting *Escherichia coli* as resistant to sulphonamide when it is sensitive, and *Staphylococcus aureus* as sensitive to penicillin when it is a penicillinase-producing organism. The technical origins of these errors ought to be well known but plainly they are not.

However, real as these laboratory deficiencies are, they are only half the story. While the microbiologist is certainly responsible for a good deal of confusion, he often simply compounds errors which are introduced by the clinician in the first place (Table 4). The microbiologist can produce results which are only as good as the material which he is given, and the clinician frequently produces specimens which are quite useless for examination in the laboratory. A good example is the surgeon who writes on the form 'Two pints of pus removed from the abdominal cavity'—and accompanies it by a dry swab with a tiny little yellow speck on the end!

TABLE 4

CONTRIBUTION OF CLINICIAN TO UNHELPFUL OR MISLEADING RESULTS

Useless specimens
- *badly selected*
  - e.g. abdominal pus
- *badly collected*
  - sputum
  - urine
- *badly transported*

The number one problem is, however, posed by those specimens which have to pass through natural passages which possess their own well-established flora to reach the outside world. Sputum and urine constitute the great bulk of specimens received in the laboratory and reports issued on them are undoubtedly responsible for a great deal of confusion. There must be many patients up and down the country who are being treated for non-existent urinary tract infection on the basis of badly collected specimens.

However well the specimen is collected in the first place, and however representative it is of the pathogens which are responsible for the infection, the results obtained will be meaningless unless it is well kept and properly transported to the laboratory so that the organisms do not overgrow or die in transit. It is perhaps worth reminding the clinicians that the microbiologist has next to no way of determining the antecedent history of the material which arrives on his bench. If you take a perineal swab and write on the form 'Conjunctivitis' I may be surprised at what I find, but I can only report it! The onus is certainly on us to give the material the best examination we can but the onus is on you to make sure it is worth examining.

We have given the mythology of the Petri dish a fairly rough going over, Harold; what about that well-known occupational therapy for physicians of 'listening to the chest'? How much credence are we expected to give to these bed-side diagnoses?

DIFFICULTIES IN PRECISE AND RAPID DIAGNOSIS

Dr. Lambert

It is a well-known British medical sport for clinician and bacteriologist to berate the other's stupidity but as Francis O'Grady has confessed to a few bacteriological deficiencies, we should be equally fair and point out how bad clinicians are at clinical medicine. Respiratory infection provides the most vivid example—an enormous field of infections caused by a vast variety of organisms, but how do clinicians actually label them? The terms we use, such as croup, bronchitis or pneumonia, are largely anatomical-pathological labels, and the various aetiological agents cut across the clinical groupings. We find the importance of the different agents depends as much on the age of the patient and on the setting in which the infection occurs as on the clinical syndrome.

This problem in precise diagnosis is no mere academic matter because it underlies the whole subject of antibiotic choice. The commonest prescription of antibiotics relate to conditions like respiratory infection, urinary infection and bowel infection in which diagnostic difficulties are greatest. Another example of inadequate clinical diagnosis is acute sore throat, where both experienced hospital doctors and general practitioners, by subjecting their findings to the discipline of controlled trial, have found that they are not much good at telling which will be streptococcal.

I wonder how this situation can be improved? There seem to me to be two general areas. One is technological advances in diagnosis such as the way in which immunofluorescent studies of respiratory infection, e.g. respiratory syncytial virus infection, has made the treatment of acute bronchiolitis more logical than it was some years ago. The other is simply to take a more analytical approach to these infections and ask where the rational field of antibiotic usage lies. The list of antimicrobial agents actually sold for use in acute gastro-enteritis includes 24 preparations in which 10 contain neomycin, 9 contain more than one antibiotic and 14 contain one or more sulphonamide.

TABLE 5

INDICATIONS FOR ANTIBIOTIC TREATMENT IN ACUTE GASTRO-INTESTINAL DISEASE

1. Septicaemic salmonella infection
2. Sick babies who might have septicaemia
3. Acute bacillary dysentery
4. Cholera
5. Enteric fever

Here, as I see it, is the residual list of indications for antibiotic treatment for acute gut disease (Table 5). As you will see there are five headings but they account for only a minute proportion of the patients with acute gastro-intestinal disturbances seen in this country today.

Difficulties in diagnosis leading to inappropriate or ineffective use of antimicrobial drugs may arise in other ways. One, for example, is that we may be too late. Most of us have blundered in, say, diagnosing tuberculous meningitis or osteomyelitis of the spine at a much later date than we should have done. Smith's figures at Oxford show just what the cost of late diagnosis may be (Smith, 1964). Instead of a survival of 93 per cent in Grade I we have a survival of 50 per cent in Grade III and many of those survivors have residual mental or neurological disabilities.

Professor O'Grady

Perhaps I could just interject to say that I think that the microbiologist should have it very much on his conscience if he is responsible for delaying the onset of treatment in patients with severe bacterial infections because of doctrinaire insistence on the necessity to have isolated the organism and discovered its sensitivities before treatment is begun. There is no question, as you have already indicated, about the crucial need to begin treatment early. For example, despite all the rude things microbiologists have said about the difficulty of establishing the diagnosis of bacterial meningitis in patients who have received antimicrobial therapy—often from the general practitioner—before the diagnosis is established, there is very good evidence that the prognosis in such patients, insofar as they have received appropriate treatment at an early stage, is better than it is in patients whose treatment is delayed even though in them the bacteriological diagnosis may have been formally established.

Blind treatment of severe infection without bacteriological assistance, and delay of treatment while the wheels of the bacteriological machine slowly turn, are both wrong. Adequate specimens should always be obtained before therapy of dangerous infections begins. However, treatment should then be instituted with what appears to be the most appropriate agent—and in making that choice, an expert eye on the Gram film can be of the greatest help.

OVERWHELMING INFECTION. HOST FACTORS

Dr. Lambert

Yes, that is true but there is also another and rather different limitation of chemotherapy which we have not yet discussed. This is not so much that the diagnosis is too late as that the disease is too rapid. We can all think of patients with apparently perfectly treatable conditions, such as staphylococcal or streptococcal septicaemia, who come into hospital early in their disease, are treated with drugs which are appropriate to the organism, and yet die of rapidly advancing septicaemia despite anything we can do.

This concept that there are patients whose disease inexorably advances in spite of treatment has been well shown by Robert Austrian's figures of the mortality from pneumococcal bacteraemia in the three eras before serum, after antipneumococcal serum, and after antimicrobial drugs (Austrian & Gold, 1964). Although there is a tremendous difference in the three curves, the interesting point is that the patients dying in the first 5 days seem to have done so at the same rate in each of these three eras. The concept here is of a point of no return at which the multiplication of bacteria has so disturbed metabolic functions that the situation is irretrievable by the time the patient has started treatment.

There are other examples in the field of pneumonia which have been calculated partly on clinical and partly on experimental grounds. In pneumonic plague the point of no return seems to be reached in 16 to 20 hours, whereas in staphylococcal and Friedlander's pneumonia we have an intermediate time of 2–3 days within which it seems to be impossible to affect the course of the disease. I think this concept of a point of no return is not merely theoretical because it defines a limitation of antibiotic usage which can presumably be removed only by advances in prevention rather than by advances in the treatment of established disease.

Our limitations in treatment, however, do not all derive from problems of diagnosis. Even with a full microbial diagnosis there are often host factors which limit the efficacy of treatment and these are becoming more and more common. We can cite the enormous subject of specific impairments of host resistance and Professor Tizard has pointed out (Tizard, 1972) that one of the unexpected results of the antibiotic era is that understanding of natural resistance has been advanced as we have been able to study children with specific immune disorders who live longer than they would previously have done.

We are also familiar with the impairments of host resistance which we impose on the patient by treatment with corticosteroids and antimitotic drugs. However, these host troubles are not really confined to rather uncommon treatments and rare diseases. They do provide dramatic examples but we are probably dealing with low resistance states much more commonly than hitherto. The syndrome of bacterial shock, for example, has attracted much interest in recent years, and there are two sets of factors which predispose to it. One is any form of medical or surgical 'operation', a urinary or venous catheter, all sorts of procedures which are much commoner than they were; and the second is the increase of vulnerable hosts, patients with chronic diseases like diabetes, cirrhosis, lymphoid disorders and malignancies, and those who are living longer than previously.

RESISTANT ORGANISMS AS LIMITATION OF TREATMENT

Professor O'Grady

It is in this sort of situation that a number of factors tend to compound one another in rendering treatment inferior. Very often the difficulties of controlling infection means that the patients have received a number of courses of chemotherapy and very soon we find that they are infected with resistant organisms. For example, Dr. Stratford's list of organisms responsible for severe infection in leukaemia shows the predominance of those outstandingly difficult organisms—pseudomonas, enterobacteria and, of course, still the staphylococcus (Stratford, 1970).

The difficulty is to decide outside this kind of patient just how much limitation of effective treatment of infection is due to antibiotic resistance. If we look at the picture produced by Dr. Thayer and his colleagues there is no doubt of its importance in gonorrhoea (Thayer *et al.*, 1965).

One of the best known pieces of evidence of the growing importance of resistant organisms in general is that of Dr. Max Finland in which he showed the considerable increase over the years in the proportion of septicaemic infections due to Gram negative rods, and particularly highly antibiotic resistant Gram negative rods (Finland *et al.*, 1959). Anti-alarmists in this country have claimed that this is essentially an American phenomenon and not something which is happening here. However it is not even necessarily something which is happening all over America and certainly marked geographical differences in the prevalence of resistance are frequently seen. If we look at what has happened in Seattle, on the other coast of America, to the resistance of staphylococci and enterobacteria over the years, we see that there has been not an increase but a decline in antibiotic resistance (Bulger *et al.*, 1967).

A similar change has been seen in this country in the resistance of haemolytic streptococci to tetracycline (Rees, 1971). This agreeable change has been attributed—I have no doubt correctly—to two factors which are of prime importance in determining the prevalence of resistant strains. The first is the usage of antibiotics: the extent to which individual agents are caused to apply a selection pressure in that particular environment. Secondly—and equally, or in some situations, more importantly—there is the capacity of resistant organisms, once they have emerged, to spread amongst the other patients.

Later on we will be hearing a good deal more of bacterial resistance and its importance and of the other factor which may seriously limit effective treatment—especially in patients infected with organisms resistant to the more widely used agents—and that is adverse reactions to the drug. That is much more in your line than mine, Harold; would you like to 'perspectivize' it for us?

UNWANTED EFFECTS OF ANTIBIOTIC THERAPY

Dr. Lambert

We tend to think of unwanted reactions and allergies as a kind of minor irritation on a generally satisfactory basis of antibiotic usage. For certain fields of treatment this is an understatement of the position and unwanted effects, quite apart from the enormous issues of drug resistance, may be very severe limitations on our freedom of action in treating important diseases.

TABLE 6

RASHES IN TREATMENT OF TUBERCULOSIS

	Incidence (%)	Severe (%)	Treatment discontinued (%)
Streptomycin, Thiacetazone, Isoniazid	17·6	20	15
Streptomycin, Isoniazid	7·7	6	6
Thiacetazone, Isoniazid	16·1	20	13

(2nd International Co-operative investigation into thiacetazone side-effects. *Tubercle*, 1971, **52**, 166.)

We also tend hopefully to think that as new drugs are found our freedom of action is inevitably increased, and our chances of getting into trouble with unwanted effects become inevitably less. This is not necessarily the case.

One could quote the treatment of tuberculosis, where drug toxicity is a very severe and general limitation and has not easily been overcome by the development of new drugs. In the treatment of tuberculosis in developing countries cheap, easy to administer drugs like thiacetazone have great importance. Table 6 is a summary of the results of the second international co-operative of 'Thiacetazone side effects' and shows a formidable incidence of 16–18 per cent of rashes in patients given various thiacetazone-containing regimens with 13 and 15 per cent of those having to discontinue treatment as a result. We have this valuable new drug rifampicin but of 105 patients given rifampicin and isoniazid, three suffered the most violent hypersensitivity reactions, 7·6 per cent developed transient rashes and 35 per cent, no less, showed disturbed tests of liver function.

It is hard to put unwanted effects into a reasonable perspective. Penicillin hypersensitivity could be considered as a rare event, with fewer than 1 per cent of unwanted reactions reported from large series originating in V.D. clinics.

TABLE 7

SEVERE REACTIONS TO ANTIBIOTICS IN U.S.A. IN 800 HOSPITALS DURING 3 YEARS

	No.	Deaths
Anaphylaxis		
Total	809	74
Penicillin	793	63
Severe angioneurotic oedema		
Total	38	5
Penicillin	37	4
Severe skin reactions		
Total	70	7
Penicillin	64	6

Penicillin production: 300 tons annually.

On the other hand, the toll of severe reactions revealed by large surveillance schemes is formidable, as shown by the survey (Table 7) of antibiotic reactions in 800 U.S. hospitals, representing 24 per cent of the hospitals in the country, over a three year period in the 1950s. How do you balance this difficult equation?

Professor O'Grady

Since we are on the subject of perspectives in antimicrobial therapy we should perhaps look at the relative importance of antimicrobials and other agents in producing particular toxic reactions. The most dreaded reaction to an antimicrobial agent must be the production of aplastic anaemia and it is interesting to compare chloramphenicol in this connection with other agents. In the list given by Professor Girdwood at a previous Beecham Symposium chloramphenicol is by no means the main offender (Girdwood, 1971). But there is perhaps no field in which it is more difficult to come by really reliable figures than when trying to establish the frequency of a toxic reaction to a particular agent. If we look at the figures produced by the American panel in 1967 you will see that chloramphenicol is easily top of the list (Best, 1967).

Or to turn to another well-known example: sulphonamides have been said to be a major cause of agranulocytosis, yet again in Professor Girdwood's list sulphonamides do not figure at all amongst the five top drugs producing agranulocytosis.

Apart from the great problems of diagnosis, proper attribution to the drug, and accurate reporting of adverse reactions, we seldom have a really solid figure to put in the denominator when we want to express the number of reactions per number of doses of drug administered. However, more of that issue in due course.

We might now just glance at the one situation in antimicrobial therapy where toxicity rather than efficacy determines the patient's treatment. That situation is the treatment of patients suffering from systemic fungal infections with amphotericin B. In this situation the patient is titrated as it were against the toxicity of the agent and just enough amphotericin is given in increasing doses each day to avoid producing more severe reactions than can be tolerated. As a basis for rational antimicrobial therapy it would be hard to think of anything more unsatisfactory and a serious attempt has been made to introduce a more microbiologically based approach (Drutz *et al.*, 1967). The minimum inhibitory concentration of amphotericin B for the infecting fungus is determined and the patient given once a day a rapid infusion of the drug calculated to produce a plasma level twice the MIC of the infecting organism. In this way, the severity of reactions, and the total dosage of this dangerous drug has been substantially reduced, and the clinical results have been just as good as those obtained by the more hazardous regimen.

This type of planned therapy opens up the whole field of our ignorance of optimum regimens for the infected patient. What, for example, is the proper dosage and duration of treatment for that very common condition urinary tract infection? Professor Brumfitt and his colleagues successfully treated some of their patients with a single dose of cephaloridine (Brumfitt *et al.*, 1970) and Dr. Williams and his colleagues some of theirs with a single dose of streptomycin (Williams and Smith, 1970). Yet nearly every patient gets several doses of drug a day for a week or more.

Without wishing in any way to diminish the great success story of antimicrobial therapy, the truth is that even in those areas where our treatment is most successful we cannot put our hands on our hearts and claim that it is based on any very clear or scientific grasp of what precisely it is that we are doing. There is obviously a great open field for prospective endeavour here—but still more so, of course, in the area of those infections for which at the moment we can do nothing.

THE EMPTY QUARTER OF CHEMOTHERAPY

Dr. Lambert

We have talked for this last spell about succcess and modified success, but what about total failure? Where is the empty quarter of chemotherapy? Obviously one of the biggest fields we have to think about is antiviral chemotherapy and this is the subject of Dr. Bauer's talk later in the Symposium. Just as an introduction one might ask which viruses a clinician would most like to be able to attack. We could each make our own list but for my part the obvious ones would be the major respiratory viruses, especially those causing acute chest infection in childhood, respiratory syncytial virus, parainfluenzal viruses and, of course, influenza itself. Also the central nervous system viruses, especially a more efficient way of treating herpes simplex infections, enteroviruses and on the world scale, the arboviruses and above all hepatitis viruses.

We are talking there of course about normal hosts, but one wonders whether progress in this direction will make much inroad on problems of infection in the abnormally vulnerable host. The enormous range of organisms which assail them—bacteria, viruses, protozoa, fungi—is it really possible that chemotherapy alone will ever achieve the sort of success it has done with normal hosts, or will they always be one jump ahead?

TABLE 8

POLIOMYELITIS ENGLAND AND WALES

	1961	*1963*	*1965*	*1967*	*1969*
Paralytic cases	707	39	55	16	9
Deaths	59	3	3	0	0

This problem serves to remind us that the chemotherapy of established disease is by no means the only method of controlling infectious disease.

There is chemoprophylaxis—what about the success of some of the isoniazid chemoprophylaxis programmes and how does their role compare with that of B.C.G.? What about vaccination? Table 8 shows the end, as we hope, of poliomyelitis in Britain, a disease which has been abolished without intervention of any chemotherapeutic agent. Where do you see the next advances?

DIRECTION OF FUTURE RESEARCH ON ANTIBIOTICS

Professor O'Grady

For my part I should most like to see a great deal of effort put into the very neglected area of the optimum use of the agents which have been put at our disposal. We have been provided relatively recently with all of these powerful agents, and we have been so swept off our feet by their tremendous capabilities that we have hardly bothered at all about the best way of using them. I think some very serious laboratory investigation, animal experimentation and above all study in patients of the most effective clinical regimens is the area where I should best like to see the effort now put. What about you Harold?

Dr. Lambert

Yes, I suppose if one was a planner of medical research on a large scale you would distinguish between tactical and strategic purposes. I agree with you, Francis, that the area you have defined is one of the most important and most likely to be fruitful immediate tactical objectives. It is interesting that the reservations about our ability to use antimicrobial drugs effectively which have followed the first dizzy successes have now led back research to aspects of host-parasite relationship which were studied before the antibiotic era. Strategically, each of us can construct his own list of world problems in which infection plays a big part and which are still unsolved. My own would include infant pneumonia, meningococcal infections, gonorrhoea, hepatitis and gastro-enteritis.

REFERENCES

AUSTRIAN, R. & GOLD, J. (1964). Pneumococcal bacteremia with especial reference to bacteremic pneumococcal pneumonia. *Annals of Internal Medicine*, **60,** 759.

BEST, W. R. (1967). Chloramphenicol-associated blood dyscrastas. A review of cases submitted to the American Medical Association Registry. *Journal of the American Medical Association*, **201,** 181.

BRUMFITT, W., FAIERS, M. C. & FRANKLIN, I. N. S. (1970). The treatment of urinary infection by means of a single dose of cephaloridine. *Postgraduate Medical Journal*, **46** (Supplement October), 65.

BULGER, R. J., ROBERTS, C. E. & SHERRIS, J. C. (1967). Changing incidence of antibiotic resistance among *Staphylococcus aureus*, *Escherichia coli*, Aerobacter-Klebsiella and Pseudomonas encountered in a teaching hospital over a 7 year period. *Antimicrobial Agents and Chemotherapy*, 1966, p. 42.

DRUTZ, D. J., SPIKARD, A. & KOENIG, M. G. (1967). New approach to therapy with amphotericin B. *Antimicrobial Agents and Chemotherapy*, 1966, p. 202.

FINLAND, M., JONES, W. F. JR. & BARNES, M. W. (1959). Occurrence of serious bacterial infections since introduction of antibacterial agents. *Journal of the American Medical Association*, **170**, 2188.

GIRDWOOD, R. H. (1971). The effects of drugs on the blood. In *The Adverse Effects of Drugs* (Ed., Hanson, G. C.), p. 70.

REES, T. A. (1971) Decline in frequency of isolation of tetracycline-resistant beta-haemolytic streptococci from ear, nose and throat 1967–71. *Lancet*, **i**, 938.

SMITH, H. V. (1964). Tuberculous meningitis. *International Journal of Neurology*, **4**, 134.

STRATFORD, B. C. (1970). Antibiotic management of septicaemia in the acute leukaemic patient. In *Advances in the Management of Pseudomonas and Proteus Infection*, p. 79. Excerpta Medical Foundation.

THAYER, J. D., SAMUELS, S. B., MARTIN, J. E. & LUCAS, J. B. (1965). Comparative antibiotic susceptibility of *Neisseria gonorrhoeae* from 1955 to 1964. *Antimicrobial Agents and Chemotherapy*, 1964, p. 433.

TIZARD, J. P. M. (1972). The use of penicillins in neonatal and paediatric practice. *Journal of the Royal College of Physicians*, **6**, 182.

WILLIAMS, J. D. & SMITH, E. K. (1970). Single dose therapy with streptomycin and sulphametopyrazine for bacteriuria during pregnancy. *British Medical Journal*, **4**, 651.

DISCUSSION

Ampicillin in glandular fever

Dr. J. Vahrman. I'd like to draw the meeting's attention to the extensive use of ampicillin which has been widely advertised as a panacea for the treatment of respiratory infections. I have found that in the part of London in which I work it is very widely used by general practitioners for the treatment of such things as sore throat. As a result, we get quite a number of patients suffering from ampicillin reactions admitted to hospital—particularly cases of glandular fever. If a patient with a sore throat is given ampicillin by a general practitioner, and doesn't respond to treatment because he has glandular fever, he is then admitted to hospital and almost invariably develops a rash. In spite of the fact that Beecham Laboratories have done a great deal of research even their recent product which has had protein removed from it seems to produce reactions. The haemolytic streptococcus is still the commonest cause of acute tonsillitis and penicillin G is still the most effective antibiotic for this organism.

Professor Sir Melville Arnott. I would endorse what you say. Ampicillin, excellent though it is, is in my experience quite often used when benzylpenicillin would be more efficient.

Professor F. W. O'Grady. I would entirely agree. What I would like to hear, perhaps this point will be taken up later on, is how do we stop general practitioners from giving patients ampicillin for a disease for which on no account is it indicated.

Sulphonamides in the gut

Mr. D. M. Hancock. If sulphonamides have lost their effect on bacilli in the GI tract, why are they so often used in combination with other drugs in bowel preparation before surgery?

Dr. H. P. Lambert. I think it is just cultural lag! It seems to take about a quarter of a century for things to happen. I don't see any reason for the frequent use of sulphonamide in this condition.

Professor Sir Melville Arnott. In the early days sulphonamides did great things in the gastro-intestinal tract. They probably saved Australia from the landing of Japanese troops because, when dysentery hit the advancing Japanese and the defending Australians in the height of the Cocoda trail in New Guinea, Hamilton-Fairley rushed sulphaguanidine up to the Australian troops which greatly helped their dysentery and they were able to hold the Japanese and that was the furthest south they penetrated in South-East Asia.

Antibiotics and host response

Dr. Hillas Smith. I was particularly interested in Dr. Lambert's statistics on the decline of various infectious diseases over a prolonged period, as I have recently used exactly the same statistics taking precisely the opposite viewpoint.

The point which comes out very clearly is that the more florid the infection, the more gross the disturbance from normal, the more likely we are to achieve a good response provided we have appropriate antibiotics. I am thinking particularly of conditions such as streptococcal and staphylococcal septicaemia. At the other end of the scale you may have a host-parasite relationship which is very subtle, as in chronic salmonella carrier states. Antibiotics then become much less useful, bringing me back to what the speaker said, that when you have immune suppression antibiotics on their own never cured anyone. We must have something more, namely of course the host response.

Dr. W. Griffel. In the list of diseases or conditions which contribute to the lowering of resistance you mentioned diabetes. What evidence is there that a well-controlled diabetic with normal sugar levels has lowered resistance? In diabetic ketosis this may be so, but in well-controlled diabetes is there really lowered resistance to infection?

Dr. H. P. Lambert. I'd accept the point completely. Diabetics, however, are often not well controlled.

Dr. J. Vahrman. Surely when a diabetic becomes infected his disease becomes unstable?

Dr. H. P. Lambert. Yes, one can quote infections that are seen virtually exclusively in diabetes or commonly only in diabetics, e.g. weird fungal infections like mucormycosis. At the extreme end of the spectrum these are clear examples but I think we should accept the questioner's point about the relative freedom from infection of well-controlled diabetics.

Dr. J. F. Munro. My experience with diabetes in Edinburgh would suggest very strongly that if a diabetic has a severe infection he is much more likely to develop bacteriaemia than a non-diabetic, and this is one way in which there is a difference in response.

2

POSSIBLE EVOLUTIONARY RELATIONSHIPS BETWEEN BETA-LACTAMASES

M. H. RICHMOND

One of the less happy aspects of the penicillin era, whose thirtieth birthday—give or take a bit—we are celebrating in this volume, is the increasing prevalence of penicillin and cephalosporin resistant organisms. The existence of such strains was well known to the pioneer workers on penicillin (see for example Abraham & Chain, 1940), but since the early days the range of different types of organisms found to express the enzyme has widened greatly (Citri & Pollock, 1966; Richmond & Sykes, 1972); and within a single species the proportion of isolates found to be lactamase producing has grown and grown to the point at which almost all the isolates of a given species may produce β-lactamase. In the early forties, for example, who would have thought of penicillinase production as a characteristic of *Staphylococcus aureus*? But these days isolates of this species made in hospitals are almost invariably β-lactamase producers.

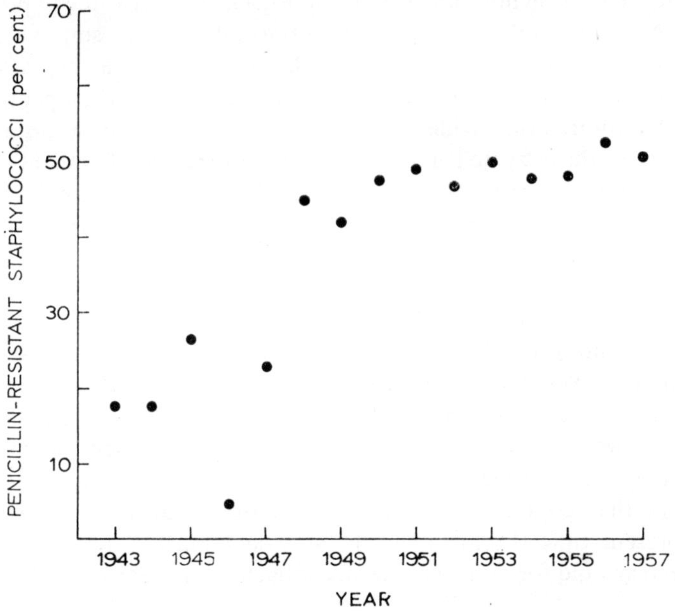

FIG. 1. The emergence of penicillinase-producing strains of *Staphylococcus aureus* following the introduction of benzyl penicillin into general therapeutic use. Redrawn from Munch-Petersen and Boundy (1962).

In practice the incidence of penicillinase production among staphylococci started to climb soon after the introduction of benzyl penicillin into clinical use (Fig. 1; Munch-Petersen & Boundy, 1962), and the process is still continuing in the sense that penicillinase production is to be found in an ever widening range of phage patterns—even if some of the patterns are now less common than hitherto (Fig. 2; see Bülow, 1971).

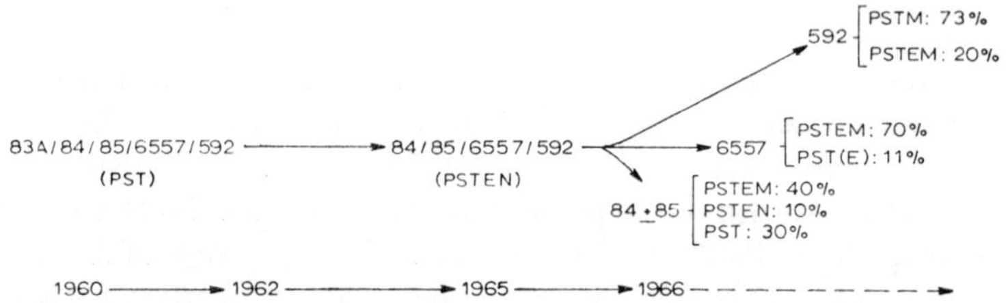

FIG. 2. The evolution of staphylococcal phage patterns and their associated antibiotic resistance characteristics. The data is confined to the 83A/84/85/6557/592 group and derived from information available in Denmark only (see Bülow, 1971). P, penicillin; S, streptomycin; T, tetracycline; E, erythromycin; N, neomycin; M, methicillin.

PENICILLIN AND CEPHALOSPORIN RESISTANCE—ROLE OF β-LACTAMASE

Resistance to penicillins and cephalosporins is primarily due to β-lactamase production in a number of clinically important species—staphylococci and many enteric species in particular—and the enzyme plays a very considerable part in undermining the value of these antibiotics as therapeutic agents. However, although the incidence of β-lactamase is now much more common than hitherto, the enzyme is not an invention of the era of penicillin therapy. Strains of *Staph. aureus* which synthesized β-lactamase are known from well before the onset of conscious penicillin use. *Staph. aureus*, strain 147, an isolate much used in the work on the nature of the genetic basis of penicillinase production (see Richmond, 1968, for a review) was isolated from a food poisoning outbreak in Omaha in 1932 (Segalove, 1947). Penicillinase production among Bacilli has certainly occurred for a much longer period: soil samples taken from herbarium specimens collected in the sixteenth Century and stored in the British Museum yielded strains of *Bacillus licheniformis* that were powerful producers of penicillinase when the spores were germinated (Sneath, 1962). Moreover the enzyme produced was indistinguishable from that commonly encountered among strains of *B. licheniformis* at the present time (Pollock, 1965). So β-lactamase is no new invention: it has been around for millenia in terms of bacterial generations.

Function of β-lactamase

Microbiologists seem to find it difficult to believe that the sole role of β-lactamases in bacterial cells is to protect them against penicillin or cephalosporin action. Always there is a tendency to look for an alternative role to provide a selective advantage for the evolution and survival of the enzyme, it being commonly assumed that selection by penicillins and cephalosporins could not have operated before β-lactamase antibiotics were used clinically. But this does not seem to be reasonable. Many of the fungi known to synthesize penicillins and cephalosporins are to be found in soil—indeed the natural environment was the source for many of the commercially-developed producing strains (Fleming, 1929; Brotzu, 1948); and if the relevance of the soil to selection pressures on *Staph. aureus* is questioned, there is always the celebrated New Zealand hedgehog whose penicillin-producing dermatophytes and commensal staphylococci could be isolated from the same lesion in many animals in the wild (Smith & Marples, 1964). Although experiments to demonstrate the presence of the β-lactam antibiotics in the natural environment have been disappointing (see Pollock, 1967, for a discussion of this point), it seems highly probable that the presence of this enzyme in bacterial strains before penicillins and cephalosporins were used therapeutically reflects the selection pressure generated by these antibiotics in Nature. And it is unnecessary to invoke alternative roles for β-lactamases in the cells that possess them.

In summary, therefore, it seems that the increase in numbers and distribution of β-lactamase reflects the operation of selection provided by therapeutic use of these compounds on a range of enzyme types initially present in a small minority of strains. There is no evidence yet for the evolution of new types of β-lactamase since penicillins and cephalosporins were used therapeutically. Wherever a detailed examination has been possible, the types of enzyme found nowadays are indistinguishable from those that had already been evolved in the pre-penicillin era (Sneath, 1962; Richmond, 1968).

Types of β-lactamase

If one examines the substrate profiles of the penicillinases and cephalosporinases from a range of bacterial species, a wide variety of individual enzyme types emerges (Citri & Pollock, 1966; Richmond & Sykes, 1972). Table 1 compares the profiles found among the enzymes from a range of Gram-positive and Gram-negative species against benzyl penicillin, ampicillin, cephaloridine, cephalexin and carbenicillin with the rate of hydrolysis recalculated against an arbitrary rate for benzyl penicillin of 100.

The enzymes range from the extreme cephalosporinases found in strains of Enterobacter (Hennessey & Richmond, 1968) and *Pseudomonas aeruginosa* (Sabath, Jago & Abraham, 1965), to the enzymes predominantly active against penicillins—for example the enzyme specified by the R-factor R 1818 (Datta & Kontomichalou, 1965; Dale, 1971). Nor are the so-called 'new penicillins'—the penicillins resistant to hydrolysis by staphylococcal penicillinase (CIBA Study Group, 1962)—universally resistant to hydrolysis. The enzyme from Bacillus for example hydrolyses cloxacillin at a significant rate (Citri & Pollock, 1966), as does the enzyme specified by R1818 (Dale, 1971).

TABLE 1

SUBSTRATE PROFILES, AND SOME OTHER PROPERTIES, OF THE β-LACTAMASES FOUND IN A RANGE OF MICRO-ORGANISMS

Species and enzyme type	*Substrate profile*					*Inhibition by*	
	Pen G	*Amp*	*CER*	*CEX*	*Clox*	*cloxacillin*	*carbenicillin*
Staphylococcus aureus	100	120	<1	—	~1	Yes	No
Bacillus cereus, Type I	100	120	35	—	~1	Yes	No
Bacillus licheniformis	100	147	7	—	4	No	No
Mycobacterium smegmatis	100	68	77	—	1	Yes	—
Enteric bacteria, Type Ia	100	0	8000	600	0	Yes	Yes
Enteric bacteria, Type Ib	100	0	350	100	0	Yes	Yes
Enteric bacteria, Type II	100	180	~5	0	0	Yes	No
Enteric bacteria, Type IV	100	140	150	0	0	Yes	No
R-factor mediated (Type III)	100	180	140	15	0	Yes	No
R-factor mediated (Type V)	100	500	50	~10	60	No	No
Pseudomonas aeruginosa (Type I)	100	10	600	80	0	Yes	Yes

Abbreviations: Pen G, benzyl penicillin; Amp, ampicillin; CER, cephaloridine; CEX, cephalexin; Clox, Cloxacillin; —, not quoted.

Minor variants

Even within a single species a superficially similar enzyme may prove to contain a number of minor variants. Three very similar variants of staphylococcal penicillinase may be detected immunologically (Richmond, 1965) and similar minor variants are to be found among strains of *Bacillus cereus*, *Bacillus licheniformis* (Citri & Pollock, 1966) and *Enterobacter cloacae* (Dr. G. Ross, unpublished experiments). Furthermore, immunological tests confirm the information available from substrate profile studies.

Although there are commonly some degree of cross-reaction between enzymes from the same species—particularly among Gram-positive bacteria—this does not extend more widely (Pollock, 1964; Richmond, 1965). There is no cross reaction, for example, between the enzymes from staphylococci on the one hand and those of *Bacillus cereus* or *Bacillus licheniformis* on the other. In Gram-negative species, cross-reaction may extend to some extent beyond species, and even generic, limits (Jack & Richmond, 1970). But in these cases the enzyme concerned is nearly always R-factor mediated; that is the enzyme is more a character of the R-factors concerned than of the species that happens to be expressing them at the time of study (Richmond, Jack & Sykes, 1971).

Differences between β-lactamases

Molecular studies on the detailed nature of the β-lactamase proteins seems also to underline the differences between the enzymes—particularly those from Gram-positive species. Table 2 shows the amino acid composition of the enzymes from *Bacillus cereus*, *Bacillus licheniformis* and *Staph. aureus*,

TABLE 2

THE AMINO ACID COMPOSITION OF β-LACTAMASES FROM *Staphylococcus aureus*, *Bacillus cereus* (TYPE I) AND *Bacillus licheniformis*

	Staph. aureus	B. cereus	B. licheniformis
Lys	44	29	22
Arg	4	14	12
His	3	6	1
Asp	40	40	28
Thr	12	27	18
Ser	16	15	10
Glu	16	29	24
Pro	11	12	9
Gly	15	22	12
Ala	18	36	19
Val	11	16	10
Met	3	4	5
Ile	18	23	9
Leu	24	23	21
Tyr	12	9	5
Phe	8	10	5
Cys	0	0	0

All values as residues/mole.

and little appears similar save the molecular weight values. The enzymes from the Bacilli are acidic proteins while the *Staph. aureus* enzyme is basic enough to migrate to the cathode at pH 8·0. Furthermore, the relative abundance of a number of the component amino acids is quite different: witness a ratio (4 arginine:44 lysine) in the staphylococcal enzyme but an equivalent ratio of (25/16) in the enzyme excreted by *Bacillus licheniformis* (Citri & Pollock, 1966).

Similarities between β-lactamases

Given these differences, therefore, it comes as a great surprise to find that there is a considerable sequence homology between the single polypeptide chains of the enzymes from *Bacillus licheniformis* and *Staphylococcus aureus* (Ambler & Meadway, 1969). Figure 3 shows a number of homologous

38
.... Lys–Arg–Phe–Ala–Tyr Ala–Ser–Thr–Ser– ....
.... Glu–Arg–Phe–Ala–Phe–Ala–Ser–Thr–Ile ....
76
.... Ala–Tyr–Ser –Pro–Ile–Leu–Glu–Lys–Tyr–Val–....
.... Val–Tyr–Asn–Pro–Ile–Thr–Glu–Lys–His–Val ....
127
.... Leu–Gly–Asp–Lys–Val–Thr–Asn–Pro–Val–Arg–Tyr....
.... Ile –Gly–Asp–Glu–Val–Thr–Asn–Pro–Glu–Arg–Phe....

FIG. 3. Some similar sequences from the β-lactamases of *Staphylococcus aureus* (top row) and *Bacillus licheniformis* (bottom row). Data from Ambler and Meadway (1969).

regions from the analyses published by Ambler and Meadway and it has been argued plausibly that about 40 per cent of the amino acid residues are in equivalent positions in these two polypeptide sequences. This fact—despite the wide difference in overall amino acid contents of the two proteins—argues

TABLE 3

THE AMINO ACID COMPOSITION OF FOUR DISTINCT β-LACTAMASES FROM ENTERIC BACTERIA

	Type Ia	*Type Ib*	*Type IIIa*	*Type IIIb*
Lys	9·1	8·2	8·5	9·4
His	2·1	1·9	1·0	1·0
Arg	4·4	5·5	5·6	5·7
Asp	13·8	9·8	13·6	11·8
Thr	7·2	6·5	7·4	7·4
Ser	4·3	4·9	4·4	6·4
Glu	12·7	14·6	15·2	12·2
Pro	5·5	5·5	5·7	3·5
Gly	3·2	4·5	3·4	4·6
Ala	5·0	6·6	6·3	6·2
Val	4·9	5·6	5·8	5·8
Met	1·9	1·9	1·9	1·9
Ile	4·0	5·6	4·2	4·1
Leu	8·8	8·8	10·0	9·1
Tyr	5·8	5·8	2·4	4·8
Phe	8·4	4·3	4·4	5·6
Cys	0	0	?	0·8

All results quoted as per cent, by weight.

strongly for their common evolutionary origin, even though this step can be proved to have taken place at least once before penicillin was used therapeutically.

Underlying similarities also seem to exist among the enzymes from Gram-negative bacteria—again despite widely different substrate profiles. Amino acid analyses of a number of the enzymes shown in Table 3 demonstrate that five of the thirteen enzymes to be found among enteric bacteria share a very similar overall amino acid composition (Jack & Richmond, 1970). Now although it is not possible to argue that a different overall analysis reflects a widely separate evolutionary origin, a similar analysis probably does represent a common underlying structure and hence a common origin. So it seems possible that the wide range of molecular types encountered among enteric bacteria and Pseudomonads may really be a cloud of molecular structures centering around a single common structure that reflects the evolutionary origin of the enzymes.

Relationship between β-lactamases from Gram-positive and Gram-negative organisms

There is no clue yet as to whether there is any relationship between the enzymes of Gram-negative species and those synthesized by their Gram-positive counterparts. Amino acid analyses are sharply different (compare Tables 2 and 3) and all the two groups have in common, apart from their ability to hydrolyse the β-lactam bond, is their universal sensitivity to I_2/KI solution. A comparison of the primary sequence of the *Bacillus licheniformis*/*Staph. aureus* structure, on the one hand, with the sequence of an enzyme from a Gram-negative species, on the other, is one of the major outstanding objectives in this field at the moment.

Possible evolutionary origins of β-lactamase

At present the structural studies summarized above point to a common evolutionary origin of many of the β-lactamases from Gram-negative species with the possibility of another—or at least a separate route—for enzymes from Gram-positives. But what of the character from which the enzymes evolved in the first place? All the evidence available at the moment suggests that the evolution of new characters takes place by the step-wise modification of old ones; so it is much more likely that the β-lactamases evolved by a relatively small number of changes in a prototype molecule rather than having been fashioned *de novo* from some completely unrelated gene.

At present there is only speculation as to the nature of the starting point for β-lactamase; and anyway it is perhaps rather meaningless to try to decide when an evolutionary sequence begins. One candidate that has been much supported is the transpeptidase molecule involved in the cross-linking reaction in mucopeptide biosynthesis (Strominger, 1968–69). This enzyme catalyses the reaction shown in Figure 4 and there is general agreement that this enzyme can be inhibited by penicillin. This last fact is the reason for the popularity of this enzyme as the putative evolutionary source of β-lactamases: it already possesses one of the properties such a molecule would need—it has a

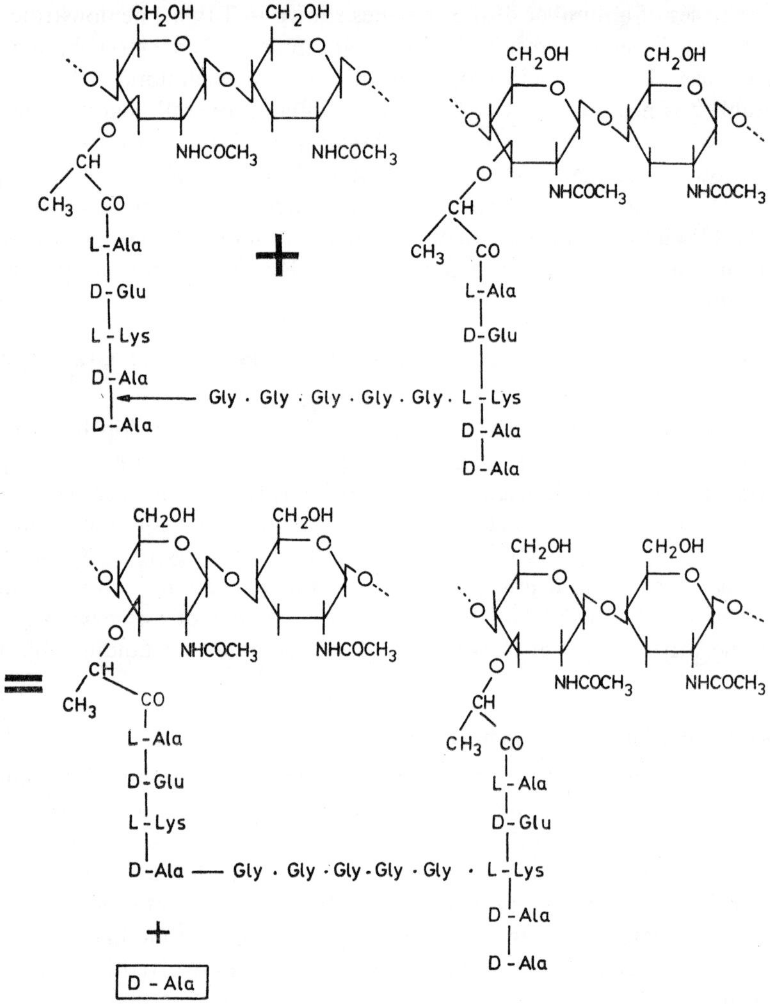

FIG. 4. Transpeptidase action. The terminal $-NH_2$ group on the pentaglycine chain attacks the peptide bond between the terminal two D-alanine residues of the pentapeptide side chain from a different mucopolysaccharide chain. The result is cross-linking with the expulsion of the terminal D-alanine distal to the point of insertion.

region on its surface that will recognize penicillins and cephalosporins. Relatively small changes, therefore, might be able to change such a protein

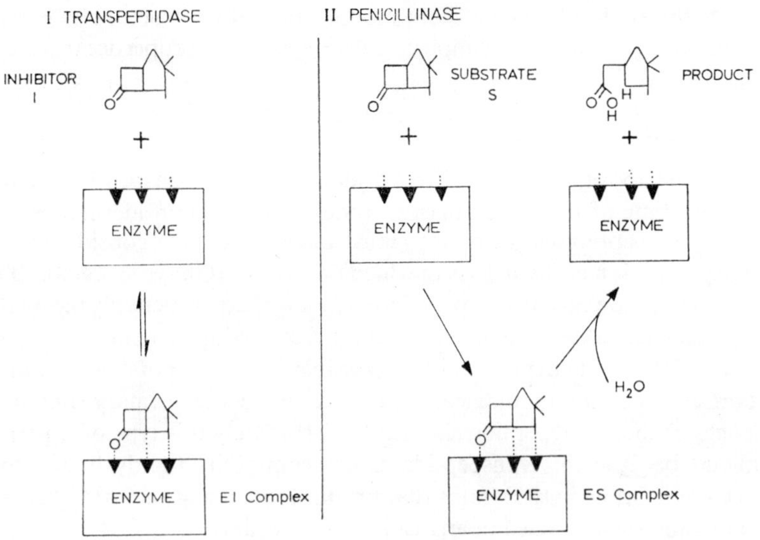

FIG. 5. A possible route for the evolution of penicillinase. I. Transpeptidase. The penicillin interacts reversibly but there is no hydrolysis of the β-lactam bond. Alternatively, according to the hypothesis of Strominger (1968–69) the penicillin (Inhibitor: I) binds irreversibly to the transpeptidase. Whatever the nature of the binding, the penicillin molecule is likely to interact with the enzyme surface at a number of points. II. Penicillinase action. The initial interaction between the penicillin (Substrate: S) and the enzyme surface may be identical with the interaction at the surface of the transpeptidase (see I). Thereafter release is accompanied by interaction with water to give penicilloic acid rather than penicillin as a released product.

from one that recognizes the β-lactam bond to one that hydrolyses it. Such a change is summarized in Figure 5.

Inhibition of β-lactamase by antibiotics

At present, although it is accepted that this enzyme is sensitive to inhibition by penicillins and cephalosporins, there is argument as to the exact way in which these inhibitors act. Strominger (1968–69) has proposed that the β-lactam antibiotics can inactivate this enzyme irreversibly by binding at the *active centre* of the enzyme, and suggests that it is aided in this reaction by a structural similarity between the antibiotic and the terminal D-alanyl-D-alanine sequence of the precursor pentapeptide (see Fig. 4). Ghuysen and his colleagues on the other hand, do not believe that penicillin interacts by binding irreversibly at the active centre (Leyh-Bouille *et al.*, 1970, 1971). Their hypothesis is that the antibiotics act by interfering at a regulatory centre on the transpeptidase enzyme.

As far as evolutionary considerations are concerned which of these two hypotheses is correct makes little difference. Whatever region of the transpeptidase it is that binds penicillin must have the necessary conformation to recognize this molecule, and a slight modification of its structure by mutation might be enough to produce a molecule with hydrolytic properties towards the β-lactam bond.

Precursor of the β-lactamases

As stressed above, there is no direct evidence that the transpeptidase enzyme is the precursor of the β-lactamases. Indeed there is considerable evidence that the transpeptidases themselves must have undergone considerable evolutionary radiation in the species in which they occur (Ghuysen, 1968). If only because of the wide variety in types of cross linkage, experimentally the relationship between these two classes of β-lactam recognizing proteins is difficult to examine. Some statements would be possible if it were possible to compare the two enzymes immunologically or to examine the primary amino acid sequences of their polypeptide chains. Unfortunately this type of experiment is difficult because the transpeptidases are commonly tightly bound to the bacterial membrane in the strains that produce them, and they are likely to be disrupted and disorganized in any isolation procedure.

CONCLUSION

In conclusion, therefore, we already know that β-lactamases from various species often show an underlying similarity—and therefore likely common evolutionary origin—despite wide differences in substrate profile. Current thinking implicates mucopeptide transpeptidase as the immediate evolutionary source of β-lactamases since evolution has already fashioned a site on the transpeptidase that can recognize the β-lactam bond. If the transpeptidase gene is indeed the source of evolutionary radiation to the β-lactamases, however, gene duplication would be an obligate step in the evolutionary sequence since loss of transpeptidase activity on mutation of its gene is likely to be lethal.

Whatever the process involved, it seems to have taken place long ago in the bacterial time scale: all the evidence suggests that the widening of the range of species that are commonly found to make β-lactamase is the consequence of the transfer of evolved β-lactamase genes between species (with possible minor modifications thereafter) rather than the major evolutionary refashioning of some gene to produce penicillin and cephalosporin destroying enzymes *de novo* in individual strains during the thirty years or so that concern us here.

REFERENCES

Abraham, E. P. & Chain, E. (1940). Enzyme from bacteria able to destroy penicillin. *Nature* (*London*), **146,** 837.

Ambler, R. P. & Meadway, R. J. (1969). Chemical structure of bacterial penicillinases. *Nature* (*London*), **221,** 24.

Brotzu, G. (1948). *Lavori Instituto Igenia, Cagliari,* 3.

BÜLOW, P. (1971). Prevalence of extrachromosomal drug resistance to Staphylococci in Danish hospitals during the last decade; factors influencing some properties of predominant epidemic strains. *Annals of the New York Academy of Sciences*, **182,** 21.

CIBA STUDY GROUP NO. 13 (1962). *Resistance of Bacteria to the Penicillins* (Eds., DeRueck, A. V. S. & Cameron, M. P.). J. and A. Churchill, London.

CITRI, N. & POLLOCK, M. R. (1966). The biochemistry and function of beta-lactamase (penicillinase). *Advances in Enzymology and related subjects of Biochemistry*, **28,** 237.

DALE, J. W. & SMITH, J. T. (1971). The purification and properties of the beta-lactamase specified by the resistance factor R-1818 in *Escherichia coli* and *Proteus mirabilis*. *Biochemical Journal*, **123,** 493.

DATTA, N. & KONTOMICHALOU, P. (1965). Penicillinase synthesis controlled by infectious R factors in Enterobacteriaceae. *Nature (London)*, **208,** 239.

FLEMING, A. (1929). On the antibacterial action of cultures of a penicillin, with special reference to their use in the isolation of *B. Influenzae*. *British Journal of Experimental Pathology*, **10,** 226.

GHUYSEN, J. M. (1968). Use of bacteriolytic enzymes in determination of wall structure and their role in cell metabolism. *Bacteriological Reviews*, December Supplement, **32,** 425.

HENNESSEY, T. D. & RICHMOND, M. H. (1968). The purification and some properties of a beta-lactamase (cephalosporinase) synthesised by Enterobacteriaceae. *Biochemical Journal*, **109,** 469.

JACK, G. W. & RICHMOND, M. H. (1970). A comparative study of eight distinct beta-lactamases synthesised by Gram negative bacteria. *Journal of General Microbiology*, **61,** 43.

LEYH-BOUILLE, M., GHUYSEN, J.-M., BONALY, R., NIETO, M., PERKINS, H. R., SCHLEIFER, K. H. & KÄNDLER, O. (1970). Substrate requirements of the *Streptomyces albus* G DD carboxypeptidase. *Biochemistry (USA)*, **9,** 2961.

LEYH-BOUILLE, M., COYETTE, J., GHUYSEN, J.-M., IDCZAK, J., PERKINS, M. R. & NIETO, M. (1971). Penicillin-sensitive DD-carboxypeptidase from Streptomyces strains R61. *Biochemistry (USA)*, **10,** 2163.

MUNCH-PETERSEN, E. & BOUNDY, C. (1962). Yearly incidence of penicillin-resistant staphylococci in man since 1942. *Bulletin of the World Health Organization*, **26,** 241.

NEW YORK ACADEMY SYMPOSIUM (1971). Problems of drug-resistant pathogenic bacteria. *Transactions of the New York Academy of Science*, **182.**

POLLOCK, M. R. (1964). Stimulating and inhibiting antibodies for bacterial penicillinase. *Immunology*, **7,** 707.

POLLOCK, M. R. (1965). Purification and properties of penicillinases from two strains of *Bacillus licheniformis:* a chemical, physiochemical and physiological comparison. *Biochemical Journal*, **94,** 666.

POLLOCK, M. R. (1967). Origin and function of penicillinase: a problem in biochemical evolution. *British Medical Journal*, **4,** 71.

RICHMOND, M. H. (1965). Wild-type variants of exopenicillinase from *Staphylococcus aureus*. *Biochemical Journal*, **94,** 584.

RICHMOND, M. H. (1968). In *Advances in Microbial Physiology* (Eds., Rose, A. H. & Wilkinson, J. F.), Vol. 2, p. 43. Academic Press, London and New York.

RICHMOND, M. H., JACK, G. W. & SYKES, R. B. (1971). Mechanisms of drug resistance. The beta-lactamases of Gram-negative bacteria including pseudomonads. *Annals of the New York Academy of Sciences*, **182,** 243.

RICHMOND, M. H. & SYKES, R. B. (1972). In *Advances in Microbial Physiology* (Eds., Rose, A. H. & Tempest, D.), Vol. 9. Academic Press, London and New York.

SABATH, L. D., JAGO, M. & ABRAHAM, E. P. (1965). Cephalosporinase and penicillinase activities of a beta-lactamase from *Pseudomonas pyocyanea*. *Biochemical Journal*, **96,** 739.

SEGALOVE, M. (1947). Effect of penicillin on growth and toxin production by enterotoxic staphylococci. *Journal of Infectious Diseases*, **81,** 228.

SMITH, J. M. B. & MARPLES, M. J. (1964). A natural reservoir of penicillin-resistant strains of *Staphylococcus aureus*. *Nature* (*London*), **201,** 844.

SNEATH, P. H. A. (1962). Longevity of microorganisms. *Nature* (*London*), **195,** 643.

STROMINGER, J. L. (1968–69). Penicillin-sensitive enzymatic reactions in bacterial cell-wall synthesis. *Harvey Lectures*, **64,** 179.

DISCUSSION

Plasmids and R factors

Dr. D. J. Lane. Could I just ask a simple point for the non-bacteriologist. Is there any difference between a plasmid and an R factor?

Professor M. H. Richmond. 'Plasmid' is the term used for any piece of DNA which can survive independently of the chromosome in a bacterial cell. An R factor, under the current definition, is a plasmid, usually transmissible, which carries resistance to various antibiotics.

Mechanisms and conditions for resistance transfer

Professor W. Brumfitt. Does transfer of resistance occur under anaerobic conditions? David Smith said that it did not and therefore it could not occur in the gut.

Professor M. H. Richmond. Dr. John Anderson in our department is at the moment studying R factor transfer under anaerobic conditions and has obtained transfer.

Professor W. Brumfitt. Does it occur as readily and how strict are the anaerobic conditions?

Professor M. H. Richmond. He says his frequencies are as high as those obtained under aerobic conditions.

Professor W. Brumfitt. Why is methicillin stable to β-lactamase? Is this because the side chain is static in relation to the rest of the molecule? Thus methicillin resistance is true steric hindrance because the side chain is unable to move, and therefore the β-lactamase is unable to make the necessary 'fit' in order to open the β-lactam ring.

Professor M. H. Richmond. No, the fascinating thing about methicillin is that it's not completely resistant to staphylococcal penicillinase. The point is an important one because it means that the enzyme can still recognize that molecule. Even so we have at the moment no β-lactamase that I know of in *Staphylococcus aureus* that can hydrolyse methicillin effectively. All the clinical problems with methicillin resistance are due to a completely different biochemical mechanism at work.

Professor W. Brumfitt. Would you care to speculate?

Professor M. H. Richmond. There are one or two hard facts and Dr. Parker knows very much more about this than I do. The first thing is that resistance to methicillin existed in the staphylococcal population before methicillin was invented. The mechanism responsible for methicillin resistance also confers resistance to benzylpenicillin and there must have been some selective advantage, a very mild one, for having this character 'underneath' penicillinase before methicillin was put on the market. As soon as you short circuit β-lactamase (the main line of defence of the staphylococcus) by using methicillin your secondary defence mechanism becomes much more important. A typical methicillin-resistant strain, when you have removed its β-lactamase so that it's just relying on what we call its intrinsic resistance, will have MIC of about 30 μg of benzylpenicillin. So it is fairly solidly resistant itself even without its first line defence of penicillinase. What the biochemical basis of that is, I still really don't know. It is a very complicated mixture of genetic selection and possible changes in the nature of the cell wall.

There is a further point on the question of transduction. It is possible that methicillin resistance is not the product of a single gene, but of more than one and therefore it is very difficult to transduce this resistance into naturally sensitive organisms. In order to do so you may have to pick up two genes which may be unlinked. What Richard Lacey has done in Bristol is to make methicillin-sensitive variants and transduce methicillin resistance back into them, but he has to make a methicillin-sensitive variant first.

Penicillinase production in staphylococci, gonococci and streptococci

Dr. N. Datta. May I comment on your point that penicillinase in staphylococci must have been vary rare before penicillin was used. It was rare, but the very fact that penicillinase-producers turned up in collections made in the 1930s shows they couldn't have been all that rare, or perhaps the alpha-toxin is linked to the penicillinase, and that that was how they came to survive?

Professor M. H. Richmond. That is a very good point. They were not as rare as, for example, neomycin-resistant enteric bacteria.

Dr. I. Phillips. Has Professor Richmond any ideas on the linked resistance that turns up in gonococci? If you test the sensitivity of gonococci and select those resistant to penicillin, we find they are often resistant to streptomycin, erythromycin, rifampicin—almost whatever you like to test, even if the antibiotic hasn't been used. I have looked at the Ugandan strains, for example, where the antibiotics have never been used.

Dr. N. Datta. David Smith of Harvard told me that some of his colleagues were extracting plasmid DNA from gonococci and that they had found these little molecules in strains which were resistant to streptomycin or tetracycline, but that they weren't particularly associated with penicillin resistance.

Dr. A. Percival. Professor Richmond says that streptococci do not become resistant to penicillin. *Strep. pyogenes* perhaps hasn't yet, but in the mouth alpha-haemolytic streptococci with considerably increased resistance to penicillin appear very rapidly during treatment with penicillin. They have come from somewhere. I've never seen anyone show that these strains do not produce penicillinase or that the so-called penicillin-resistant gonococci do not produce penicillinase. I'd like to be assured about that.

Professor M. H. Richmond. The second point is technically a little difficult to deal with because it is always difficult to get large quantities of gonococcus to examine biochemically; but *Strep. viridans* has not, in my hands ever shown lactamase activity. That's based, however, on just one or two experiments on substantially resistant strains.

Resistance of Bacteroides Spp

Dr. J. G. Lewis. How does Bacteroides figure in this because it is still fairly sensitive to tetracycline and does play, volume-wise, quite a part in the gut. This is an extension of your question—why some and not others.

Professor M. H. Richmond. We've looked for R factors in Bacteroides and for the ability to transfer them to Bacteroides; but so far haven't succeeded in either. Some Bacteroides strains do destroy penicillins and others cephalosporins. Has Dr. Datta has any information about this.

Dr. Datta. No.

Professor W. Brumfitt. Have you isolated the enzyme yet?

Professor M. H. Richmond. We've got one of the enzymes in cell-free form and know something about the molecular characteristics as far as the substrates are concerned.

3

TRANSMISSIBLE ANTIBIOTIC RESISTANCE

NAOMI DATTA

THIS symposium is on 'Antibiotics After 30 Years'. Thirty years is only about one human generation but for bacteria it could be over a million generations—a number which would take us, on our scale, back more than 300,000 years. It is not surprising, therefore, that we can observe, during our working lives, evolution in bacteria actually taking place. One example is penicillinase production by *Staphylococcus aureus*. This was a rare phenomenon 25 years ago and limited to a particular phage type (Barber, 1947) but now 92 per cent of strains of *Staph. aureus* isolated from nose swabs of patients in London hospitals are penicillin resistant (Stokes *et al.*, 1972). We actually observed the change, but were unfortunately powerless to stop it. The introduction of the penicillinase resistant semi-synthetic penicillins provided an answer to the problem, but bacterial evolution continues.

ANTIBIOTIC RESISTANCE RESULTING FROM MUTATION

The study of microbial genetics has developed in the last 30 years and has been able to explain, though not control, the acquisition of antibiotic resistance by bacteria. Bacteria can become resistant to drugs by mutation: for instance, in any large population of drug-sensitive bacteria (10^9 or more), there will probably be a few spontaneous mutants, resistant to streptomycin. If the population is exposed to streptomycin, the mutants will continue to multiply, while the rest of the population is killed. That resistance is caused by spontaneous mutation and not by any direct effect of exposure to streptomycin, can be conclusively proved (Lederberg & Lederberg, 1952).

This is an extreme example of Darwinian evolution, the selection of those variants best able to survive in any particular environmental conditions, and has important clinical relevance. It is well known that treatment of an infection with streptomycin alone, especially long-continued treatment, often leads to the appearance of streptomycin-resistance in the infecting bacteria. Nalidixic acid is another drug to which resistance can be acquired by a single mutational event, but the same is not true of most antibiotics. Penicillin-resistant *Staph. aureus* can be obtained in the laboratory by culturing a sensitive strain on gradually increasing concentrations of penicillin, that is by multiple mutations, each one slightly increasing the level of resistance. The result is quite different from naturally occurring resistant strains. The laboratory-cultivated ones are slow-growing, no longer produce typical golden colonies and are penicillinase-negative (Barber, 1962).

ANTIBIOTIC RESISTANCE DETERMINED BY PLASMIDS

Antibiotic resistance in naturally occurring bacteria seems usually to have resulted not from mutation, but from acquisition of ready-made resistance genes, which can be transferred from one bacterium to another. The elements transferred are DNA molecules, known as episomes or plasmids. Encoded in their DNA is the genetic information which confers drug-resistance. Most is known about the R factors or transmissible resistance plasmids of the Enterobacteriaceae.

R factors

R factors were discovered in Japan in 1959. They were first found in *Shigella flexneri* and conferred resistance to streptomycin, the tetracyclines, chloramphenicol and the sulphonamides (Watanabe, 1963). Resistance to all four drugs was transmissible from the resistant Shigella to sensitive strains of Shigella, Salmonella, Escherichia, Klebsiella, Proteus etc. in fact all the Enterobacteriaceae. It was also transferable to *Vibrio cholerae* and *Yersinia pestis* but not to Gram positive bacteria (Datta, 1965). During the 1960s, transmissible resistance to kanamycin and neomycin appeared. It was first identified in *Salmonella typhimurium* (Lebek, 1963) and rapidly became common among strains of *Escherichia coli* causing gastroenteritis of infancy (Rozansky *et al.*, 1964).

R factors giving resistance to the penicillins, including ampicillin and carbenicillin were the next ones in order of appearance (Anderson & Datta, 1965). In the 1970s, R factors conferring resistance to gentamicin (Witchitz & Chabbert, 1971) and trimethoprim (Fleming, Datta & Grüneberg, 1972) have been discovered.

No R factor yet identified gives resistance to all these drugs simultaneously. There is a great variety of patterns of transmissible resistance. Resistance to sulphonamide or tetracycline, singly, is often carried by R factors, but multiple resistance is commoner and is transmissible *en bloc*. Some resistance patterns determined by R factors are given in Table 1.

TABLE 1

SOME R FACTOR PATTERNS

R Factor	*Resistance pattern*	*Reference*
R222	STCSu	Watanabe, 1963
R5	STCSuK	Lebek, 1963
R1	ASCKSu	Meynell & Datta, 1966
R2	STSu	Datta, 1962
R57b	ACSuKG	Witchitz & Chabbert, 1971
R389	STCSuTp	Fleming *et al.*, 1972

Symbols. Resistance to:

A = ampicillin	S = streptomycin	T = tetracycline
C = chloramphenicol	Su = sulphonamides	K = kanamycin/neomycin
G = gentamicin	Tp = trimethoprim	

Resistance plasmids of staphylococci

These are analogous to R factors, although not identical. Resistance genes which are at least sometimes plasmid-borne in *Staph. auerus* are listed in Table 2. Although the spread of penicillinase production in *Staph. aureus* was observed earlier than the discovery of R factors, its plasmid nature was only recognized later (Novick, 1963; Novick & Richmond, 1965). The study of staphylococcal plasmids is more difficult than the study of R factors because much less is known about the genetics and biochemistry of staphylococci than of *Esch. coli.*

TABLE 2

ANTIBIOTICS TO WHICH STAPHYLOCOCCAL PLASMIDS DETERMINE RESISTANCE

Antibiotic	*Reference*
Penicillin	Novick, 1969
Tetracycline	Novick, 1969
Chloramphenicol	Shaw, Bentley & Sands, 1970
Erythromycin	Novick, 1969
Kanamycin	Evans & Waterworth, 1966
Fusidic acid	Evans & Waterworth, 1966
Neomycin	Lacey, 1971a

Transfer of resistance genes

R factors carry genes determining their own transmissibility, as well as genes for drug resistance. They are examples of bacterial sex factors, since they bring about conjugation, with transfer of DNA from one bacterium to another. The mechanism of mating is not fully understood. Male or donor bacteria (i.e. ones possessing the sex factor) produce on their surface hair-like outgrowths in the form of protein tubes, approximately 100 Å in diameter, known as sex pili (Lawn, 1966). Sex pili are necessary for conjugation and DNA transfer, but whether they are ducts through which linear DNA molecules pass from one cell to another is not known (Brinton, 1965; Curtiss, 1969).

Not all resistance plasmids determine their own transfer. In both Gram negative and Gram positive bacteria there are also plasmids which confer drug resistance but cannot be transmitted from one bacterium to another except by the intervention of another element, either a sex factor (or transfer factor) or a bacterial virus.

In the case of staphylococci, transfer of resistance plasmids by means of bacteriophage has been extensively used in the laboratory, but did not seem to provide a mechanism of high enough efficiency to account for the great spread of antibiotic resistance among hospital staphylococci which took place during the 1950s (Richmond, 1969). However, transfer of resistance between staphylococci in mixed culture, or upon human skin, has been demonstrated recently (Lacey, 1971a, b) at frequencies similar to those found with R factors in *Esch. coli.* The transfer seems to be brought about by bacteriophage, not by sex factors of the kind known in Gram negative bacilli, but the mechanism is different from, and more efficient than transfer (transduction) by phage particles isolated from their bacterial hosts.

INCIDENCE AND SPREAD OF R FACTORS

In Salmonella and Shigella

During the 1960s R factors spread in Salmonella and Shigella *spp* all over the world. Multiple resistance was unknown in *Shigella flexneri* in Japan before 1955, when one single strain with the R factor pattern (STCSu) was identified. There has been a great increase since (Table 3). Very much the same

TABLE 3

Shigella flexneri IN JAPAN

Per cent of multi-resistant strains	
1957	0.08
1960	9
1965	55
1970	70

happened with *Shigella sonnei* in London, where studies have been made by Dr. Joan Davies and her colleagues. Multiple resistance first appeared in the late 1950s and increased in frequency until, in 1970, 70 per cent of strains were resistant to at least three drugs. Resistance to ampicillin, streptomycin, tetracycline and sulphonamides are the commonest; resistance to kanamycin/neomycin has begun to appear in the last few years (Farrant & Tomlinson, 1966; Davies, Farrant & Uttley, 1970).

The incidence of R factors in Salmonella has been studied in this country by Anderson (1968a, b) and in Holland by Manten and his colleagues (Manten, Guinée & Kampelmacher, 1966). In both countries, the incidence rose steeply, from about 2 per cent at the beginning of the 1960s to about 60 per cent by the mid-60s. The distribution of resistance in different serotypes is uneven. In *Salmonella typhimurium* a particular phage type, type 29, was shown by Anderson (1968a) to be of especial interest. It is a bovine strain, which was fairly unusual, and always drug-sensitive, until 1963. The strain was the cause of extensive outbreaks of infection in the 1960s (Fig. 1) during which time it acquired transmissible resistance first to streptomycin and sulphonamides, later to the tetracyclines and later still to ampicillin, kanamycin/neomycin and chloramphenicol. The strain spread widely among calves and in the human population, becoming commoner as it acquired multiple resistance. It appeared that its spread was encouraged by the prophylactic administration of antibiotics to calves. The calves were collected from the farms where they were born, herded together and taken to centres in various parts of the country to be reared. Deaths from scours were common. The prophylactic use of antibiotics, far from being effective, resulted in the acquisition of resistance by the causative organism, *S. typhimurium* type 29, to the particular drugs being used (Anderson, 1968b).

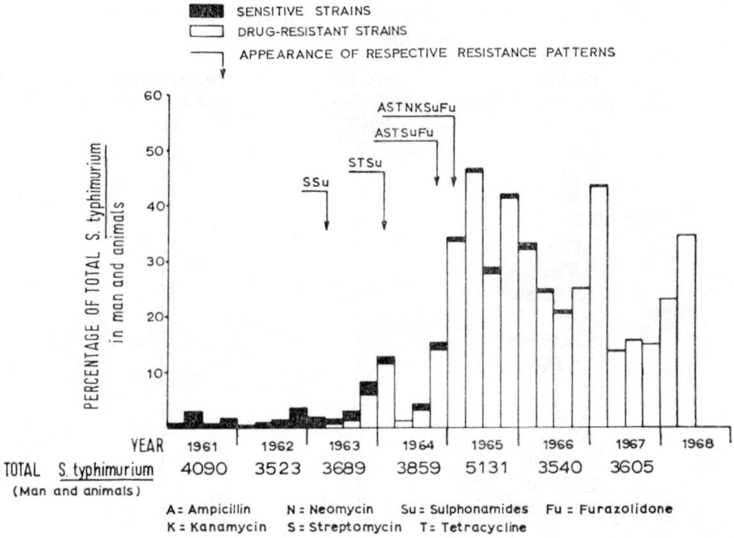

FIG. 1. Incidence of type 29 as a percentage of total *S. typhimurium* infection in man and animals, 1961–1968. (By kind permission of E. S. Anderson.)

Salmonella panama has had a rather similar history. It was a rare serotype in 1960, but spread widely in the past decade all over north-west Europe, incidents of infection becoming more frequent as the organism acquired antibiotic resistance (Manten *et al.*, 1966).

In the normal bowel flora

My colleagues and I have studied R factors in normal faecal bacteria, and shown that about 50 per cent of adults, outside hospitals, harboured R^+ bacteria. In about 30 per cent, R^+ bacteria were present in very large numbers. The drugs to which the normal bowel bacteria were most often resistant were streptomycin, tetracycline and the sulphonamides (Datta, 1969a; Datta *et al.*, 1971 and unpublished observations, 1971) (Table 4). Becoming a hospital inpatient had only a slight effect in increasing the numbers of R^+ bacteria carried (Datta, 1969a, b). Oral administration of ampicillin or sulphonamides had small effect, but a course of tetracycline therapy had a highly significant effect, leading to the excretion of *Esch. coli* resistant not only to the tetracyclines but also, in statistically significant numbers, to ampicillin, streptomycin, chloramphenicol and the sulphonamides. The effect, however, had disappeared a month after the course of treatment (Datta *et al.*, 1971). The findings are summarized in Table 5.

R factors are carried even more frequently by normal babies (Moorhouse, 1969) and young children (Linton *et al.*, 1971) than by adults.

TABLE 4

RESISTANCE PATTERNS OF FAECAL *Esch. coli* FROM PATIENTS OUTSIDE HOSPITAL

Pattern (in order of frequency)	*No. of isolations*	*No. transferring R to* Esch. coli *K12*
T	16	11
Su	10	4
SSu	10	4
TSu	8	5
ST	6	6
STSu	6	5
ASSu	4	1
ASTCSu	4	3
A	3	1
STCSu	3	3
ASTSu	3	3
AT	2	2
ASu	2	1
AS	1	1
ASCSu	1	1
STKSu	1	1
STCKSu	1	1
Total	81	53 (65 per cent)

TABLE 5

PROPORTION (PER CENT) OF PATIENTS EXCRETING R^+ *Esch. coli*

Hospitalized	*Antibiotic treatment*	*In any numbers (10^{-5} detectable)*	*In large numbers (> 25 per cent of yield)*
No	No	54	29
Yes	No	55	38
No	Ampicillin	62	27
No	Sulphonamide	61	50
No	Tetracycline	100	100

Figures from Datta (1969) and Datta *et al.* (1971)

In parenteral infections

R factors in the normal bowel flora are harmless, but they provide a reservoir from which enteric pathogens may acquire resistance. Even more important, bacteria which are commensals in the bowel can play a pathogenic role in urinary and other parenteral infections.

Among strains of bacteria (usually *Esch. coli*) causing urinary infection outside hospital, about 25 per cent are resistant to one or more antibacterial drugs. As with the bowel flora, the commonest resistances are against tetracycline, streptomycin and the sulphonamides (Brumfitt *et al.*, 1971; Robertson, 1971; E. J. Shaw, personal communication). At present, therefore, there remains a choice of effective drugs for the treatment of infection, even when the bacteria carry R factors, but the frequency of resistance shows how desirable it is for infections to be diagnosed by urine culture and for sensitivity tests to be made at the outset.

Urinary infections in hospital practice tend to be caused by more resistant strains belonging to a wider variety of bacterial genera. Urinary pathogens cultured from inpatients at Hammersmith Hospital during 1970 are compared with those from general practice in Table 6. During our 1970 survey (Anderson, Datta & Shaw, 1972) we found, however, that less than 1 per cent of 326 urinary strains of Enterobacteriacae were resistant to all four of the drugs sulphonamide, ampicillin, trimethoprim and nalidixic acid; the multiplicity

TABLE 6

Escherichia coli ISOLATED FROM URINARY TRACT INFECTIONS

Patient group	*Total No.*	*Sensitive*	*Resistant to one or more drugs (per cent)*		*Resistant to ampicillin (per cent)*	
Domiciliary[a]	50	40	10	(20)	1	(2)
Hospital (medical)[b]	52	29	23	(44)	14	(27)
Hospital (surgical)[b]	45	23	22	(49)	15	(33)

[a] Figures from Shaw *et al.*, 1972.
[b] Figures from Anderson *et al.*, 1972.

of resistance was thus seldom so great as to leave the clinician without a suitable antibacterial drug for treatment. Our survey covered all 'Gram negative' infections, not only urinary ones, and it was generally true that, in spite of a high incidence of R factors, multiplicity of resistance was never so great as to render effective therapy impossible. Infections with *Pseudomonas aeruginosa* were, as expected, the ones in which choice of antibacterial therapy was most limited. Although R factors conferring a high level of carbenicillin-resistance have been identified in *Ps. aeruginosa* (Sykes & Richmond, 1970; Fullbrook, Elson & Slocombe, 1970) none was found either during our 1970 survey, or since, at Hammersmith Hospital.

This is the position in a general hospital in London. In particular situations, however, the incidence of R factors and the breadth of their resistance spectra have caused greater concern. In hospital environments where antibiotics are used intensively, and particularly if they are used prophylactically, outbreaks of infection with Klebsiella *spp* more resistant than those we have encountered at Hammersmith Hospital have occurred. The resistance has been R-factor determined. Examples are reported by Gardner and Smith (1969) in Massachusetts General Hospital and by Price and Sleigh (1970) in a Scottish neuro-surgical unit. In the latter instance, the outbreak ceased upon the withdrawal of all antibiotics.

CONCLUSIONS

The importance of transferable antibiotic resistance obviously reflects the importance of antibiotic treatment of infection caused by various groups of organisms. Multiple resistant staphylococci have presented serious therapeutic problems. How much resistance was due to acquisition of plasmids (i.e. transfer of resistance) is not known but it was probably a major factor. In diarrhoeal infections, R factors are common, but the importance of antibacterial therapy is disputable. In parenteral infections of all kinds, antibacterial therapy is called for and may be life-saving. Antibiotic-resistance, usually plasmid-determined, has spread and has made it necessary to seek and develop new drugs. The pharmaceutical industry has, for the most part, kept just ahead. In the last few years the penicillinase-resistant penicillins and cephalosporins, together with gentamicin and trimethoprim, have provided effective defences against most resistant bacteria. Bacterial evolution shows signs of overcoming these defences, and it is unlikely that a state of equilibrium has been reached.

REFERENCES

ANDERSON, E. S. (1968a). Drug resistance in *Salmonella typhimurium* and its implications. *British Medical Journal*, **3,** 333.

ANDERSON, E. S. (1968b). The ecology of transferable drug resistance in the enterobacteria. *Annual Review of Microbiology*, **22,** 131.

ANDERSON, E. S. & DATTA, N. (1965). Resistance to penicillins and its transfer in Enterobacteriaceae. *Lancet*, **i,** 407.

ANDERSON, F. M., DATTA, N. & SHAW, E. J. (1972). R factors in hospital infection. *British Medical Journal*, **3,** 82.

BARBER, M. (1947). Staphylococcal infection due to penicillin-resistant strains. *British Medical Journal*, **ii,** 863.

BARBER, M. (1962). Coagulase-positive staphylococci resistant to benzylpenicillin, methicillin and other penicillins. *Resistance of Bacteria to Penicillins.* CIBA Foundation Study Group No. 13. Churchill, London.

BRINTON, C. C. (1965). The structure, function synthesis and genetic control of bacterial pili and a molecular model for DNA and RNA transport in Gram negative bacteria. *Transactions of the New York Academy of Sciences*, **27,** 1003.

BRUMFITT, W., FAIERS, M. C., REEVES, D. S. & DATTA, N. (1971). Antibiotic-resistant *Escherichia coli* causing urinary tract infection in general practice. *Lancet*, **i,** 315.

CURTISS, R. (1969). Bacterial conjugation. *Annual Review of Microbiology*, **23,** 69.

DATTA, N. (1962). Transmissible drug resistance in an epidemic strain of *Salmonella typhimurium. Journal of Hygeine* (Cambridge), **60,** 30.

DATTA, N. (1965). Infectious drug resistance. *British Medical Bulletin*, **21,** 254.

DATTA, N. (1969a). Drug resistance and R factors in the bowel bacteria of London patients before and after admissions to hospital. *British Medical Journal*, **2,** 407.

DATTA, N. (1969b). Drug resistance of bowel bacteria (letter). *British Medical Journal*, **ii,** 697.

DATTA, N., FAIERS, M. C., REEVES, D. S., BRUMFITT, W., ØRSKOV, F. & ØRSKOV, I. (1971). R factors in *Escherichia coli* in faeces after oral chemotherapy in general practice. *Lancet*, **i,** 312.

DAVIES, J., FARRANT, W. N. & UTTLEY, A. (1970). Antibiotic resistance of *Shigella sonnei*. *Lancet*, **ii**, 1157.

EVANS, R. J. & WATERWORTH, P. M. (1966). Naturally-occurring fusidic acid resistance in Staphylococci and its linkage to other resistances. *Journal of Clinical Pathology*, **19**, 555.

FARRANT, W. N. & TOMLINSON, A. J. H. (1966). Some studies on the epidemiology of Sonne dysentery. Changes in colicine type and antibiotic resistance between 1956 and 1965. *Journal of Hygiene (Cambridge)*, **64**, 287.

FLEMING, M. P., DATTA, N. & GRÜNEBERG, R. N. (1972). Trimethoprim resistance determined by R factors. *British Medical Journal*, **1**, 726.

FULLBROOK, P. D., ELSON, S. W. & SLOCOMBE, B. (1970). R-factor mediated β-lactamase in *Pseudomonas aeruginosa*. *Nature (London)*, **226**, 1054.

GARDNER, P. & SMITH, D. H. (1969). Studies on the epidemiology of resistance (R) factors. I. Analysis of *Klebsiella* isolates in a general hospital. II. A prospective study of R factor transfer in the host. *Annals of Internal Medicine*, **71**, 1.

LACEY, R. W. (1971a). High-frequency transfer of neomycin resistance between naturally-occurring strains of *Staphylococcus aureus*. *Journal of Medical Microbiology*, **4**, 73.

LACEY, R. W. (1971b). Transfer of tetracycline-resistance between strains of *Staphylococcus aureus* in mixed cultures. *Journal of General Microbiology* (in the press).

LAWN, A. M. (1966). Morphological features of the pili associated with *Escherichia coli* K 12 carrying R factors or the F factor. *Journal of General Microbiology*, **45**, 377.

LEBEK, G. (1963). Uber die Entstehung mehrfachresistenter Salmoneller. Ein experimenteller Beitrag. *Zentralblatt fur Bakteriologie, Parasitenkunde, Infektionskrankheiten und Hygiene, Erste Abteilung: Originale (Stuttgart)*, **188**, 494.

LEDERBERG, J. & LEDERBERG, E. M. (1952). Replica plating and indirect selection of bacterial mutants. *Journal of Bacteriology*, **63**, 399.

LINTON, K. B., RICHMOND, M. H. & GILLESPIE, W. A. (1971). Influence of employment with livestock on antibiotic-resistant *E. coli* in the faeces of healthy people. *Journal of Clinical Pathology*, **24**, 767.

MANTEN, A., GUINÉE, P. A. M. & KAMPELMACHER, E. H. (1966). Incidence of resistance to tetracycline and chloramphenicol among Salmonella bacteria found in the Netherlands in 1963 and 1964. *Zentralblatt fur Bakteriologie, Parisitenkunde, Infektionskrankheiten und Hygiene, Erste Abteilung: Originale (Stuttgart)*, **200**, 13.

MEYNELL, E. & DATTA, N. (1966). The relation of resistance transfer factors to the F-factor (sex-factor) of *Escherichia coli* K 12. *Genetical Research (Cambridge)*, **7**, 134.

MOORHOUSE, E. C. (1969). Incidence of transferable drug resistance in Enterobacter isolates from urban infants. *British Medical Journal*, **ii**, 405.

NOVICK, R. P. (1963). Analysis of transduction of mutations affecting penicillinase formation in *Staphylococcus aureus*. *Journal of General Microbiology*, **33**, 121.

NOVICK, R. P. (1967). Penicillinase plasmids of *Staphylococcus aureus*. *Federation Proceedings: Federation of American Societies for Experimental Biology (Bethesda)*, **26**, 29.

NOVICK, R. P. (1969). Extrachromosomal inheritance in bacteria. *Bacteriological Reviews*, **33**, 210.

NOVICK, R. P. & RICHMOND, M. H. (1965). Nature and interactions of the genetic elements governing penicillinase synthesis in *Staphylococcus aureus*. *Journal of Bacteriology*, **90**, 467.

PRICE, D. J. E. & SLEIGH, J. D. (1970). Control of infection due to *Klebsiella aerogenes* in a neurosurgical unit by withdrawal of all antibiotics. *Lancet*, **ii,** 1213.

RICHMOND, M. H. (1969). Extrachromosomal elements and the spread of antibiotic resistance in bacteria. *Biochemical Journal*, **113,** 225.

ROBERTSON, M. H. (1971). A 6-year study of resistance patterns of urinary tract pathogens in general practice. *Postgraduate Medical Journal*, **47,** 111.

ROZANSKY, R., BERANT, M., ROSENMANN, E., BEN-ARI, Y. & STERK, V. V. (1964). Enteropathogenic *Escherichia coli* infections in infants during the period from 1957 to 1962. *Journal of Pediatrics*, **64,** 521.

SHAW, W. V., BENTLEY, D. W. & SANDS, L. (1970). Mechanism of chloramphenicol resistance in *Staphylococcus epidermidis*. *Journal of Bacteriology*, **104,** 1095.

SHAW, E. J., DATTA, N. & BRUMFITT, W. (1971). Antibiotic resistance patterns in Enterobacteriaceae causing urinary tract infections in general practice. *Proceedings of the VII International Congress of Chemotherapy* (In press).

STOKES, J., BRADLEY, J., THOMPSON, R. E. M., HITCHCOCK, N., PARKER, M. & WALKER, J. (1972). Hospital staphylococci in three London teaching hospitals. *Lancet*, **i,** 84.

SYKES, R. B. & RICHMOND, M. H. (1970). Intergeneric transfer of a β-lactamase gene between *Pseudomonas aeruginosa* and *Escherichia coli*. *Nature* (*London*), **226,** 952.

WATANABE, T. (1963). Infective heredity of multiple drug resistance in bacteria. *Bacteriological Reviews*, **27,** 87.

WITCHITZ, J. L. & CHABBERT, Y. A. (1971). High level transferable resistance to gentamicin. *Journal of Antibiotics*, **24,** 137.

DISCUSSION

Clinical factors determining resistance

Professor O. L. Wade. The permissive sex life of *Esch. coli* is fascinating! What worries me is that Dr. Ayliffe said that they had found this multiple resistance in one hospital and not in another. Are you able to pin down any particular factors in a hospital, e.g. clinician's behaviour or use of antibiotics, or the type of patients, which determines that that hospital has a high incidence of R factors?

Dr. N. Datta. Only in the most general terms. A very intensive use of antibiotics, particularly prophylactic use of antibiotics, leads to a greater incidence of resistant infections.

Clinical significance of resistance

Dr. A. W. Asscher. Could I ask Dr. Datta the level of resistance to which she is referring in relation to urinary pathogens as we know that with most drugs the MIC is greatly exceeded in the urine. Are the levels of resistance due to R factors of the sort of magnitude where the drug would be ineffective in the urine?

Dr. N. Datta. Yes, but not necessarily with tetracycline, although most doctors would not use tetracycline when treating urinary tract infections. Tetracycline resistance levels are often low. With sulphonamides we don't count them as resistant unless MICs are greater than 1000 μg/ml, and in fact they are always over 500 μg/ml. With ampicillin they vary quite a lot but 125 is about the usual and they go up to well over 1000 μg/ml.

Dr. N. A. Simmons. My question follows on from that. About six years ago Watanabe wrote that within the foreseeable future, because of the R factors, we could be plunged back into the pre-antibiotic era. Do you agree?

Dr. N. Datta. If it were not for the pharmaceutical industry, yes! (But this applies to the Gram-negative bacilli, not to all bacterial infections.)

Gentamicin resistance of pseudomonas

Dr. D. Shanson. Did the French workers demonstrate resistance transfer factors for gentamicin to *Pseudomonas aeruginosa*?

Dr. N. Datta. No—we have tried to transfer the gentamicin-resistance factors found in Paris to *Ps. aeruginosa* without success. In fact, the only R factors we have been able to transfer to *Ps. aeruginosa* are those which Dr. Lowbury and Dr. Ayliffe mentioned. Dr. Lowbury mentioned that the same kind had been found in Glasgow and in one other Birmingham hospital. I have had some strains from South Africa which appear to carry the same kind of R factors which we have called P, for Pseudomonas.

Dr. Chabbert has recently found R factors conferring gentamicin resistance in *Ps. aeruginosa* (Witchitz & Chabbert, 1972. *Annals of the Institute Pasteur*, **122** 367.)

DISCUSSION

4

ASSESSMENT OF RESISTANCE†

G. N. ROLINSON

WITHIN the field of antibiotic chemotherapy the question of bacterial resistance forms an important aspect. The terms sensitive and resistant however can be used in two rather different ways.

BACTERIOLOGICAL DEFINITION OF RESISTANCE

In a purely bacteriological sense, bacteria can be said to be sensitive if the level of antibiotic required for inhibition is similar to the concentration required to inhibit the majority of strains of that particular species, irrespective of the actual level concerned. In other words, the criterion is whether the bacterium shows *typical* sensitivity. For example, penicillin-sensitive strains of staphylococci are typically inhibited by benzylpenicillin at a concentration of 0·01 μg/ml, or less, and strains which require for inhibition a level of 1 or 2 μg/ml would certainly be considered resistant. However, strains of staphylococci showing minimum inhibitory concentrations of 1 to 2 μg/ml with methicillin are considered sensitive because this value is a typical level of sensitivity for staphylococci with this particular antibiotic. The sensitivity of the gonococcus to benzylpenicillin also provides an example in which the minimum inhibitory concentration may itself be quite low yet strains can be resistant if this minimum inhibitory concentration is significantly higher than that shown by typically sensitive strains. For example, sensitive strains of gonococci are inhibited by benzylpenicillin at a concentration of 0·005 μg/ml or less and therefore strains with a minimum inhibitory concentration even as low as 0·1 μg/ml may be considered penicillin resistant, or at least relatively resistant. This does not mean, however, that infections with such strains may not be successfully treated with benzylpenicillin. It may mean only that higher and perhaps more prolonged dosage is required to inhibit such strains.

CLINICAL SIGNIFICANCE OF 'RESISTANCE'

From the chemotherapeutic point of view the definition of sensitivity and resistance is rather different. In terms of the treatment of infection, bacteria may be said to be sensitive if the concentration of antibiotic required for inhibition is one which can readily be achieved in the body, at the site of infection, and this is the question which must be answered when sensitivity testing is carried out on clinical isolates in order to assist in the choice of antibiotic

† This paper was read by R. Sutherland.

for treatment. From the clinical point of view, sensitivity becomes a question of whether the minimum inhibitory concentration of the pathogen is likely to be reached at the site of infection and this will depend on where the site of infection is, and on the pharmacokinetic properties of the antibiotic and the dose and route of administration to be used.

Certain sites of infection are not readily accessible to certain antibiotics and pathogens present at such sites may be judged resistant for this reason. Other sites are potentially accessible but the level of antibiotic actually reached at these sites may vary greatly. For example, in the case of an antibiotic excreted largely through the kidneys, a level of over 1000 μg/ml might easily be reached in the urine, whereas the level in the tissues might not exceed 1 or 2 μg/ml. A pathogen showing a minimum inhibitory concentration of 5 μg/ml might therefore be judged sensitive if present at the one site but resistant in the other. This situation might be changed, however, by dosage and route of administration. In the case of a relatively non-toxic drug a higher dose, and intramuscular or intravenous administration, might result in tissue levels which clearly exceed the minimum inhibitory concentration. The same pathogen might now be considered sensitive whereas formerly it was considered resistant.

Sensitivity in a clinical sense means the ability to achieve an inhibitory concentration of antibiotic at the site of infection and this may be limited by toxicity. For example, if a strain of *Pseudomonas aeruginosa* was encountered in the tissues showing a minimum inhibitory concentration as high as 10 μg/ml with gentamicin this would certainly be considered resistant because toxicity does not allow this concentration of gentamicin to be reached with safety in the body. On the other hand, strains of *Ps. aeruginosa* showing minimum inhibitory concentrations as high as 50 or even 100 μg/ml with carbenicillin may be considered sensitive because carbenicillin is extremely non-toxic and such levels can safely be reached in the body with appropriate dosage.

Antibiotic levels in the patient

Sensitivity is therefore a relative term and is only meaningful in relation to the antibiotic levels in the body. The measurement of such levels in certain body fluids such as blood and urine is relatively simple. Determination of tissue levels of antibiotic, however, presents certain difficulties. Assay of homogenized tissue does not necessarily reflect the drug levels in the tissue fluid since they may be contaminated with blood or, in the case of kidney, with urine. The use of plasma levels as an index of tissue levels also has limitations. Firstly, certain antibiotics may diffuse poorly from the vascular system into the tissues and, secondly, the diffusion may be influenced by the extent of protein binding. With most antibiotics, and certainly with the penicillins, binding to plasma proteins is readily reversible and as unbound drug molecules diffuse out from the vascular system, bound drug dissociates rapidly. However, protein binding does have the effect of confining within the vascular system a proportion of the drug in a temporarily inactive and non-diffusible form. In this system the unbound drug molecules are quite free to diffuse into the tissues but the concentration gradient for this diffusion will be set by the level of unbound drug in the plasma and not by the level of total drug. For this reason, when the infection is present in the tissues, it is probably best to consider the sensitivity of the organism in relation to the levels of free antibiotic reached in the plasma rather than in relation to the total level of bound and free drug.

LABORATORY METHODS FOR DETERMINING SENSITIVITY OF BACTERIA

Minimum inhibitory concentrations

Determination of the sensitivity of the pathogens in terms of the minimum inhibitory concentration also presents some difficulties both practical and theoretical. The sensitivity of the organism at the site of infection may not be the same as that shown *in vitro*. Such factors as the number of bacteria present, the pH and the presence of proteins and other substances may influence markedly the concentration of antibiotic required for inhibition. From the practical point of view, determination of the minimum inhibitory concentration by a serial dilution procedure is also considered by most clinical laboratories to be too time-consuming for routine sensitivity testing and it is for this reason that the disc sensitivity test is by far the most widely used method.

Disc sensitivity testing

In practice the disc test is extremely simple to carry out. Paper discs, impregnated with antibiotic, are placed on the surface of an agar plate which has been inoculated with the test organism. After incubation, a zone of inhibition is obtained around the disc and the diameter of this zone is used as an index of the sensitivity of the organism. The size of the inhibition zone, however, is influenced by a number of factors including inoculum size, the conditions of incubation, the depth of agar and the medium composition, etc., and these factors must be controlled in order to obtain reliable and reproducible results.

Recommendations for the standardization of disc testing have been made, notably by Ericsson (1960), Bauer, Kirby, Sherris and Turck (1966) and by Ericsson and Sherris (1971). However, these recommendations involve such rigid control of the test conditions that the simplicity of the disc test is to some extent lost and many laboratories may feel unable to adopt these recommendations in full. If the Ericsson or Kirby-Bauer methods are not followed completely the laboratory should at least make use of standard organisms so that inhibition zones can be compared with those obtained with organisms of known sensitivity (Barber & Stokes, 1966).

METHOD COMBINING SIMPLICITY OF DISC TEST WITH QUANTITATIVE SENSITIVITY DETERMINATION

Because of the problems associated with the standardization and interpretation of disc sensitivity testing we have devised a test method (Rolinson & Russell, 1971) which retains the simplicity of the disc test but which allows determination of sensitivity to be made to known concentrations of drug as is the case in a serial dilution test. In this method, known concentrations of antibiotic are obtained by placing papers impregnated with antibiotic on to the surface of small volumes of agar contained in a plastic tray and allowing the antibiotic to diffuse into the agar until a uniform concentration is achieved. By using a relatively shallow layer of agar, uniform distribution of the antibiotic in the agar is achieved in a surprisingly short period of time and for most antibiotics a period of 3 hours diffusion is sufficient. The papers are then removed and the agar surface inoculated with the test organism. After incubation, bacterial growth, or inhibition of growth, is observed directly.

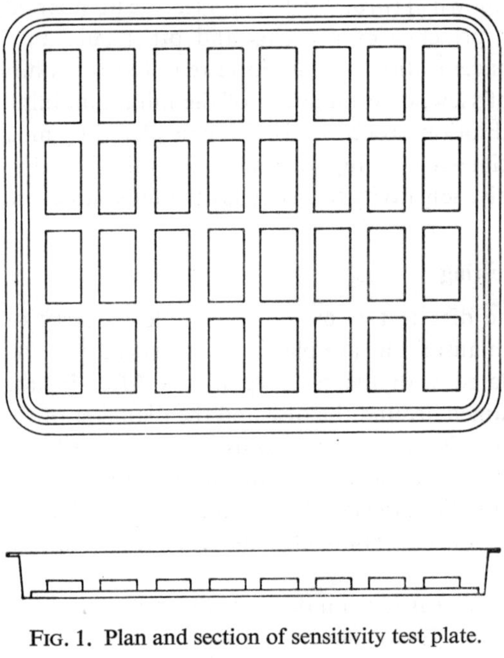

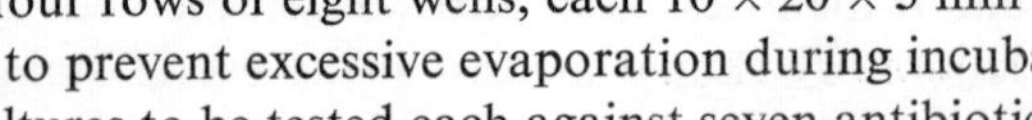

FIG. 1. Plan and section of sensitivity test plate.

The plastic tray containing the wells which are filled with agar may be of any suitable shape and a drawing of one design is shown in Figure 1. This plate provides four rows of eight wells, each $10 \times 20 \times 3$ mm in depth with a close fitting lid to prevent excessive evaporation during incubation. The tray enables four cultures to be tested each against seven antibiotics with one well containing drug-free agar for control growth. It is envisaged that the tray itself would be made available commercially, pre-poured with agar ready for use. Paper strips, 1 cm wide, impregnated uniformly with individual antibiotics would also be supplied commercially. The quantity of antibiotic on the paper strips would be such that the correct amount was available for diffusion into each agar well to give the desired concentration.

The diffusion of antibiotics into such wells of agar has been measured in the following way. Papers impregnated with antibiotic were placed on the surface of blocks of agar 10 × 20 × 3 mm and the papers then removed after intervals of time. The residual amount of antibiotic in each paper after removal was then assayed. In addition, the concentration of antibiotic at both the upper and lower surfaces of the agar block was also assayed. This was carried out by applying drug-free paper to both surfaces and allowing the papers to absorb liquid from the agar. By this means a standard volume of liquid was obtained in which the antibiotic concentration was representative of that present at

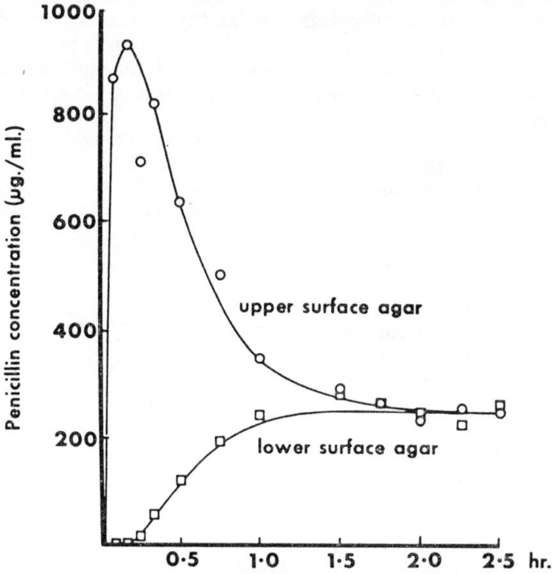

FIG. 2. Diffusion of penicillin G through a 3 mm layer of agar. Concentration of penicillin in the upper surface of agar ○—○; concentration of penicillin in the lower surface of agar □—□. Blocks of agar 1 cm × 1 cm × 3 mm were prepared and 1 cm squares of filter paper containing 100 μg penicillin G were applied to the upper surface of the blocks. After intervals of time the concentration of penicillin in the upper and lower surfaces of agar was assayed. This was carried out by removing the antibiotic paper and applying a 1 cm square of filter paper to the upper and lower surfaces of the blocks. A fixed volume of liquid is thus taken up by the paper from the agar surfaces and the concentration can be assayed against standards prepared from agar containing known concentrations of antibiotic.

the upper and lower agar surface. The papers were then placed on an agar assay plate seeded with a suitable test organism. After incubation the resulting zones of inhibition were used to calculate the antibiotic concentration by reference to regression lines prepared using blocks of agar containing known concentrations of antibiotic.

An example of these experiments is shown in Figure 2. This shows the diffusion of benzylpenicillin and it will be seen that the antibiotic diffused rapidly from the paper into the agar. Assay of the antibiotic concentration at the upper and lower surfaces of the agar block showed that essentially uniform distribution throughout the agar was achieved in approximately $1\frac{1}{2}$–2 hours.

TABLE 1

RATE OF DIFFUSION OF ANTIBIOTICS IN AGAR

1 cm squares of Whatman no. 1 paper impregnated with 100 μg antibiotic were placed on the upper surface of blocks of Blood Agar Base (Oxoid), 1 cm × 1 cm × 3 mm thick and the diffusion of the antibiotic into the agar was measured after intervals of time. The diffusion time is the time taken for the concentration of antibiotic at the lower surface of the agar to reach 95 per cent of the concentration at the upper surface. Results given are the mean of at least two determinations.

Antibiotic	*Diffusion time (minutes)*
Cephaloridine	90
Benzylpenicillin	110
Ampicillin	120
Methicillin	130
Cloxacillin	140
Fusidic acid	150
Streptomycin	160
Kanamycin	160
Gentamicin	190
Lincomycin	200
Erythromycin	220
Tetracycline	230
Novobiocin	270
Vancomycin	300
Polymyxin	480

The diffusion time for a number of other antibiotics is shown in Table 1. The diffusion time referred to in this table is the time taken for the antibiotic concentration at the lower agar surface to reach 95 per cent of that present at the upper surface, that is to say, essentially uniform distribution. It will be seen that the diffusion time of the penicillins and cephaloridine was rapid, the diffusion time being approximately 2 hours. With fusidic acid, streptomycin, kanamycin, gentamicin and lincomycin, diffusion was essentially complete after approximately 3 hours, while in the case of erythromycin, tetracycline, novobiocin and vancomycin 4–5 hours was required. Polymyxin required approximately 8 hours for 95 per cent uniform distribution but after only 3 hours the concentrations at the upper and lower surfaces differed by less than a factor of two and in practice a 3 hour period of diffusion has proved adequate to give reliable results with all the antibiotics shown in this table.

A comparison of minimum inhibitory concentrations determined using the test method described here, with the values obtained by conventional serial dilution of the antibiotics in agar is shown in Table 2. It will be seen that the results are in very close agreement and they confirm that the antibiotic concentrations obtained by this method are valid. In these experiments the paper strips impregnated with antibiotic were left in contact with the agar for 3 hours.

TABLE 2

COMPARISON OF NEW METHOD AND CONVENTIONAL SERIAL DILUTION METHOD

		Minimum inhibitory concentration (μg/ml)	
Antibiotic	*Organism*	*Conventional serial dilution in agar*	*New method*
Cloxacillin	*Staph. aureus*	0·1	0·25
Ampicillin	*E. coli*	2·5	2·5
Carbenicillin	*Ps. aeruginosa*	25	25
Cephaloridine	*E. coli*	2·5	2·5
Tetracycline	*E. coli*	5·0	5·0
Chloramphenicol	*Salm. typhi*	1·0	1·0
Erythromycin	*Staph. aureus*	0·1	0·1
Sulphamethoxazole	*E. coli*	2·5	2·5

When using this plate for routine sensitivity testing if diffusion is allowed to take place during the morning the plate is ready for use in the afternoon. Alternatively, diffusion can be allowed to proceed overnight.

After the period of diffusion the papers are removed and the plate inoculated using a swab, each specimen being streaked across the plate from one side to the other. After overnight incubation, bacterial growth or inhibition of growth can be seen directly.

The sensitivity test method described here is not significantly more time consuming than the conventional disc test and has certain advantages. Firstly, the test is a direct one which avoids completely the interpretation of a zone of inhibition and, secondly, it is less influenced by inoculum size than is the disc test. This is because diffusion of the antibiotic and growth of the test organism do not proceed simultaneously as they do in the disc test. The main advantage of the method, however, is that organisms can be tested for sensitivity to known concentrations of antibiotic and these concentrations can be chosen to correspond to the levels of antibiotic likely to be achieved in the body.

REFERENCES

BARBER, M. & STOKES, E. J. (1966). Association of Clinical Pathologists Broadsheet, No. 55.

BAUER, A. W., KIRBY, W. M. M., SHERRIS, J. C. & TURCK, M. (1966). Antibiotic susceptibility testing by a standard single disk method. *American Journal of Clinical Pathology*, **45,** 493.

ERICSSON, H. M. (1960). Rational use of antibiotics in hospitals. *Scandinavian Journal of Clinical and Laboratory Investigation*, **12,** Supplement 50.

ERICSSON, H. M. & SHERRIS, J. C. (1971). Antibiotic sensitivity testing. *Acta Pathologica et Microbiologica Scandinavica*, Supplement 217.

ROLINSON, G. N. & RUSSELL, E. J. (1971). A new method for antibiotic sensitivity testing. *Lancet*, **2,** 745.

DISCUSSION

Comments by the bacteriologists

Dr. Joan Stokes. I think that this is an extremely good way of getting over the difficulty which all laboratories have of making dilutions in media. It does save adding quantities of drug to molten agar which is a tricky thing to do and also gets over the inaccuracies of dilution techniques. One thing that worries me slightly is that it's rather more difficult to control and I think that whatever method you adopt you should compare with a sensitive control. This of course could be done in this method but then you would have to do it for each drug on each batch of plates. This can be overcome and I think that it holds great promise. I would be interested to try it out and would like to know when the plates and strips will be commercially available?

Mr. R. Sutherland. They won't be commercially available until trial runs show that people are interested in the method. Dr. Rolinson is hoping that some plates will be prepared and some paper strips will be available fairly soon so that certain laboratories can try the method. We are not ourselves directly concerned with routine sensitivity testing so this is largely a theoretical exercise. We'd like to see how it works in the routine laboratory.

Miss P. M. Waterworth. I think the only answer is that the proof of the pudding must be in the eating. When Professor Garrod read the original paper he was very much afraid that this was being put out as a 'do it yourself' kit, such as is so often done in America. I think there is a point that you could make clear and that is that it has only been recommended for use in laboratories—not for people to give to their general practitioners to inoculate and use for themselves. Apart from this I look forward to trying it.

Dr. G. M. Williamson. I certainly am not greatly enamoured with the FDA's recommendations on the Kirby-Bauer technique.

Professor W. Brumfitt. Do the audience know what the Kirby-Bauer technique is? Would you mind briefly describing the technique.

Dr. G. M. Williamson. Briefly, if you plot the range of MIC's on one axis against the zone of inhibition against a standard disc on the other axis there is a straight line relationship. Kirby and his collaborators have gone into this in great detail and have drawn up limits of zones of inhibition in which you can define that an organism is either sensitive or resistant. It is a very tricky technique. If one attempts to do it as the FDA laid down against barium sulphate standards I can't see any routine laboratory using this technique. I have always got at the back of my mind, having worked in a diagnostic laboratory, that the busy clinical bacteriologist can't work with these highly refined techniques.

Professor W. Brumfitt. So that in summary this is an attempt by a disc method to produce an MIC by comparing disc zone with accurate MIC's and then from this plot reading them off?

Dr. G. M. Williamson. Yes, that is right. Like Professor Garrod I was very interested in the original paper on the present technique, and I am sure our speaker has given us only one or two examples. My criticism is that you are only using one concentration of a particular antibiotic. I still feel that the method that the Oxoid Group produce, of a high and low disc, is the most practical but I may be out of date.

Professor W. Brumfitt. Would you use control organisms?

Dr. G. M. Williamson. I am a great believer in a control organism.

Mr. R. Sutherland. The only comment that I would make is that Dr. Gould tried the Kirby-Bauer method a long time ago, but it didn't become fashionable presumably as it involved too much work on the part of the laboratory.

Dr. J. C. Gould. I think that all of this discussion really centres around the question of the desirability of a strictly quantitative, or what one might imagine as a quantitative, estimation of the sensitivity of an organism as opposed to qualitative estimations. One must ask the question, as I'm sure Mr. Sutherland and others are continually asking themselves, whether we are in a position to benefit from these more exact estimations? One benefit of the diffusion tests, whether they are carried out carelessly or carefully is that you do get a range of values. I admit that there are a large number of variables but all tests have variables and they must be controlled. It is certainly a very interesting method and well worth evaluating in the laboratory. Dr. Williamson has said, however, if you have a large routine laboratory you must evaluate this also against the time available. I accept at its face value what you say about it in comparison with the simple disc diffusion tests in requiring no more time. I would like to try that in practice.

Comment by a physician

Dr. J. G. Lewis. As far as I am concerned, sensitivity tests with organisms from sputum, which are what I deal with most commonly, are valueless, as invariably a non-pathogen is isolated and the sensitivity test is religiously done on the organism which couldn't possibly be doing any harm to the patient.

5

USE OF ANTIBIOTICS AND RESISTANCE

G. A. J. Ayliffe

The well-known adaptability of micro-organisms to toxic agents has been clearly demonstrated by the emergence of resistance to most antibiotics introduced over the past 30 years. The organisms particularly involved in the emergence of resistance are *Staphylococcus aureus*, gram negative bacilli (Enterobacteria and *Pseudomonas aeruginosa*) and also tubercle bacilli, which are not considered in this paper.

Benzylpenicillin was introduced as a therapeutic agent in 1940 and the clinical problem of penicillin-resistant *Staph. aureus* became apparent in the late nineteen-forties when Mary Barber and others described the increasing incidence of resistant-strains in hospitals (Barber & Rozwadowska-Dowzenko, 1948). From this time and during the nineteen-fifties a number of other antibiotics active against staphylococci were introduced, i.e. chloramphenicol, tetracyclines, erythromycin, novobiocin, kanamycin, neomycin, vancomycin and ristocetin. Resistance emerged to all these antibiotics except vancomycin and ristocetin which are toxic antibiotics and were infrequently used.

A high incidence of resistant-strains in hospital patients or in the environment was often related to usage of a particular antibiotic (Knight & Holzer, 1954; Alder & Gillespie, 1967), although sometimes there was a long delay before resistance emerged (Forfar *et al.*, 1966); resistant-strains of *Staph. aureus* did not appear for over nine years after the introduction of neomycin (Lowbury *et al.*, 1964). A reduction in usage of the antibiotic was often associated with a corresponding reduction in the frequency of isolation of resistant-strains (Kirby & Ahern, 1953) and sometimes a plasmid controlling resistance was lost (Ayliffe, 1970).

The introduction from 1960 onwards of methicillin, other penicillinase resistant penicillins and the cephalosporins was followed by a decline in importance of staphylococcal infections, and since then gram negative bacilli have played a dominant role in hospital infection. However, the late Mary Barber and other microbiologists considered that methicillin-resistant staphylococci would become a therapeutic problem in the future, particularly as a few naturally methicillin-resistant strains had already been described. The incidence of methicillin-resistant staphylococci is now high in some countries, e.g. Denmark (Rosendal, 1971), and appears to be increasing in this country (Parker & Hewitt, 1970). The influence of antibiotic usage on the resistance of gram negative bacilli is more difficult to determine, since a number of genera and species are involved, methods of typing are less readily available, and some organisms show a natural resistance to certain antibiotics. Nevertheless, there is considerable evidence of selection of resistant species following antibiotic treatment.

In the present study, the resistance of *Staph. aureus* and Gram negative bacilli and the use of antimicrobial agents in hospitals of the Birmingham Region is considered.

SURVEYS OF ANTIBIOTIC-RESISTANT ORGANISMS IN BIRMINGHAM

Cross-sectional surveys of hospital infection have been made in over thirty hospitals of varying size and type in the Birmingham Region since 1967 (Ayliffe *et al.*, 1969). In a survey, a team visits all the wards in a hospital and records the number of infections, details of ward structure and practices, which include the number of patients receiving antimicrobial agents at the time of the visit. Swabs are taken from the noses of all patients and from lesions.

Bacteriological methods

Bacteriological swabs from noses were cultured on nutrient agar containing 1 per cent serum, 10 μg/ml tetracycline and phenolphthalein diphosphate (Barber & Kuper, 1951). Nose swabs were screened for tetracycline-resistant staphylococci since these are mainly hospital strains and are still uncommon in the general population. Presumptive colonies of *Staph. aureus* were confirmed by slide or tube coagulase tests. Antibiotic sensitivities of *Staph. aureus* and some of the Gram negative bacilli were determined by the ditch-plate method. Methicillin-resistance was detected initially by the use of 5 per cent salt agar, and for the past two years by the presence of growth of staphylococci when cultured for 18 hours at 30°C (Annear, 1968). Other samples were cultured on blood agar and McConkey plates and antibiotic sensitivities were determined by a disc method (Oxoid multodiscs). Strains showing a reduced zone of inhibition by either method when compared with a standard sensitive organism were reported as resistant. Minimum inhibitory concentrations of antibiotics were determined by broth or agar dilution methods on many strains, particularly if resistance appeared to be doubtful by the other methods, or was otherwise unusual.

Incidence of resistant organisms related to antibiotic use

The incidence of usage of antibiotics and resistance of *Staph. aureus* from patients' noses are shown in Table 1. Similar patterns of resistance were obtained from wounds and lesions. Resistance to benzylpenicillin is excluded from the table since resistance is now frequently found in strains isolated from the general community. The incidence of methicillin-resistant strains has increased since 1968, but usage has remained the same. The increased incidence is mainly a measure of cross-infection in some hospitals and is not

TABLE 1

USE OF ANTIBIOTICS AND RESISTANCE OF *Staph. aureus* ISOLATED FROM NOSES OF PATIENTS IN HOSPITALS OF THE BIRMINGHAM REGION 1967–1970

		Per cent of patients treated				*Per cent incidence of resistance of* Staph. aureus *in noses*			
Year	*Number of patients*	*Tet.*[a]	*Meth. or Clox.*	*Ery.*	*Nov.*	*Tet.*	*Meth.*	*Ery.*	*Nov.*
1967	1478	5·4	1·1	0·2	0·14	10·7	0·14	3·6	0·5
1968	2319	7·2	2·9	0·5	0	9·1	1·0	5·1	2·3
1969	2181	4·8	2·8	0·4	0	9·4	2·4	4·6	3·0
1970	2321	5·1	2·4	0·1	0	6·2	2·7	4·6	2·2

[a] Tet.—tetracycline; Meth.—methicillin; Clox.—cloxacillin; Ery.—erythromycin; Nov.—novobiocin.

TABLE 6

RESISTANCE TO ANTIMICROBIAL AGENTS OF ROUTINE LABORATORY ISOLATES OF GRAM NEGATIVE BACILLI IN TWO HOSPITALS

			Per cent of strains resistant to						
Organism	*Source of organisms*	*Number isolated*	*Amp.*	*Kan.*	*Tet.*	*Strep.*	*Nit.*	*Nal.*	*Trim.*
Proteus mirabilis	1. Burns Unit	268	52·6	70·9	93·7	11	98	3	14·9
	2. A General Hospital	282	24	4	88	36	64	6	—
Klebsiella aerogenes	1. Burns Unit	215	75·8	55·8	72·1	30	77	4	12·1
	2. A General Hospital	167	98	9	46	38	19	23	—

Amp.—ampicillin; Kan.—kanamycin; Tet.—tetracycline; Strep.—streptomycin; Nit.—nitrofurantoin; Nal.—nalidixic acid; Trim.—trimethoprim; — Not tested.

necessarily related to the amount of antibiotic used in those hospitals, but could also be related to an overall increase in the use of penicillins. Most of the methicillin-resistant strains whether isolated in the same or different hospitals, showed a similar phage pattern (29/77/88 or various combinations of these phages).

Erythromycin and particularly novobiocin were rarely used for treating patients yet resistant-strains were frequently isolated. Resistance to these antibiotics appears to be stable and may be linked to that of penicillin and tetracycline and sometimes to neomycin and methicillin. Resistance and usage of other antibiotics, e.g. fucidin, lincomycin, chloramphenicol was low during the period of study shown in this table. The level of neomycin (or kanamycin) resistance (3·2 per cent) during the four years was presumably due mainly to topical use, although this was difficult to assess. An increased incidence of fusidic acid and lincomycin-resistance was found in surveys of dermatological wards during the past year (Table 2). The minimum inhibitory concentration

TABLE 2

INCIDENCE OF *Staph. aureus* RESISTANT TO FUSIDIC ACID AND LINCOMYCIN IN NOSES OR ON SKIN OF PATIENTS IN DERMATOLOGICAL WARDS

Date of survey	*Number of patients sampled (nose & skin)*	*Number of patients carrying strains resistant to*	
		Fusidic acid	*Lincomycin*
September 1970	40	2 (5%)	0
April 1971	51	13 (26%)	1 (0·5%)
December 1971	30	13 (43%)	11 (37%)

of fusidic acid ranged from 4 to 32 μg/ml and that of lincomycin was >256 μg/ml. The use of topical preparations of fusidic acid in these wards had increased from 1902 g of ointment during a period of April to September 1970 to 3550 g during a similar period in 1971. Lincomycin or clindamycin was commonly used but no obvious increase in use was found. It is probable that other factors, e.g. cross-infection, susceptibility to colonization and age of patient are as or more important than the use of antibiotics in the establishment of an antibiotic-resistant flora in a hospital.

TABLE 3

THE INCIDENCE OF TETRACYCLINE-RESISTANT *Staph. aureus* IN NOSES, ANTIBIOTIC USAGE AND LENGTH OF STAY OF PATIENTS IN BIRMINGHAM HOSPITALS 1967–70

Type of patient	*Number of patients*	*Per cent showing Tet. res.* Staph. aureus *in noses*	*Per cent treated with antibiotics*	*Mean length of stay (days)*
Geriatric	165	13·3	8·5	77
Surgical	1253	10·6	30	17
Medical	1081	9·9	26	17
Paediatric	249	3·6	38	18
Obstetric	398	3·5	10	8

Table 3 shows several relevant factors and indicates that the incidence of tetracycline-resistant strains in noses of patients varies with the type of ward, age and length of stay of patient as well as with the use of antibiotics. Geriatric patients show a high carriage rate and although few are treated with antibiotics the average length of stay in hospital is far longer than any other patient. In contrast, obstetric patients are young, in hospital for a short time and have a low carriage rate; the number treated with antibiotics is also low.

Linked resistance and antibiotic use

The changes in the use of other antibiotics and antimicrobial agents from 1967–8 to 1969–70 are shown in Table 4. Although the overall incidence of

TABLE 4

USE OF ANTIMICROBIAL AGENTS IN HOSPITALS OF BIRMINGHAM REGION 1967–70

Agent	*Per cent of patients treated* 1967–8	1969–70
Ampicillin	7·6	10·4
Tetracycline	6·5	5·0
Penicillin	5·2	4·2
Streptomycin	2·0	1·6
Sulphonamides	1·2	0·8
Nitrofurantoin	1·4	0·8
Co-trimoxazole	0·0	1·6
Others	<0·5	<0·5
Total	25·7	26·3

1967–8—3797 patients: 1969–70—4502 patients.

patients treated remained unchanged, more were treated with ampicillin and fewer with tetracycline and other antibiotics. The possible effect of these changes on resistance of gram negative bacilli is clearly of importance. A single survey of the number of patients treated with antimicrobial drugs in one

TABLE 5

USE OF ANTIMICROBIAL AGENTS AND RESISTANCE OF ROUTINE LABORATORY ISOLATES OF *Esch. coli*

Antibiotic	*Per cent of resistant strains*[a]	*Per cent of patients treated*[b]
Ampicillin	35	12
Tetracycline	36	5·2
Sulphonamide	31	2·2
Streptomycin	31	1·4
Kanamycin	4	0·1
Nitrofurantoin	6	1·4
Nalidixic acid	5	0·4

[a] Total isolates in Dudley Road Hospital July–September 1971—853.

[b] Survey of 709 patients—August 1971.

hospital was made by the Dudley Road Infection Control staff in August 1971, and is shown with the resistance of routine laboratory isolates of *Escherichia coli* from July to September 1971 in Table 5. The pattern of use is fairly similar to that in the Region as a whole. The incidence of resistance to sulphonamides and streptomycin was the same as that of resistance to ampicillin and tetracycline, although the former were used much less, and the similarity of the incidence of resistance between these four agents suggests that resistance may be linked and probably controlled by a resistance ('R') factor. Resistance to ampicillin, tetracycline, sulphonamides and streptomycin is a common pattern of resistance controlled by an 'R' factor and in laboratory experiments using some of these strains, resistance to all four agents could usually be transferred together to a sensitive strain of *Esch. coli* K12

Nitrofurantoin was used as often as streptomycin, but resistance to it was much less common and was not transferable, although strains of *Proteus mirabilis* were usually resistant and may have been selected by its use (Table 6, page 55). The use of trimethoprim is increasing and although resistance is not yet a problem in most hospitals, resistant strains have been isolated in the burns unit of the Birmingham Accident Hospital and have increased since the previous survey in that unit (Roe & Lowbury, 1972).

The spread in a ward or unit of an 'R' factor controlling resistance to several antibiotics may be due to the predominant use of one of these antibiotics; cross-infection with the multiple-resistant organism will lead to a further increase of bacteria showing this resistance pattern through transfer of the 'R' factor to the same or other species.

Table 6 shows a comparison between resistance patterns of *P. mirabilis* and *Klebsiella aerogenes* isolated in the burns unit of Birmingham Accident Hospital 1969–71 and from routine specimens in a general hospital (Dudley Road) from July to September 1971. The main differences between the two hospitals are the much higher incidence in the burns unit of resistance of both organisms to kanamycin, and of *P. mirabilis* to ampicillin. The ampicillin-resistant strains from the burns unit were also mainly resistant to carbenicillin, and carried an 'R' factor controlling resistance to ampicillin, carbenicillin, tetracycline and kanamycin. A much smaller percentage of strains from the general hospital were resistant to kanamycin suggesting this particular 'R' factor occurs infrequently. The 'R' factor was also unusual in that it could be transferred to *Ps. aeruginosa* (Roe & Lowbury, 1972). After transfer of carbenicillin-resistance to sensitive strains of *Ps. aeruginosa* had taken place in the unit (Lowbury *et al.*, 1969) carbenicillin, one of a limited number of antibiotics available for treating Pseudomonas infections, was of much less therapeutic value in the unit.

PRESENT TRENDS IN ANTIBIOTIC RESISTANCE

Although in some hospitals there is evidence of a reduction in the incidence of antibiotic resistance in isolates of *Staph. aureus* over the past ten years

(Bulger *et al.*, 1968; Ridley *et al.*, 1970), this is not so in hospitals without an antibiotic policy or with no measures for controlling cross-infection (Stokes *et al.*, 1972). Methicillin-resistant strains are isolated with increasing frequency and strains resistant to the 'reserve' antibiotics, fusidic acid and lincomycin, emerge when these antibiotics are used. Restriction of antibiotics which were widely used in the past, i.e. erythromycin and novobiocin, has not obviously been followed by an associated loss of resistance or by the disappearance of resistant strains; if resistance to several antibiotics is sometimes linked in *Staph. aureus*, use of any one of several antibiotics will tend to select the strain. From the results obtained in this Region, it seems possible that within a few years there may be no effective non-toxic antibiotics available for treating hospital-acquired staphylococcal infection in some hospitals.

A similar situation arises with gram negative bacilli, although as with *Staph. aureus*, evidence of increasing incidence of resistance varies in different countries, regions, or hospitals. In one study from four hospitals, there appeared to be little evidence of increasing resistance to ampicillin from 1961 to 1967 (Slocombe & Sutherland, 1969). Other studies have shown an increasing incidence of ampicillin-resistant strains and some reports suggest *Klebsiella* sp. were probably selected by the prophylactic use of ampicillin (Price & Sleigh, 1970). Superinfection or colonization with resistant strains is commonly observed in patients treated with broad spectrum antibiotics. In a study of our own (J. Noy—personal communication), ampicillin-resistant *Klebsiella* sp. were isolated from the faeces of 43/47 (92 per cent) neonates treated with ampicillin or 'ampiclox' and from 101/242 (42 per cent) in untreated infants.

CONCLUSION

The high incidence and disturbing prospects of antibiotic resistance as described in this paper are influenced by the consideration only of hospitals and by the inclusion of special units where cross-infection is difficult to prevent and resistant organisms are particularly likely to emerge. Resistant organisms in the general population are not yet a major problem and some organisms, e.g. Lancefields' Group A haemolytic streptococci, have remained sensitive to benzylpenicillin after 30 years exposure to the antibiotic. Nevertheless, strains of *Staph. aureus* (and gram negative bacilli) resistant to five or six antibiotics are present in many of the thirty hospitals surveyed; it seems likely that similar resistant strains are present in many other hospitals throughout the country (Hale & Selkon, 1970), despite reports indicating a much lower incidence in some individual hospitals. Treatment problems due to infection with these resistant strains already exist and measures are required to prevent the emergence of resistance to 'reserve' or newly introduced antibiotics and to prevent the spread of resistant strains both within and between hospitals.

Effective use of an antibiotic policy and the provision of adequate isolation facilities for infected patients in all hospitals are urgent requirements.

I wish to thank Mrs. K. Brightwell, S.R.N., Dr. E. J. L. Lowbury and Dr. J. D. Williams for their collaboration in this study.

REFERENCES

ALDER, V. G. & GILLESPIE, W. A. (1967). Influence of neomycin sprays on the spread of resistant staphylococci. *Lancet*, **ii**, 1062.

ANNEAR, D. I. (1968). The effect of temperature on resistance of *Staphylococcus aureus* to methicillin and some other antibiotics. *Medical Journal of Australia*, **1**, 444.

AYLIFFE, G. A. J. (1970). Stability of neomycin resistance in *Staphylococcus aureus*. *Journal of Clinical Pathology*, **23**, 19.

AYLIFFE, G. A. J., BRIGHTWELL, K. M., COLLINS, B. J. & LOWBURY, E. J. L. (1969). Varieties of aseptic practice in hospital wards. *Lancet*, **ii**, 1117.

BARBER, M. & KUPER, S. W. A. (1951). Identification of *Staphylococcus pyogenes* by phosphatase reaction. *Journal of Pathology and Bacteriology*, **63**, 65.

BARBER, M. & ROZWADOWSKA-DOWZENKO, M. (1948). Infection by penicillin-resistant staphylococci. *Lancet*, **ii**, 641.

BULGER, R. J. & SHERRIS, J. C. (1968). Decreased incidence of antibiotic resistance among *Staphylococcus aureus*. A study in a University Hospital over a 9 year period. *Annals of Internal Medicine*, **69**, 1099.

FORFAR, J. O., KEAY, A. J., MACCABE, A. F., GOULD, J. C. & BAIN, A. D. (1966). Liberal use of antibiotics and its effect in neonatal staphylococcal infection with particular reference to erythromycin. *Lancet*, **ii**, 295.

HALE, J. H. & SELKON, J. B. (1970). Multiple resistant staphylococci. *Lancet*, **ii**, 528.

KIRBY, W. M. M. & AHERN, J. J. (1953). Changing pattern of resistance of staphylococci to antibiotics. *Antibiotic and Chemotherapy*, **3**, 831.

KNIGHT, V. & HOLZER, A. R. (1954). Studies on staphylococci from hospital patients; predominance of strains of Group III phage patterns which are resistant to multiple antibiotics. *Journal of Clinical Investigation*, **33**, 1190.

LOWBURY, E. J. L., BABB, J. R., BROWN, V. L. & COLLINS, B. J. (1964). Neomycin-resistant *Staphylococcus aureus* in a burns unit. *Journal of Hygiene (Cambridge)*, **62**, 221.

LOWBURY, E. J. L., KIDSON, A., LILLY, H. A., AYLIFFE, G. A. J. & JONES, R. J. (1969). Sensitivity of *Pseudomonas aeruginosa* to antibiotics: Emergence of strains highly resistant to carbenicillin. *Lancet*, **ii**, 448.

PARKER, M. T. & HEWITT, J. H. (1970). Methicillin-resistance in *Staphylococcus aureus*. *Lancet*, **i**, 800.

PRICE, D. J. E. & SLEIGH, J. D. (1970). Control of infection due to *Klebsiella aerogenes* in a neurosurgical unit by withdrawal of all antibiotics. *Lancet*, **ii**, 1213.

RIDLEY, M., BARRIE, D., LYNN, R. & STEAD, K. C. (1970). Antibiotic-resistant *Staphylococcus aureus* and hospital antibiotic policies. *Lancet*, **i**, 230.

ROE, E. & LOWBURY, E. J. L. (1972). Changes in antibiotic sensitivity patterns of Gram-negative bacilli in burns. *Journal of Clinical Pathology*, **25**, 176.

ROSENDAL, K. (1971). *Proceedings of International Conference on Nosocomial Infections, August*, 1970, p. 11. Waverley Press, Baltimore.

SLOCOMBE, B. & SUTHERLAND, R. (1969). Sensitivity of Gram-negative bacilli to ampicillin after six years clinical use. *Journal of Clinical Pathology*, **22**, 644.

STOKES, E. J., BRADLEY, J. M., THOMPSON, R. E. M., HITCHCOCK, N. M., PARKER, M. J. & WALKER, J. S. (1972). Hospital staphylococci in three London teaching hospitals. *Lancet*, **i**, 84.

DISCUSSION

Carbenicillin resistance of pseudomonas

Dr. E. J. L. Lowbury. Dr. Ayliffe spoke about the peculiar flora and resistance patterns that we have experienced in the Burns Unit at the Birmingham Accident Hospital. Figure 1 illustrates the appearance of strains of *Pseudomonas aeruginosa*, highly resistant to carbenicillin, which appeared in that Unit in March 1969, three years after we started using carbenicillin—a three year period in which numerous strains were tested and found sensitive to carbenicillin. In the upper histogram, the black columns show the resistant and the dotted columns the sensitive isolates of *Ps. aeruginosa.* Within the two months from March to May, sensitive strains were completely replaced by resistant strains. The most interesting fact, however, was that within a very short period of time several different unrelated types of *Ps. aeruginosa* (as shown by serological and phage typing) showed this high degree of resistance, which was associated also with 'carbenicillinase' activity (a feature not previously found in any strains of *Ps. aeruginosa*).

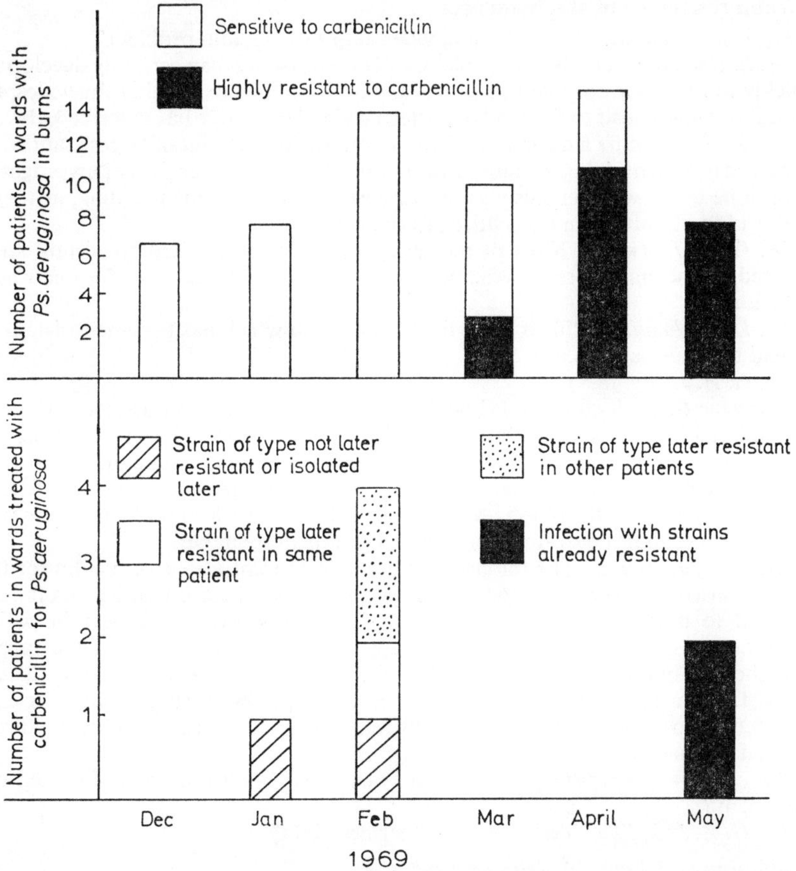

FIG. 1. Emergence of carbenicillin-resistant pseudomonas strains—Birmingham Accident Hospital (Courtesy of the Editor, *The Lancet*).

This gave us the idea that these organisms were carrying an R factor. Work by Professor Richmond and his colleagues in Bristol and by the team at the Beecham Research Laboratories quickly confirmed that this was the case, and in fact implicated enterobacteria such as *Escherichia coli*, proteus and klebsiella as a potential source from which the pseudomonas had acquired this R factor. The R factor carried linked resistance to tetracycline, kanamycin, carbenicillin, ampicillin and cephaloridine, and we found that it could be transferred between enterobacteria and *Ps. aeruginosa* in mouse burns.

Since then we have examined strains from eleven hospitals in addition to our own and have found that there was only one other hospital, apart from our own, where a pseudomonas of the same sort as ours was found—also a hospital with a burns unit. The same two hospitals and one other hospital in Birmingham were also the only ones where strains of proteus carrying an R factor which could transfer carbenicillin resistance to *Ps. aeruginosa* via an *Esch. coli* K12 was also found. From the other hospital in Birmingham, only one of the strains of proteus sent to us for examination carried an R factor, and so far as I am aware no problem of pseudomonas resistance to carbenicillin has been reported in that hospital.

Fucidin resistance of staphylococci

Professor Brumfitt. Dr. Goldman, what about the fucidin problem?

Dr. L. Goldman. Yes, it is a problem. Fucidin resistance can certainly develop very quickly in the laboratory and there has always been the anxiety that the widespread topical use might lead to the kind of pattern which Dr. Ayliffe has described. I would like to ask Dr. Ayliffe a question. These 13 out of 30 or 30 out of 50 resistant strains appeared in a dermatological unit. Presumably phage-typing and other investigations were done to see whether this was one organism or one strain spreading, as they do in this kind of unit, from one patient to the next?

Dr. G. A. J. Ayliffe. Most of the phage patterns of the fucidin-resistant strains isolated in the unit were very similar and there is evidence of widespread cross-infection.

Dr. L. Goldman. So this is quite likely one strain which has become resistant and spread to other patients.

Dr. G. A. J. Ayliffe. Yes.

Professor G. R. F. Hilson. I'd like to follow up the fucidin question. You were determining I presume bacteriological resistance to fucidin. This is one of the cases where there is a difference between bacteriological resistance and clinical resistance. The first-step mutation in fucidin is from about two to three micrograms up to about twelve or twenty but the blood level is about 100. What I would like to know is was there evidence that the strain as such was clinically untreatable?

Dr. G. A. J. Ayliffe. The minimum inhibitory concentrations of fucidin for these strains varied between 8 and 64 μg/ml. There is no evidence that lesions failed to respond to treatment, but resistant organisms did sometimes appear in patients after the end of treatment. A topical preparation of fucidin was used and presumably there were areas of skin adjacent to lesions in which levels of fucidin fell below the M.I.C. for the organism. In which case, strains of low resistance may be selected, but there is no evidence that they actually remained in the presence of fucidin directly applied to the skin.

Professor W. Brumfitt. How do you know they didn't become re-infected post-treatment?

Dr. G. A. J. Ayliffe. Yes, this is another possibility.

Ampicillin resistance of *Proteus mirabilis*

Miss P. M. Waterworth. Does Dr. Lowbury know if all ampicillin resistance in *Proteus mirabilis* is on an R factor. Is it always transferable? Penicillinase-producing

Pr. mirabilis has existed from the beginning but I have never heard of it transferring resistance before.

Dr. E. J. L. Lowbury. We have described one particular R factor which determines a linked resistance to carbenicillin, ampicillin, tetracyline, cephaloridine and kanamycin. I was not referring to any other types of R factor or other types of resistance unrelated to R factors. Ampicillin-resistance unrelated to R factors does undoubtedly exist.

Dr. G. A. J. Ayliffe. As far as I am aware, most penicillinase-producing strains of *Pr. mirabilis* do not transfer resistance. This does seem to be an unusual strain.

6

VETERINARY USES OF ANTIBIOTICS

G. C. Brander

In any discussion of the use of antibiotics in animals, one has to consider why they are used and what part they play in the maintenance of animal health and also in the successful management of animals being reared for human consumption.

TREATMENT OF INFECTIONS IN ANIMALS

In the treatment of the diseases of horses, dogs, cats and the adult cow and pig, antibiotics are prescribed for the individual animal on the basis of a specific

Table 1

BACTERIAL INFECTIONS OF DOMESTIC ANIMALS

	Disease	*Bacteria involved*
Cattle	Calf scours and pneumonia	*Esch. coli*
		Staphylococci
	Calf enteritis and septicaemia	*Salmonella* species
	Mastitis	*Staphylococci*
		Streptococci
		Esch. coli
		Pseudomonas
	Metritis	*Esch. coli*
		Staphylococci
		Streptococcus faecalis
		Proteus species
	Pyelonephritis	*Cornebacterium renale*
Pigs	Enteritis and pneumonia	*Esch. coli*
		Salmonella
	Erysipelas	*Erysipelothrix rhusiopathiae*
	Metritis	*Esch. coli*
		Staphylococci
Horses	Enteritis and septicaemia in the young foal	*Esch. coli*
		Proteus
		Staphylococci
	Metritis	*Esch. coli*
		Staphylococci
	Pneumonia	*Staphylococci*
		Pasteurella species
	Strangles	*Streptococcus equi*
Dogs	Enteritis	*Esch. coli*
	Ear infections	*Staphylococci*
		Streptococci
		Esch. coli
		Pseudomonas
	Leptospirosis	*Leptospira canicola*
	Respiratory infections	*Staphylococci*
		Streptococci

disease diagnosis. Whereas in the control of the diseases associated with the intensive management of poultry and pigs, it is usual to base the treatment regimen on the diagnosis made following the examination of a batch of animals. The antibiotic selected is then given to the animals in the food or the water supply. Since the findings of the Swann Report on antibiotics, it is usual for therapeutic agents to be given in the food or the water for a 5 to 7 day treatment period.

Table 1 gives an indication of some of the major diseases of animals which are associated with bacterial infections and which have been found to respond to antibiotic therapy.

ANTIBIOTIC USE IN ANIMAL PRODUCTION

In considering present and past use of antibiotics and antibacterials in animal production, it is useful to consider some of the developments which have followed the introduction of antibiotics to the animal field and what had led to our present thinking on their use.

Prior to the development of the sulphonamides and antibiotics in the 1940s, animal diseases such as mastitis, pneumonia and enteritis caused continual heavy losses in livestock, and without antibiotics to control these problems, it would not have been possible to have upgraded the whole animal industry in the U.K. and the U.S.A. In the majority of cases, antibiotics are used for the treatment of specific disease entities, but it was found, particularly in pigs and poultry, that the addition of penicillin and tetracyclines to the food of young growing animals caused better growth, and a reduction of chronic subclinical disease. These antibiotics were therefore developed in special feed formulations for growth promotion and the control of subclinical disease. The majority of antibiotics and antibacterials commonly used in human medicine are also employed in animal treatments—a logical development in that in many cases both species suffer from similar types of bacterial invasion. The disease manifested however, may show different symptoms and virulence; for instance, infections due to *Salmonella typhimurium* or *Salmonella dublin* can cause acute systemic disease in both young and adult cattle, whereas the same organisms in man usually cause only an enteritis.

EMERGENCE OF RESISTANT ORGANISMS

As in the human field, the general use of antibiotics and antibacterials has led to an increase in resistant strains of bacteria found in certain specialized areas of management. Strains of resistant staphylococci have proved to be a problem in individual dairy units as in certain hospital wards. Strains of resistant *Escherichia coli* have become a problem in intensive pig units; likewise the same type of organism has proved a problem in urological and other wards of hospitals.

The possible implications of the development of resistant strains of bacteria in animals have been reviewed at regular intervals, both in the United Kingdom and by the World Health Organisation. A Joint Committee of the Agricultural Research Council and the Medical Research Council (Netherthorpe Committee Report, 1962) reviewed the problem from 1960 to 1962 and reported that 'it saw no reason to discontinue the permitted usage of feed additives, and recommended that the use of feed additives be extended to calves'.

After 1960 a new factor arose in the use of antibiotics; the phenomenon of infectious or transferable drug resistance, which was reported in shigella organisms recovered from man in Japan. This factor led the A.R.C./M.R.C. subcommittee to reconsider the problem of resistant strains of bacteria in man and animals. The subcommittee reported in 1966, and agreed that there was some cause for concern at the emergence of multiple resistant strains of bacteria and of infectious resistance, but did not find evidence to suggest that the use of penicillin and the tetracyclines in pig and poultry feeding had played a part in bringing about the new situation. It recommended, however, that a body with wider terms of reference be set up to review the total use of antibiotics in animal husbandry and veterinary medicine.

THE SWANN COMMITTEE

Such a committee was formed under the chairmanship of Professor Swann, and submitted its report to Parliament in November 1969 (Swann Committee Report, 1969). In the report the committee discussed the real and potential dangers to man of antibiotic usage in animals under the following headings:

(a) *Residues in food*
  i. Milk
  ii. Other animal products
  iii. Residues arising from food preservation.

(b) *Antibiotic resistance*

Under (a) it was concluded that the efforts of the Milk Hygiene Subcommittee of the Ministry of Agriculture to control antibiotic residues in milk had been remarkably successful, but they felt that there was still a need for a 'suitable marker' to be included in intramammary antibiotic and antibacterial formulations—so that residues could be readily detected by the farmer and the Milk Marketing Board. Residues in other animal products following antibiotic therapy did not appear to be harmful, and even if residues were present in tissues, such as the kidney or liver, they were generally destroyed by cooking.

Under (b) it was concluded that if antibiotics are used unwisely in animal treatment, a rapid propagation of antibiotic-resistant strains can occur, and some of these strains may prove a hazard to man. Because of this, the committee felt that it would be wise to reduce as far as possible the actual and potential dangers to man which may result from the giving of antibiotics to animals.

Recommendations

In summary the committee considered antibiotic usage in animals under two headings, (a) Antibiotics for growth promotion, and (b) Antibiotics for specific therapy. They recommended that penicillin and the tetracyclines should *not* be used for growth promotion, and that they should be replaced by antibiotics which are (i) of economic value to livestock, (ii) have little or no application as therapeutic agents in animals and man, (iii) are not likely to impair the efficacy of prescribed therapeutic antibiotics through the development of resistant strains or organisms. Three antibiotics have been approved for this method of usage—Zinc Bacitracin, Virginiamycin and Flavomycin.

They recommended that a full range of antibiotics should be available for use in animals, but only when prescribed by a member of the veterinary profession who had the animals under his care.

The major recommendations of the Swann Committee have been accepted by the Government, and are now being implemented.

FUTURE USES OF ANTIBIOTICS IN ANIMALS

The publication of the Swann Report and the discussions which followed its acceptance and the subsequent implementation of the Medicines Act should ensure that in future antibiotics and antibacterials will be used in the animal field in a controlled manner. It must be realized, however, that antibiotic usage in the United Kingdom for animal treatment has always been of a higher standard than that in other countries such as the U.S.A., Eire and South Africa, in that, apart from growth promotion, all were under veterinary control and therefore used only after the diagnosis of an infection.

As previously mentioned, the use of antibiotics has made possible present day systems of animal management and reduced the overall loss and suffering from disease. It seems likely in the future that developments in disease control will be related very closely to the economic value of therapy and also the relationship of therapy to the epidemiology of the diseases being treated. In the control of one of the major diseases of the dairy herd, mastitis, an effort is being made to ensure that when antibiotics are used therapeutically they are administered at the most effective time both for the control of bacteria and when the likelihood of milk residues is at a minimum. A system is in use in which the teats of the cows are treated following milking with an antibacterial, either an iodophor or a hypochlorite, to prevent cross infection from cow to cow during milking. The same cows when they are dried off are then treated with an antibiotic which will eliminate most of the staphylococci and streptococci which have established themselves in the udder during the lactation period.

This method of control is an example of how antibiotics and antibacterials can be used in the control of other diseases. Because of the bacterial burden carried by animals and the potential danger of some of these bacteria to humans it will be necessary in the foreseeable future for most antibiotics to be available for animal as well as human therapy.

REFERENCES

Report of the Joint Committee on Antibiotics in Animal Feeding (Chairman: Lord Netherthorpe). H.M.S.O., London, 1962.

Report of the Joint Committee on the Use of Antibiotics in Veterinary Medicine and Animal Husbandry (Chairman: Professor M. M. Swann). H.M.S.O., London, 1969, Cmnd 4190.

7

ANTIBIOTIC USE IN OBSTETRIC PATIENTS

J. D. WILLIAMS AND E. K. SMITH

LIFE threatening infections are now rare in obstetric patients. Puerperal fever was at one time the most prominent cause of maternal death but several factors have combined to make this condition much less common. Aseptic and antiseptic precautions had been steadily reducing the incidence of this disease since the realization that this was an infectious process; however in 1935 at the time of the introduction of sulphonamides the maternal mortality rate from sepsis in England and Wales was still 1·34 per 1000. By 1950 this figure had fallen to 0·12 per 1000 live and still births (Lewis, 1964). Since then it has continued to fall but deaths still occur and each time one does it is an individual tragedy. In the three years, 1964 to 1966, 123 maternal deaths occurred from sepsis, 28 following delivery, 66 following abortion and 29 following surgical intervention in pregnancy. (Confidential enquiries into maternal deaths, 1969.)

Despite the dramatic part which antibiotics have played in the reduction of the maternal death rate the present low incidence of infection combines with other factors to ensure that patients in obstetric wards receive less antibiotics than patients in other hospital wards. Furthermore when one looks at the antibiotics which pregnant women are receiving one finds they are usually given for some condition unrelated to the pregnancy such as tuberculosis, chest infection or diarrhoea. Only one in ten obstetric patients receive an antibiotic during their stay in hospital compared to 40 to 50 per cent of patients in general medical or surgical wards (Ayliffe & Williams, unpublished data).

The reasons for the low usage of antibiotics are seen if one examines the changes which have occurred in the main conditions for which pregnant women in hospital receive antibiotics. Acute pyelonephritis has become less common since the association between bacteriuria and pyelonephritis was established (Kass, 1962). Most ante-natal clinics now have screening procedures to detect bacteriuric women and eradicate the bacteriuria before pyelonephritis occurs (e.g. Sleigh *et al.*, 1963; Williams *et al.*, 1965a). Demonstration of the association between catheterization in labour and puerperal urinary tract infection (Brumfitt, Davies & Rosser, 1961) means that catheterization is used less frequently and for shorter periods of time.

Puerperal pyrexia has dwindled to such small numbers that it ceased to be a notifiable disease in 1968. The low prevalence of group A Beta-haemolytic streptococci contributes to this low incidence of pyrexia. Antibiotics have played some part in this reduced prevalence but infection control measures such as isolation of infected patients, exclusion of attendants with sore throats from labour wards and the growth of hospital sterile supply units also play a large part in keeping the incidence low. Interauterine sepsis has also diminished with the falling into disfavour of 'membrane sweeps' and of difficult manipulations during labour.

Administration of prophylactic antibiotic therapy to patients undergoing surgical induction of labour has been widely practised and a variety of regimens have been suggested (Lennon, 1957; Theobald, 1959). Women with membranes ruptured for 24 hours or more appear more likely to develop pyrexia (Parker, 1957) and it was common practice to give antibiotics to women in this situation. Pharmacological studies with ampicillin have shown delay in passage of the antibiotics into the liquor (Belcher *et al.*, 1966; Williams & Felton, 1966) and antibiotic administration to women after 24 hours with ruptured membranes does not appreciably alter the incidence of pyrexia (Felton & Williams, 1967). Only if adequate concentrations are present in the liquor at the time of surgical induction can any protection from puerperal pyrexia be noted and even then this protection does not extend for more than 24 hours (Felton & Williams, 1967). The obvious corollary to this is to ensure that women with induced labour are delivered within 24 hours and oxytocics make this possible reducing sepsis without exhibition of antibiotics (Cope, 1967).

These changes in obstetric practice have led to a reduction in the number of pregnant women requiring antibiotics. Not only has a reduction in numbers occurred but also a reduction in the length of administration. Prophylactic antibiotics are usually given for only 2–3 days, patients with urinary tract infections seldom receive more than 7 days treatment and most patients with puerperal sepsis require only 5 days of antibiotic therapy. Thus the total quantity of antibiotics received by pregnant women is small.

Interest in antibiotics in pregnancy today is mainly concerned with teratogenicity, pharmacology and urinary tract infection and this paper will deal briefly with these subjects and also give some suggested regimes of treatment for the more frequently occurring infections.

TERATOGENICITY AND TOXIC EFFECTS OF ANTIBIOTICS

The choice of which antibiotic to use for a particular condition is more limited for the obstetrician than for the general physician or surgeon because of the presence of the foetus. As with all new drugs, the effects on pregnant rats and rabbits can be determined in the laboratory but there remains a variation in species which cannot be overcome. The final test therefore is what effect, if any, a particular antibiotic has on the foetus of a mother given that compound during pregnancy.

Antibiotics, in common with most new drugs arrive with the advice, 'to be used with caution in women of childbearing age', which is of little value in attempting to weigh up the possible toxicity to the foetus. This type of warning provides little guidance to the doctor faced with a woman requiring antibiotic therapy and who may be pregnant, or with a woman who has become pregnant during the course of treatment.

Relationship of toxicity to stage of pregnancy

Pregnancy can be divided into three periods which determine the type of abnormality, if any, that a drug may produce (Fig. 1). The first period is that before implantation, the time between the fertilization of the ovum and its embedding in the uterus. In the human, fertilization normally takes place in the fallopian tube and, while active division of the cells is proceeding to form a blastocyst, the cellular mass is propelled by the cilia of the tube into the uterus. This period lasts for about six days and during this stage, any toxic effect on the blastocyst is likely to lead to destruction rather than teratogenesis.

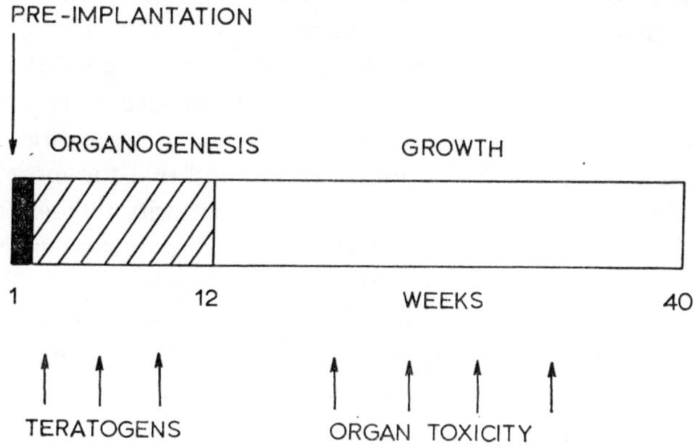

FIG. 1. Relationship of possible untoward effects of drugs to the stage of pregnancy.

The second period, that of organogenesis, lasts from the time of implantation to about the twelfth week of pregnancy. This is the most crucial period of development and the time when most harm can be done to organogenesis.

From the twelfth week onwards the main processes are maturation, functional development and increase in size. Even during the last weeks of pregnancy the foetus may be adversely effected by drugs but these correspond to the toxic effects in newborns in that teratogenic effects are unlikely.

Difficulties in assessing teratogenesis

There are obvious ethical objections to performing clinical trials in pregnant women to assess teratogenic effects. One is therefore left with assessment of the results of animal experiments and analysis of the effects of the drug on the foetuses of women given the drug either accidentally or for a justifiable reason during pregnancy. Extensive animal experiments are performed before compounds are available clinically and it can be assumed that any which have produced teratogenic effects in animals is unlikely, now, to elude the screening procedure of the pharmaceutical industry. For example, the long acting sulphonamide, sulphadimethoxypyrimidine which produced skeletal malformations in rats was withdrawn (Green, 1963).

In assessing results in humans the incidence of congenital abnormalities in the normal population must be taken into account as well as the known predisposing factors such as heredity, maternal age, parity and some viral infections. Additionally one must consider the stage of pregnancy at which the drugs were administered.

In several groups of pregnant women who have been treated with different antibiotics for bacteriuria, we have maintained observation of control groups of untreated women to assess the effect, if any, of bacteriuria on the pregnancy. Following the reported abortions in pregnant rats given large doses of trimethoprim (Udall, 1969) assessment of women treated with co-trimoxazole was carried out more intensively (Williams *et al.*, 1969). It was found that only 10 (8 per cent) of 120 women receiving the drug were less than 16 weeks pregnant when treated, foetal abnormalities were just as common in the control patients as in the treated patients, that the abnormalities had arisen at a time unrelated to the drug administration and that the most prominent features of the mothers were high parity and seniority. Thus even in this relatively large group of patients treated no clear result emerged. It is unlikely that it will ever be possible to categorically assert that a given compound is free from teratogenic effects but when one considers the large amounts of antimicrobial agents which over the past 30 years have been taken by pregnant women the dangers from these compounds must be very small.

Toxic effects of antibiotics in pregnancy

The evidence of toxicity to the foetus of antibiotics given during pregnancy is better documented than teratogenicity. The foetus may be adversely effected by toxic agents but as stated earlier these correspond to toxic effects in new-borns and teratogenic effects are unlikely.

Nitrofurantoin is not teratogenic (Fingold *et al.*, 1968). However, the use in pregnancy is often limited by troublesome side effects such as nausea and vomiting. It is not recommended for use in neonates. The adverse effects of tetracycline on the foetus was first reported by Kline *et al.* (1964). Tetracyclines chelate with calcium and cross the placenta in sufficient quantity to stain the deciduous teeth if given after the fourth month of pregnancy. It should not be given to young children as it has a similar effect on the permanent teeth.

Meuwissin *et al.* (1967), claim that streptomycin is one of the chief causes of iatrogenic deafness. However, Sakula (1954) showed that the concentration of streptomycin in the foetal circulation was half or less than that in the maternal circulation. In this series patients on prolonged therapy, including those treated during the first three months of pregnancy, produced normal infants. In the review of Adamsons and Joelsson (1966), a very low incidence of neonatal deafness was found in the children of mothers on prolonged therapy for tuberculosis. It would appear therefore that a short course of streptomycin given during pregnancy will not adversely effect the foetus.

Kanamycin does not pass the placenta in significant amounts (Pulaski *et al.*, 1959). Ototoxic effects on the mother can be avoided in most cases by keeping the blood level below 20 μg/ml. As with streptomycin only short courses of treatment should be used.

Nalidixic acid is best avoided because of the neurotoxicity in neonates.

Although the controversy about the toxicity of chloramphenicol in adults persists, it does not adversely effect the foetus (Adamsons & Joelsson, 1966). This seems surprising because in neonates it produces the well-known grey syndrome (Garrod & O'Grady, 1971).

There has been considerable discussion over the role of sulphonamides in the pathogenesis of neonatal jaundice. Dunn (1964) found that nine babies whose mothers had received prophylactic sulphonamides for ruptured membranes for 2–28 days before delivery, developed jaundice within 26 hours of delivery. However 6 of these babies were of low birth weight and 7 were less than 36 weeks gestation. The suggested mechanism for the jaundice is that of competition by the sulphonamide with bilirubin for conjugation with glucuronic acid. However it is unlikely that enough sulphonamide could cross the placenta to block sufficient binding sites to produce jaundice (Adamsons & Joelsson, 1966). Most obstetricians do not use sulphonamides after the 38th week of pregnancy because of this, mainly theoretical, possibility.

There are some antibiotics which appear to be quite safe in pregnancy. The penicillin group have not been shown to have adverse effects on the foetus despite wide use and the cephalosporins are closely related. Erythromycin has no adverse effects (Ross *et al.*, 1968) and although no reports on the toxicity of lincomycin in pregnant humans have appeared experimental dosage in pregnant rats produced negative results (Gray *et al.*, 1964).

The use of these compounds together with nitrofurantoin (in reduced dosage) sulphonamides (before 38 weeks gestation) and short courses of aminoglycosides should enable us to adequately treat the majority of infections which arise in pregnancy.

PHARMACOLOGY OF ANTIBIOTICS IN PREGNANCY

Information on the behaviour of antibiotics in the foetus during the early months of pregnancy is lacking but several studies have been made during the last trimester. It is known that sulphonamides appear rapidly in the foetal circulation after administration to the mother (Speert, 1943) and penicillins pass into the liquor in addition (Wolz & Wiley, 1946; Charles, 1954). Streptomycin appears in the cord blood within 5 minutes (Sakula, 1954) but apparently, like tetracyclines and chloramphenicol, at a reduced level compared to the mother and negligible amounts appear in the liquor (Charles, 1954). More recently studies on newer penicillins and cephalosporins have appeared. Ampicillin passes in a similar manner to penicillin into the foetus and liquor (Belcher *et al.*, 1966) but after oral administration there is considerable delay in the attainment of adequate levels in the liquor (Williams & Felton, 1966). Cephalosporins have been shown to pass in and out of the liquor readily (MacAulay & Charles, 1968) but there is some discrepancy in the concentrations found in the foetus (Morrow, Palmisano & Cassidy, 1968; Paterson *et al.*, 1970).

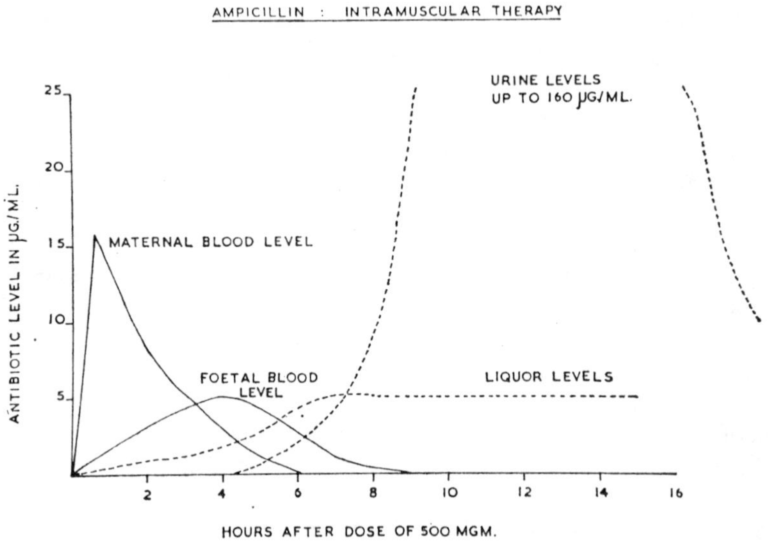

FIG. 2. *Ampicillin.* Maternal blood and liquor levels; foetal blood and urine levels following a dose of 500 mg intramuscularly 6 hourly.

With Mr. Ken Stewart, Senior Registrar in Obstetrics, one of us (J. D. Williams) has recently been studying the passage of ampicillin, cephaloridine and cephalothin into the liquor and the foetal blood and urine in a series of women undergoing surgical membrane rupture and requiring antibiotic therapy. We found that ampicillin and cephaloridine behaved in a similar manner to each other (Figs. 2 and 3). Foetal blood levels are found to rise slightly more slowly than maternal levels and reach approximately half the level found in the mother. Evidence that considerable quantities of antibiotic pass into the foetus is also shown by the high levels obtained in the foetal urine. Both compounds showed a slower passage into the liquor amnii; 6 hours elapsed before levels of 4–5 µg/ml were reached.

Cephalothin (Fig. 4) on the other hand showed very rapid passage in and out of the foetus. Blood levels were transient and the highest recorded level

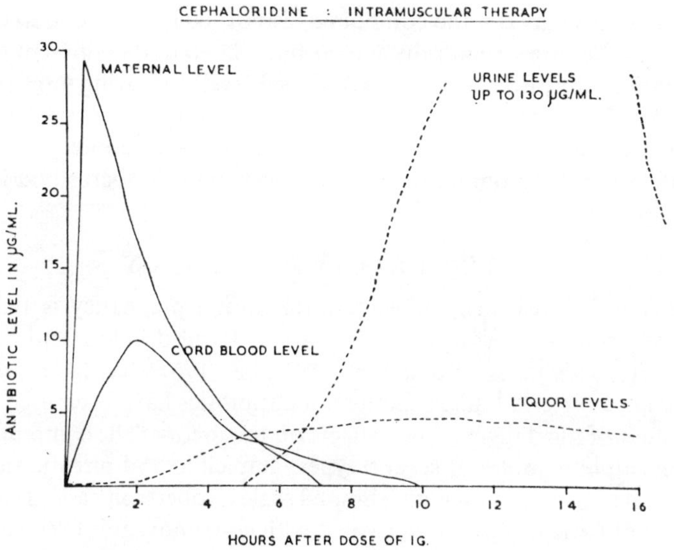

FIG. 3. *Cephaloridine.* Maternal blood and liquor levels; foetal blood and urine levels following a dose of 1 g intramuscularly 12 hourly.

following 1 g of cephalothin was 4 µg/ml. Similarly relatively low levels were seen in foetal urine. However passage into the liquor amnii was very rapid appearing within 15 minutes and reaching 4–5 µg/ml in one hour.

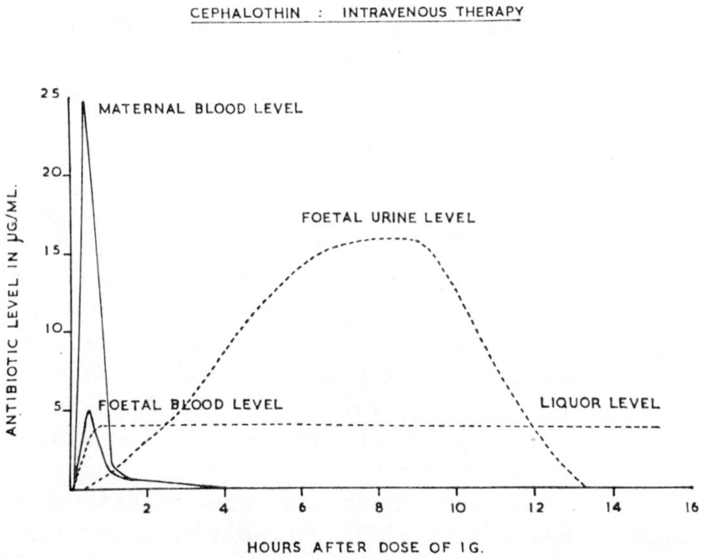

FIG. 4. *Cephalothin.* Maternal blood and liquor levels; foetal blood and urine levels following a dose of 1 g intravenously 12 hourly.

The differences between the compounds is not likely to be due to chemical differences as they are structurally similar but related to the different routes of administration, the lower and more prolonged levels following intra-muscular injection helping passage into the foetus. One might assume from these studies that the quickest way to treat severe intra-uterine infection is to use both routes at once to obtain therapeutic levels both in foetus and liquor as rapidly as possible.

BACTERIURIA IN PREGNANCY

The reason for treatment of bacteriuria during pregnancy is that 25–30 per cent of bacteriuric women if left untreated will develop acute pyelonephritis during pregnancy (Kass, 1960; Whalley, 1967; Savage *et al.*, 1967; Condie *et al.*, 1968). A limited number of antibiotics have been used in treatment because of the danger of side effects on the foetus. The compounds used have been sulphonamides of several types, ampicillin and nitrofurantoin but cycloserine has also been used on a limited scale (Robertson *et al.*, 1968) and a small series of patients have been treated with co-trimoxazole (Williams *et al.*, 1969) and cephalosporins (Brumfitt *et al.*, 1970). Wide variation has occurred in the duration of treatment given to patients. Treatment has been given in some series throughout pregnancy (Savage *et al.*, 1967; Robertson *et al.*, 1968), in others for 30 days (Little, 1966), 3 weeks (Pathak *et al.*, 1967) or for 8 days (Williams *et al.*, 1965b). The cure rates obtained with these different regimes of treatment are rather similar because bacteriuric women are not a homogeneous group but contain a wide variety of conditions. Some patients will respond to the simplest of treatment whereas others with abnormal urinary tracts have infections which are not amenable to chemotherapy alone.

Some efforts have been made to find the smallest amount of chemotherapy which will produce a high cure rate in women with uncomplicated bacteriuria and leave only the complicated cases for more intensive treatment and follow up. The use of single dose of sulphormethoxine produced different cure rates in London where most organisms are sulphonamide sensitive (79 per cent clear of infection 6 weeks after treatment) and in Birmingham where approximately 40 per cent of bacteriuric women have a sulphonamide resistant organism (52 per cent clear of infection 6 weeks after treatment) (Williams *et al.*, 1968). More recently we have been treating patients in Birmingham with a single dose of streptomycin in addition to sulphonamide in an effort to deal with these sulphonamide resistant strains (Williams & Smith, 1970). The results are summarized in Table 1. Using single doses of 1 g cephaloridine Professor Brumfitt and his colleagues (1970) obtained a cure rate of 44 per cent.

Acute pyelonephritis can have a dramatic onset in pregnancy and because it is frequently accompanied by vomiting and because of the variable absorption of oral antibiotics in pregnancy it is best treated with parenteral antibiotics. The majority of organisms are sensitive to ampicillin and a dose of 500 mg 6 hourly should be commenced. Oral treatment with 500 mg 8 hourly can be substituted when the fever has settled and treatment continued for a total of 10 days.

TABLE 1

SINGLE DOSE OF BACTERIURIA IN PREGNANCY

	Dose	*Cure rate at 6 weeks*	*Reference*
Sulphadoxine	2 g oral	79 per cent (London) 52 per cent (Birmingham)	Williams *et al.* (1968)
Sulphametopyrazine	2 g oral	62 per cent	Williams & Smith (1970)
Sulphametopyrazine and Streptomycin	2 g oral 1 g I.M.	70 per cent	Williams & Smith (1970)
Cephaloridine	1 g I.M.	44 per cent	Brumfitt *et al.* (1970)

TREATMENT OF PUERPERAL SEPSIS AND POST ABORTAL SEPSIS

These conditions may be considered together because the organisms concerned and the treatment required are similar. The causative organisms are usually bacteroides and various types of streptococci (non-haemolytic streptococci, Beta-haemolytic streptococci or anaerobic streptococci) derived from the woman's own vaginal flora. More rarely is infection due to *Clostridium welchii* or *Staphylococcus pyogenes*. The role of gram negative bacilli remains obscure but these are probably only colonists in the majority of patients.

In the severe cases, one should start treatment with intramuscular penicillin 2 million units followed by 1 million units 4 hourly together with streptomycin 500 mg twice daily. This therapy usually results in a marked improvement and after 48 hours the dosage of penicillin can then be decreased. A 5-day course of both antibiotics is usually sufficient. There is not usually a requirement for newer broad spectrum antibiotics as the organisms are relatively sensitive; hospital-acquired infections with multiple resistant strains are unusual. The one new antibiotic which may be helpful is lincomycin because of its activity against bacteroides (Geddes, 1967; Tracey *et al.*, 1972). Intramuscular ampicillin is widely used at a dose of 500 mg 6 hourly; beta-haemolytic streptococci are sometimes resistant to the tetracyclines and these should therefore be avoided. Similarly kanamycin and gentamicin are not active against streptococci and if they are thought to be necessary they should not be used alone but together with a penicillin.

EFFECT OF MATERNAL ANTIBIOTIC ADMINISTRATION ON COLONIZATION OF THE FOETUS

One often unrecognized side-effect of treatment is the way in which maternally administered antibiotics leads to the colonization of the foetus with antibiotic resistant organisms. These organisms may subsequently give rise to infection in the neonate. Felton and Williams (1967) showed the relationship of membrane rupture to the colonization of the birth passages with gram negative bacilli. The longer the membranes are ruptured the higher is the incidence of colonization. Before membrane rupture 5 per cent of women have gram-negative bacilli in the vagina but if the membranes have been ruptured for longer than 48 hours the incidence rises to 90 per cent. If antibiotics are given to the mother this colonization of the vagina is more likely to occur with antibiotic-resistant strains and these strains subsequently colonize the baby. In Table 2 are shown the results of vaginal swab cultures

TABLE 2

COLONIZATION OF VAGINA IN WOMEN RECEIVING ANTIBIOTICS DURING LABOUR AND SUBSEQUENT COLONIZATION OF THE UMBILICAL CORD OF BABIES DELIVERED FROM THESE WOMEN

Vaginal swab	*Antibiotics given before delivery*	*No antibiotic given*
Number tested	67	69
G.N.B. present	33 (49 per cent)	15 (22 per cent)
G.N.B. resistant to ampicillin	18 (27 per cent)	9 (13 per cent)
Cord swab		
Number tested	65	70
G.N.B. present	22 (33 per cent)	15 (22 per cent)
G.N.B. resistant to ampicillin	15 (23 per cent)	7 (10 per cent)

(G.N.B. = Gram-negative bacilli.)

in women with and without antibiotics in labour. Ten per cent of women not receiving antibiotics become colonized with ampicillin-resistant bacteria compared to 25 per cent colonization of women who did receive antibiotics. The same pattern was also seen in the results of umbilical swab cultures 2 days after delivery (Table 2).

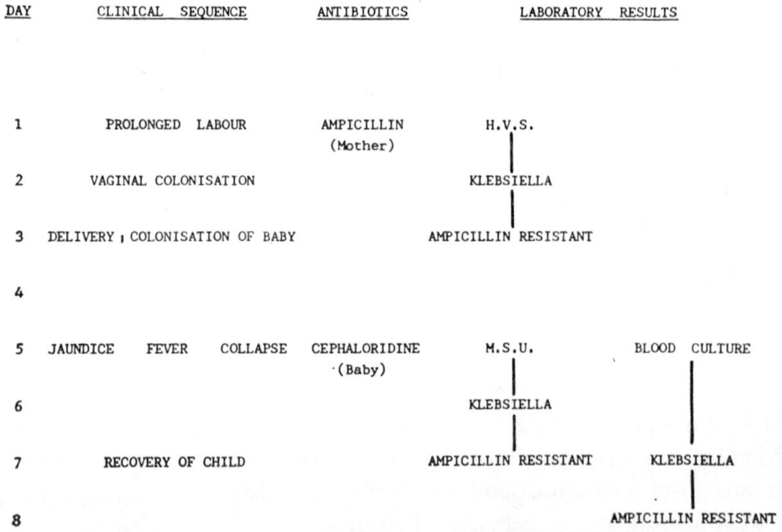

FIG. 5. Course of infection and treatment in a mother and child and the relation to antibiotic therapy.

This colonization has more than theoretical interest as the sequence of events in Figure 5 shows. In this example a child developed a urinary tract infection the day after delivery with jaundice, fever and septicaemia. The mother had previously been treated with ampicillin during labour and the vagina had become colonized with an ampicillin resistant strain of klebsiella. This organism was subsequently isolated from the urinary tract and blood stream of the child. The bacteriological findings are 2 days behind the clinical sequence and are therefore only of retrospective value to the paediatrician. However the policy of using an antibiotic for treatment of the foetus which is different to that used in the mother produced a successful outcome in this case.

We would like to thank the consultant obstetricians at Dudley Road Hospital, Mr. W. Macdougall, Mr. G. Mitchell and Miss A. Reynolds, for their continuing help and co-operation in many fields and Mr. K. Stewart for this co-operation in the pharmacological studies with antibiotics. Mrs. J. Andrews, F.I.M.L.T. performed much of the laboratory work and Mrs. S. Austin, S.R.N. collected many of the specimens examined.

REFERENCES

ADAMSONS, K. & JOELSSON, J. (1966). The effects of pharmacological agents upon fetus and new born. *American Journal of Obstetrics and Gynecology*, **96,** 437.

BARR, W. & GRAHAM, R. M. (1967). Placental transmission of cephaloridine. *Postgraduate Medical Journal*, August supplement, **43,** 101.

BELCHER, T. E., EDGAR, W. M., MELVILLE, H. A. H. & PEEL, K. R. (1966). Transplacental passage of ampicillin. *British Medical Journal*, **1,** 137.

BRUMFITT, W., DAVIES, B. I. & ROSSER, E. (1961). Urethral catheter as a cause of urinary tract infection in pregnancy and the puerperium. *Lancet*, **ii,** 1059.

BRUMFITT, W., FAIERS, M. C. & FRANKLIN, I. N. S. (1970). The treatment of urinary infection by means of a single dose of cephaloridine. *Postgraduate Medical Journal*, October supplement, **46,** 65.

CHARLES, D. (1954). Placental transmission of antibiotics. *Journal of Obstetrics and Gynaecology of the British Commonwealth*, **61,** 750.

CONDIE, A. P., WILLIAMS, J. D., REEVES, D. S. & BRUMFITT, W. (1968). Complications of bacteriuria in pregnancy. In *Urinary Tract Infections* (Eds., O'Grady, F. & Brumfitt, W.), p. 148. Oxford University Press.

Confidential Enquiries into Maternal Deaths in England and Wales 1964–66, p. 89. H.M.S.O., London, 1969.

COPE, E. (1967). Induction of labour. *Practitioner*, **198,** 207.

DUNN, P. M. (1964). The possible relationship between the maternal administration of sulphamethoxypyridazine and hyperbilirubinaemia in the newborn. *Journal of Obstetrics and Gynaecology of the British Commonwealth*, **71,** 128.

FELTON, D. J. C. & WILLIAMS, J. D. (1967). Prophylactic ampicillin in the surgical induction of labour. *Journal of Obstetrics and Gynaecology of the British Commonwealth*, **74,** 862.

FINGOLD, S. M. & ZIMENT, I. (1968). Sulphonamides, Nitrofurans and Nalidixic acid. *Paediatric Clinics of North America*, **15,** 95.

GARROD, L. P. & O'GRADY, F. (1971). In *Antibiotic and Chemotherapy*, 3rd edition, p. 142. Livingstone, Edinburgh and London.

GEDDES, A. M., MUNRO, J. F., MURDOCH, J. McC., BEGG, K. J. & BURNS, B. A. (1967). In *Proceedings of the Fifth International Congress of Chemotherapy*, Vol. I, p. 361. Vienna, Wiener Medizinische Academie, 1967.

GRAY, J. E., PUMALIS, A. & FIENSTRA, E. S. (1964). Animal toxicity studies of a new antibiotic—Lincomycin. *Toxicology and Applied Pharmacology*, **6,** 476.

GREEN, K. G. (1963). Bimez and teratogenic action. *British Medical Journal*, **1,** 56.

KASS, E. H. (1960). Bacteriuria and pyelonephritis of pregnancy. *Archives of Internal Medicine*, **105,** 194.

KASS, E. H. (1962). Pyelonephritis and bacteriuria; a major problem in preventive medicine. *Annals of Internal Medicine*, **56,** 46.

KLINE, A. H., BLATTNER, R. J. & LUNIN, M. (1964). Transplacental effect of tetracyclines on teeth. *Journal of the American Medical Association*, **188,** 178.

LENNON, G. G. (1957). Induction of labour in pre-eclampsia and eclampsia. *Proceedings of the Royal Society of Medicine*, **50,** 793.

LEWIS, T. L. T. (1964). *Progress in Clinical Obstetrics and Gynaecology*, p. 3. Churchill, London.

LITTLE, P. J. (1966). The incidence of urinary tract infection in 5,000 pregnant women. *Lancet*, **ii,** 925.

MACAULAY, M. A. & CHARLES, D. (1968). Placental transfer of cephalothin. *American Journal of Obstetrics and Gynecology*, **100,** 940.

MEUWISSEN, H. G. & ROBINSON, G. C. (1967). The ototoxic antibiotics. *Clinical Paediatrics*, **6,** 262.

MORROW, S., PALMISANO, P. & CASSIDY, G. (1968). The placental transfer of cephalothin. *Journal of Paediatrics*, **73,** 262.

PARKER, R. B. (1957). The results of surgical induction of labour. *Journal of Obstetrics and Gynaecology of British Empire*, **64,** 94.

PATERSON, L., HENDERSON, A., BURNETT, L. C. & McGURK, S. (1970). Transfer of cephalothin sodium to the fetus. *Journal of Obstetrics and Gynaecology of the British Commonwealth*, **77,** 565.

PATHAK, U. N., TANG, A. & STUART, K. L. (1967). Bacteriuria of pregnancy: results of treatment. In *Symposium on Pyelonephritis*, p. 28. Edinburgh, 1966.

PULASKI, E. J. & TUBBS, R. S. (1959). Inhibitory effects of kanamycin and its diffusion into various body fluids. *Antibiotic Medicine*, **6,** 589.

ROBERTSON, J. G., LIVINGSTONE, J. R. B. & ISDALE, M. H. (1968). The management and complications of asymptomatic bacteriuria in pregnancy: report of a study on 8275 patients. *Journal of Obstetrics and Gynaecology of the British Commonwealth*, **75,** 59.

ROSS, S. (1968). Erythromycin, oleandomycin and triacetyloleandomycin. *Pediatric Clinics of North America*, **15,** 119.

SAKULA, A. (1954). Streptomycin and the foetus. *British Journal of Tuberculosis*, **48,** 69.

SAVAGE, W. E., HAJJ, S. N. & KASS, E. H. (1967). Demographic and prognostic characteristics of bacteriuria in pregnancy. *Medicine (Baltimore)*, **46,** 385.

SLEIGH, J. D., ROBERTSON, J. D. & ISDALE, M. H. (1963). Asymptomatic bacteriuria in pregnancy. *Journal of Obstetrics and Gynaecology of British Commonwealth*, **71,** 74.

SPEERT, H. (1943). Placental transmission of sulphathiazole and sulphadiazine and its significance for fetal chemotherapy. *American Journal of Obstetrics and Gynaecology*, **45,** 200.

THEOBALD, G. W. (1959). The choice between death from postmaturity or prolapsed cord, and life from induction of labour. *Lancet*, **i,** 59.

TRACY, O., GORDON, A. M., MORAN, F., LOVE, W. C. & MCKENZIE, P. (1972). Lincomycins in the treatment of Bacteroides infections. *British Medical Journal*, **1**, 280.

UDALL, V. (1969). Toxicology of sulphonamide—trimethoprim combinations. *Postgraduate Medical Journal*, November supplement, **45**, 42.

WHALLEY, P. (1967). Bacteriuria of pregnancy. *American Journal of Obstetrics and Gynecology*, **97**, 723.

WILLIAMS, J. D., LEIGH, D. A., ROSSER, E. I. & BRUMFITT, W. (1965a). The organisation and results of a screening programme for the detection of bacteriuria of pregnancy. *Journal of Obstetrics and Gynaecology of the British Commonwealth*, **72**, 327.

WILLIAMS, J. D., BRUMFITT, W., LEIGH, D. A. & PERCIVAL, A. (1965b). Eradication of bacteriuria in pregnancy by a short course of chemotherapy. *Lancet*, **i**, 831.

WILLIAMS, J. D., BRUMFITT, W., CONDIE, A. P., REEVES, D. S., FRANKLIN, I. S. N. & LEIGH, D. A. (1968). The treatment of bacteriuria of pregnancy. In *Urinary Tract Infection* (Eds., O'Grady, F. & Brumfitt, W.), p. 160. Oxford University Press.

WILLIAMS, J. D., BRUMFITT, W., CONDIE, A. P. & REEVES, D. S. (1969). The treatment of bacteriuria in pregnant women with Sulphamethoxazole and trimethoprim. *Postgraduate Medical Journal*, November supplement, **45**, 71.

WILLIAMS, J. D. & FELTON, D. J. C. (1966). Passage of ampicillin into foetal blood and liquor amnii. *Journal of Obstetrics and Gynaecology of British Commonwealth*, **73**, 654.

WILLIAMS, J. D. & SMITH, E. K. (1970). Single dose therapy with streptomycin and sulphamethopyrazine for bacteriuria during pregnancy. *British Medical Journal*, **4**, 651.

WOLZ, J. H. E. & WILEY, M. M. (1946). The transmission of penicillin to the previable fetus. *Journal of the American Medical Association*, **131**, 969.

DISCUSSION

Follow up and controls. Single dose of streptomycin

Dr. A. W. Asscher. Dr. Smith said that it would be preferable to have a 10-year radiological follow up on chronic bacteriuric women. I have done this over 5 years and found no change. You have not got a control series and I believe it is very important to have a control group as the effect of age on creatinine clearance and blood urea and other criteria is very marked over a 10-year period. I feel that you might not be all that much wiser unless this particular group is matched with controls.

I am not a bacteriologist, but I am a little worried about a single injection of streptomycin and what this might do, if anything, to your immigrant population's tuberculosis. There is an incompatibility in what you say. On the one hand you have this population of difficult women and you want to get the drug into them there and then. Difficult as they are, you seem to have got very extensive data on them and I wonder how you can make these two things compatible.

Dr. E. K. Smith. We have a resident interpreter in the clinic. All our instructions in the antenatal clinic and in the wards are written out in four different languages (and that's just to cover the Indians and Pakistanis) which helps to get the message over. If all else fails we give a note to take to the husband, and overcome it this way. Eventually we get the correct specimen and attendances.

Dr. J. D. Williams. Patients are not very good at taking tablets. I don't think anybody has ever taken a full 8-day course of sulphonamides. Most people feel better after two or three days and don't complete the course. Therefore, I do not think you can really object to us trying to give the whole of the course in one dose. It is nothing to do with an immigrant population. No one likes taking tablets and single dose therapy is well established in the treatment of gonorrhoea.

There are two problems with regard to tuberculosis. Firstly, there are the effects which this treatment is going to have on resistance. The tuberculosis physicians don't give one dose; they give 6-month courses of anti-tuberculous treatment. Thus, the contribution to the problem of streptomycin resistance which we are making with one single dose is very small. Secondly, there are the diagnosis difficulties but I do not believe that one dose of streptomycin is going to turn a person with pulmonary tuberculosis from sputum positive to sputum negative.

Significance of studies of bacteriuria in pregnancy

Professor R. G. Petersdorf. One has to take particular care in generalizing from the kind of data that Dr. Smith has presented. Whether one deals with Asian immigrants in this country, or with indigenous blacks in America, we may forget that most pregnant women do not belong to either of these categories. Therefore, the data which in both parts of the world has been derived from these populations are not generally applicable. I don't disagree with anything that you have said that is applicable to Dudley Road Hospital. I do think however that the incidence of bacteriuria in pregnancy in these populations is about three times the incidence in middle class populations that receive average obstetric care. Since the risk is much lower I wonder whether this type of treatment with antimicrobials is indeed warranted.

One statement that does raise my hackles, because I have worked in this area for 10 years, is the fact that bacteriuria of pregnancy increases foetal wastage and prematurity. When you review the literature on this subject, the data really doesn't hold up except in an indigenous population. This is the very population in whom risks of prematurity from many factors, such as malnutrition or other infections, is highest and it is difficult to separate out bacteriuria as being an important causative factor in prematurity. I simply would like to leave these cautions with you because the whole problem of over-treatment and over-reaction to bacteriuria in pregnancy has become a world-wide phenomenon and I for one would like to stem it.

Dr. J. D. Williams. I am sure that we don't over-react to bacteriuria in pregnancy or over-treat the patients. The reason for treating bacteriuria in pregnancy is that if patients are not treated, 30 per cent of these women will develop acute pyelonephritis. One doesn't have to raise prematurity or maternal anaemia in order to justify treatment of bacteriuria in pregnancy. And all we are giving is one dose of antibiotic.

Role of beta-haemolytic streptococci

Dr. M. T. Parker. I am a little distressed that Dr. Williams might give the impression that Group A Streptococci are losing virulence. A few unfortunate women pay with their lives every year because of this misconception on the part of young practitioners. What probably happens is that almost everybody who gets fever in the puerperium has a little penicillin and the diagnosis doesn't get made.

Dr. J. L. Honigman. One point which Dr. Williams made at the beginning was that he attributed the reduction in antibiotic use to decreased streptococcal virulence. It is worth noting historically that a major fall in puerperal pyrexia occurred in the early forties with the introduction of effective anti-streptococcal antiseptics into midwifery. Is this still significant?

Dr. J. D. Williams. I quite agree there are still very virulent strains of Beta-haemolytic streptococci. There has however been some reduction in prevalence. With regard to asepsis, antisepsis and general measures to control infection. I would agree that these are of prime importance.

Other indications for antibiotics in pregnancy

Professor R. E. O. Williams. I am surprised you didn't have anything to say about infection in abortions, whether therapeutic or convenience.

Dr. E. K. Smith. There hasn't been enough time, but the problems are the same as in the puerperium.

Professor O. L. Wade. I value your data on adverse reactions during pregnancy, but I would like to see more information from larger series. Clearly nobody wants to give drugs to women during pregnancy, especially in the first 3 months, unless there is a good reason for treatment. I don't want to see drugs which these women need being denied them, and sometimes I have seen this happen.

Do you use prophylactic antibiotics in heart disease in pregnancy?

Dr. J. D. Williams. Yes we do, but if you give prophylactic therapy it has to be given properly. Many clinicians give a small dose for a short period, often the wrong period. If you wish to use it for cover during delivery in a woman with a heart lesion you must give an intramuscular antibiotic. The absorption of many antibiotics is not complete at the best of times and is decreased in pregnancy. The second point is that the serum antibiotic levels have to be adequate at the time of delivery and therefore treatment should be started some hours before delivery. In extracting teeth one is mainly worried about *Streptococcus viridans* but in obstetrics the enterococcus must also be considered. This organism may not be very sensitive to benzylpenicillin but is a little more sensitive to ampicillin. Therefore, we recommend that the patient is given ampicillin in a dose of at least 500 mg 6-hourly as soon as labour starts and this should be continued for a day or two after delivery. The cardiologists like to continue this therapy for longer—perhaps for up to 10 days.

8

NEONATAL INFECTIONS

K. B. ROGERS

INFECTIONS in older babies, children and adults present in a manner very different from that of similar infections in the first few days of life, when the time between an infection becoming manifest and a baby being moribund can be as short as a few hours. Strictly speaking neonatal covers the first month, but most of what I shall describe will be concerned with the practical diagnostic and therapeutic problems of the first 10–14 days of life.

UNDIAGNOSED SEVERE INFECTIONS IN NEONATES

When a neonate becomes ill a blood culture and cerebrospinal fluid should be obtained before therapy is started, even though it is essential that treatment is started before the identity of the aetiological agent is fully established. Cultures of the throat, umbilicus, urine and conjunctival sacs may also help to establish the cause of the infection. There is always a septicaemia when a patient has meningitis, and in the neonate there can be several thousand organisms per ml in the blood culture. A neonate with meningitis often has a pneumonia as well. The organisms which most frequently cause such infections are members of the enterobacteriaceae, streptococci and *Listeria monoctyogenes*.

My choice of antibiotics for these babies, before the organisms have been identified, is gentamicin and ampicillin. Smears of the centrifuged deposit of the cerebrospinal fluid will allow enterobacteriaceae and streptococci to be seen. We frequently have difficulty finding Listeria in the centrifuged deposit of the C.S.F. but as this is a relatively uncommon organism and as it is sensitive to both gentamicin and to ampicillin, it will be covered by the suggested therapy. The results of the C.S.F. culture and sensitivities will not be available for at least 8 hours, when the pour plate blood culture will also probably be showing growth. Up to the present time I have not yet isolated a strain of *Escherichia coli*, *Proteus spp.* or of the Klebsiella group, which has been resistant to gentamicin. The few strains of Listeria I have isolated have all been sensitive to that antibiotic but the Lancefield Group B and A strains, *Streptococcus agalactiae* and *Strep. pyogenes*, have been relatively resistant. I suggest ampicillin rather than penicillin because some of the enterobacteriaceae are sensitive to it and the Lancefield Group B and A streptococci are sensitive to both of these penicillins. The cost of gentamicin is relatively unimportant if the therapy saves a baby's life and a change can be made after a day if the cultures show that other antibiotics can be substituted.

CONTRAINDICATIONS TO ANTIBIOTICS IN NEONATES

Certain antibiotics should be used with great care in neonates (Dunne, 1972; Wood, 1972), particularly those which are albumin bound as they then displace bilirubin; sulphonamides, co-trimoxazole, novobiocin, nitrofurantoin and fucidic acid are probably the most dangerous of these. There are other antibiotics which will kill the organisms for which each of these is effective, so although some workers may consider the displacement of bilirubin only to be a theoretical danger, it is possible to avoid using these agents. Chloramphenicol may cause the 'grey baby' syndrome but if the standard dose is reduced this can be avoided. Tetracyclines are deposited in growing teeth and bones and they should not be used in neonates. Streptomycin in particular, and more rarely gentamicin and kanamycin may affect the eighth nerve.

STAPHYLOCOCCAL INFECTIONS

Since I started working as a paediatric bacteriologist the pattern of bacterial disease has changed markedly. Some infections that were common in 1948 have become rarities and since the introduction of methicillin and its related penicillinase resistant penicillins, severe staphylococcal infections of neonates have become increasingly uncommon, especially osteomyelitis and pneumonia. Thrush oesophagitis, which was usually followed by staphylococcal aspiration pneumonia (Wolff *et al.*, 1955), has not been seen in my hospital since 1960.

One must assume, until a sensitivity test proves otherwise, that all staphylococcal infections in neonates will be due to penicillinase-producing staphylococci and this applies to lesions amongst discharged patients as well as those in hospital. By 1970, 86 per cent of all staphylococci isolated from the patients attending Birmingham Children's Hospital, Casualty and Out-patient departments, were penicillin resistant and this could have been predicted from the slow and steady rise we have seen over the last 20 years (Heider & Rogers, 1972). We have seen a few cloxacillin resistant staphylococci in these out-patients (Skirrow & Rogers, 1971), but have not yet had a neonate admitted with such a staphylococcus, although the local maternity unit has isolated five cloxacillin resistant strains from babies, and three from members of the staff, in the last three years.

Superficial infections of the skin and eyes are not now usually of a serious nature. Pemphigus is rare, compared with the incidence 14 years ago, but sometimes it is diagnosed when a baby has a generalized *Herpes simplex* infection with skin lesions; when staphylococci have not been isolated from the blisters, the diagnosis of herpes should always be considered. The immuno-fluorescence technique and tissue culture establishes the correct diagnosis of herpes quickly: therapy with 2-deoxy-5-iodouridine has not been successful.

OPHTHALMIA NEONATORUM

In recent years the majority of eye infections are due to staphylococci, nearly all of which are penicillin resistant but which will usually respond to other antibiotics, given locally or parenterally. Ophthalmia neonatorum due to *Neisseria gonorrhoeae* has become uncommon (although it may already be increasing again) and it is worth identifying the neisseria isolated from an ophthalmia: our last three infections responded well to local chloramphenicol and systemic penicillin therapy, but two were caused by *N. meningitidis* and the third by *Neisseria catarrhalis*. Other ophthalmia infections have been due to enterobacteriaceae, pneumococci and *Haemophilus influenzae*, which have responded to correctly chosen therapy. A few cases of ophthalmia have been due to *Candida albicans* which can be diagnosed on the direct smear examination and confirmed by the cultures: these infections were cured by local amphotericin B or nystatin therapy.

INTESTINAL INFECTIONS

Specific bacterial intestinal infections are relatively uncommon in the neonate and can be due to any of the recognized pathogens such as salmonellae and shigellae or enteropathogenic strains of *Esch. coli*. The last is uncommon except in a premature baby unit which admits babies from hospitals in a wide area (Stulberg *et al.*, 1955). This is because few mothers carry a strain of enteropathogenic *Esch. coli* and, especially if the baby is breast fed, it is unlikely to develop enteritis (Mortimer, P. R.—to be published). Should it do so and, if the strain is sensitive to neomycin, neomycin-kaopectate is probably the best therapy. If the strain is neomycin resistant, gentamicin should be given orally and parenterally (Coetzee & Leary, 1971).

Salmonella infections

A baby ill with salmonellosis should be treated, as some neonates with salmonellosis develop meningitis (Brown, G. L., 1972—personal communication). Chloramphenicol, ampicillin and co-trimoxazole are the best agents, but the dosage of the first must be kept low and the sulphonamide component of the last could cause an undesirable hyperbilirubinaemia. This means that there are drawbacks to the use of the two most effective agents, so it is best to give large doses of ampicillin.

Shigella infections

Shigella infections of neonates are uncommon and therapy will depend on the sensitivity of the causal strain: if it is sensitive, oral streptomycin or paromycin are ideal. Neomycin is surprisingly ineffective compared with the response to paromomycin (Rogers *et al.*, 1956; Coles *et al.*, 1960).

Fungal infections

Candidal enteritis is also uncommon but it may occur in a ward where candidosis is endemic even if the affected baby is not receiving antibiotic therapy (Rogers, 1966 & 1971). The infection will respond to oral nystatin or amphotericin B. We have found it very difficult to prevent the active ingredient of the nystatin suspension from sedimenting to form a very firm caked deposit at the bottom of the bottle issued to the ward (Leach R. H.—personal communication). We therefore changed to amphotoricin B suspension for the treatment of intestinal candidosis. Unfortunately this has not been available recently as the makers have had difficulty producing a new formulation of the amphotericin B oral suspension, but it should be available for use in hospitals very soon.

Candidal enteritis will also respond to oral gentian violet but the widespread staining of the napkins, clothes and buttocks is sometimes unpopular. The appearance of the faeces of a baby with candidal enteritis is very characteristic, looking dark green and slimy, like meconium; direct smears of the faeces will provide the diagnosis when many hyphae and spores of candida are seen. We have not yet had a neonate with giardiasis but if we do we shall treat it with metronidazole as there were no side effects when we employed that to treat a 13-day old neonate who had trichomonas vaginitis.

NEONATAL URINARY TRACT INFECTIONS

Urinary tract infections are relatively uncommon but may be severe; some are associated with septicaemia, and even meningitis, the same sero-type being isolated from urine, blood and meninges. The treatment is the same as that of the meningitis, due to the same organisms. The use of an indwelling catheter has allowed some of our neonates to become infected with *C. albicans* and some of them have had a candidal bacteraemia, the organism being recovered from the blood probably because of movement of the catheter (Rogers, 1966). Most of these infections have occurred in boys with congenital urethral values. We have treated the majority of these babies with systemic amphotericin B, but before this treatment was available more than one baby died with a metastatic candidal abscesses in the kidney, brain and lung. A very few of these bladder infections have been successfully treated with bladder washes using amphotericin B.

INFECTIONS WITH *PSEUDOMONAS AERUGINOSA*

Pseudomonas aeruginosa can cause septicaemia, meningitis and pneumonia and it is probably the most dangerous of all the Gram negative bacilli causing such infections: fortunately we have had few of these infections. Nearly every strain of this organism is fully sensitive to gentamicin so the initial therapy referred to earlier in this paper, would cover such an infection. The diagnosis is helped by the very characteristic rash which is most often present on the limbs and trunk and consists of circumscribed macular-papular indurated areas which vary between 0·5 and 2 cm in diameter. If the child survives these areas will undergo necrosis and take a considerable time to heal. *Ps. aeruginosa* infections of the eye can be treated with local installation of polymyxins but great care must be taken not to damage the conjunctiva as a panophthalmitis may develop if the organism penetrates the conjunctiva.

PORTALS OF ENTRY

There are several portals of entry by which neonates become infected. Probably the commonest are inhalation and aspiration which may occur *in utero*, or during delivery and this particularly applies to the infections due to the enterobacteriaceae, Lancefield Group B streptococci and Listeria. Epidemiological studies show that the organism isolated from the baby is usually the same as that isolated from the mother. This raises the question as to whether there should be a screening programme of pregnant women to identify vaginal carriers of Listeria and *Strep. agalactiae*. Such a programme would take a great deal of time and probably a large number of babies would be treated unnecessarily. A few lives might be saved as fewer babies would be infected because the institution of very early therapy prevents septicaemia and meningitis.

REFERENCES

COETZEE, M. & LEARY, P. M. (1971). *Esch. coli* gastroenteritis. *Archives of Diseases of Childhood*, **46,** 646.

COLES, H. M. T., MACNAMARA, B., MUTCH, L., HOLT, R. J. & STEWART, G. T. (1960). Paromomycin in the treatment of Shigella and Salmonella infections in children. *Lancet*, **i,** 944.

DUNNE, J. F. (1972). Toxic effects of drugs. In *The Therapeutic Choice in Paediatrics* (Eds., Burland, N. L. & Laurance, B. M.), p. 75. Churchill and Livingstone, Edinburgh and London.

HEIDER, Y. & ROGERS, K. B. (1972). Unpublished data.

ROGERS, K. B. (1966). Candida infections in paediatrics. In *The Symposium on Candida Infections* (Eds., Winner, H. I. & Hurley, R.), p. 179. E. & S. Livingstone, Edinburgh and London.

ROGERS, K. B. (1971) Role of Candida in infantile gastroenteritis. *13th International Congress of Paediatrics*, **6,** 111.

ROGERS, K. B., BENSON, R. P., FOSTER, W. P., JONES, L. F. & WILLIAMS, T. C. (1956). Phthalylsulphacetamide and neomycin in the treatment of infantile gastroenteritis. *Lancet*, **ii,** 599.

SKIRROW, M. B. & ROGERS, K. B. (1971). Cloxacillin resistant staphylococci in a children's hospital. *Journal of Clinical Pathology*, **24,** 48.

STULBERG, C. S., ZUELZER, W. W., NOLKE, A. C. & THOMPSON, A. L. (1955). *Escherichia coli* 0127.B8 a pathogenic strain causing infantile diarrhoea. *American Journal of Diseases of Childhood*, **90,** 125.

WOLFF, O. H., PETTY, B. W., ASTLEY, R. & SMELLIE, J. M. (1955). Thrush oesophagitis with pharyngeal inco-ordination treated with hydroxystilbamidine. *Lancet*, **i,** 991.

WOOD, B. S. B. (1972). Choice of drugs in clinical paediatrics. In *The Therapeutic Choice in Paediatrics* (Eds., Burland, W. L. & Laurance, B. M.), p. 75. Churchill and Livingstone, Edinburgh and London.

9

MANAGEMENT OF URINARY TRACT INFECTION IN WOMEN

A. W. Asscher

The aims of treatment of urinary tract infection are to reduce morbidity and prevent mortality. The extent of the morbidity which arises from urinary tract infection is illustrated by the findings of Logan and Cushion (1958) who showed that 11 per 1000 consultations in general practice are on account of symptoms suggestive of urinary tract infection. The extent of the mortality associated with urinary tract infection is less well documented. It is not known with what frequency, if any, untreated or inadequately treated urinary tract infections lead to progressive kidney damage, rise of blood pressure and kidney failure. It has been established that the urinary tract is a common source of gram negative septicaemia particularly in patients in whom defensive mechanisms are impaired (Altemeier *et al.*, 1967; Freid & Vosti, 1968).

The two aims of treatment, avoidance of morbidity and prevention of mortality, are interrelated. Thus, if urinary tract infections lead to progressive kidney damage, asymptomatic infections need to be detected and treated. In contrast, if this were not the case, asymptomatic episodes of infection could be left untreated, and clinicians could reassure patients concerning the effect of repeated infections on kidney function. Such reassurance *per se* would constitute an important part of the management of the patient.

REDUCTION OF MORBIDITY FROM URINARY TRACT INFECTION

Since the usual source of urinary pathogens is the normal bowel flora (Grüneberg *et al.*, 1968), primary prevention of urinary tract infection is unlikely to be successful. Stamey *et al.* (1971) showed that the establishment of bladder bacteriuria in patients with recurrent urinary tract infections is preceded by colonization of the perineal floor with the same strain of *Escherichia coli* which can later be recovered from the bladder urine. This would suggest that recurrent urinary tract infections are attributable to a breakdown of the defensive mechanisms of the perineal floor. Observations such as these have prompted the use of antiseptic applications to the perineal floor in order to reduce morbidity. Such regimes have proved unrewarding.

The ascent of micro-organisms to the bladder is thought to be facilitated by the shortness of the female urethra, the existence of a retrograde flow of urine in the female urethra, the fact that infection may be present in the female analogue of the prostate gland (peri-urethral glands) and the possibility that the organisms may enter the bladder during bathing, or perhaps most important of all, as a result of sexual intercourse.

Relationship of infection to sexual intercourse

An opportunity recently arose to obtain pre- and post-sexual intercourse mid-stream urine specimens from a medical practitioner who had for some time suffered from recurrent attacks of frequency and dysuria following sexual intercourse. This patient had been most carefully instructed in urine collection technique and on many occasions had been shown to have a negative urine culture. We were able to show by the 'dip-slide' technique that a 6 hour post-intercourse specimen contained a pure growth of 10^3 *Esch. coli* per ml, whereas the pre-intercourse specimen had shown no growth. Clearly observations of this kind must be extended, but the difficulties are obvious. The role of sexual intercourse in the pathogenesis of the frequency and dysuria syndrome is well known to clinicians as implied in the term 'honeymoon cystitis'. The frequency and dysuria syndrome is more commonly precipitated by sexual intercourse in the younger than in the older woman. This may be on account of their greater sexual activity but poor sexual technique may also be a contributing factor.

Table 1 shows my experience during the year 1971 of 88 patients who presented in the out-patient department, with the frequency and dysuria syndrome. Forty of the patients (45 per cent) were found to have significant bacteriuria and in 36 of the patients (41 per cent) the symptoms were precipitated by sexual intercourse. In the patients in whom a relationship to sexual

TABLE 1

RELATION OF FREQUENCY AND DYSURIA SYNDROME TO SEXUAL INTERCOURSE (S.I.) IN PATIENTS SEEN IN HOSPITAL PRACTICE

Number of patients	*Urine culture*		*Symptoms precipitated by S.I.*	*Response to treatment*			
				Good		*Nil*	
	Pos.	*Neg.*		*Culture Pos.*	*Culture Neg.*	*Culture Pos.*	*Culture Neg.*
88	40	48	36	18	12	2	4
				(Not significant)		(Not significant)	

intercourse existed, simple instruction in sexual technique and advice to empty the bladder after intercourse and to take a single dose of an anti-bacterial agent at this time, resulted in relief of symptoms in 30 (83 per cent of the patients). There was no significant difference between the success rate obtained in patients with positive urine cultures as compared with those in whom the bacteriological findings had been negative on first attendance.

It follows, that the chance of relieving morbidity from the frequency and dysuria syndrome is high when the syndrome is related to sexual intercourse and a direct enquiry into the relationship of the symptoms to sexual intercourse should not be omitted.

Other precipitating factors

In patients in whom such a relationship does not exist, other precipitating factors may be discovered. The onset of symptoms may be related to the menstrual periods, childbirth, previous gynaecological operations or instrumentation of the urinary tract or the use of an intra-uterine contraceptive device or diaphragm. In some 50 per cent of the patients, however, no precipitating factor was obvious. In these patients, provided urine culture is positive, the approach to treatment should depend on whether or not one is dealing with a *relapse* of infection, i.e. a recurrence of infection due to the same organism which was isolated before treatment, or a *re-infection*, i.e. a recurrence due to a different micro-organism from that originally isolated. Relapses signify ineffective treatment whereas re-infections indicate failure of the host defensive mechanisms.

Approach to treatment

The approach to treatment of these two types of recurrence should be different. Thus, with relapsing infection, an attempt should be made to eradicate infection once and for all by high dosage treatment using bactericidal agents. Should this fail, long-term suppressive therapy with urinary antiseptics or low doses of antibacterial agents may prove successful in ridding the patient of recurrent symptoms. Reinfections may be dealt with as they arise and the patient should be given an antibacterial agent to take home with instructions to take a 1-week course of the drug at the first sign of symptomatic reinfection. At the same time she should send an inoculated dip-slide to the laboratory so that in case of failure to respond to treatment a further course of treatment may be prescribed on the basis of the sensitivity of the infecting micro-organism to antimicrobial agents.

Asymptomatic bacteriuria

The value of screening for and treating asymptomatic infections in reducing morbidity must also be considered. The outcome of these asymptomatic infections in pregnancy has been extensively studied. Some 20 per cent of women who enter pregnancy with asymptomatic infection later develop symptomatic infection either during pregnancy or the puerperium. This risk is largely avoided if the asymptomatic bacteriuria (a.s.b.) is eradicated (Kass, 1960). This relationship of a.s.b. in early pregnancy to the emergence of symptomatic infection at a later stage of pregnancy has received widespread confirmation (Whalley, 1967) and forms the basis for advocating bacteriuria screening in antenatal clinics.

It would clearly be an advantage if treatment of a.s.b. in pregnancy could be confined to the 20 per cent of pregnant bacteriuric women who go on to develop symptomatic infection. As yet there is no reliable means of doing this.

The value of screening non-pregnant women for a.s.b. in the prevention of morbidity is much less clear since the natural history of a.s.b. in the non-pregnant woman differs from that in the pregnant woman in two important respects (Asscher *et al.*, 1969). Firstly, bacteriuria in non-pregnant women shows a high spontaneous cure rate and secondly, although bacteriuria in the non-pregnant woman pre-disposes to urinary symptoms these are milder than in the pregnant woman and are usually confined to the lower urinary tract. Asscher *et al.* (1969), showed that in the non-pregnant woman with a.s.b. a short course of treatment did not lead to a lasting cure and that the reinfections which followed 'successful' treatment were more commonly associated with a bout of symptoms than the persistent infections in untreated bacteriuric subjects. It seems, therefore, that the bacteria in the urinary tract of asymptomatic adult bacteriuric women are living in a kind of peaceful symbiosis with their host and are better left undisturbed.

PREVENTION OF MORTALITY FROM URINARY TRACT INFECTION

The role of urinary tract infection in the pathogenesis of progressive kidney damage, raised blood pressure and eventual kidney failure has not so far been settled beyond doubt. Evidence from prospective and retrospective studies of the natural history of urinary tract infection indicates that in the adult urinary tract infection rarely leads to progressive kidney damage in the absence of obstruction (Asscher & Waters, 1971). Although it is not possible to prove such a negative finding, it is clear that even if urinary tract infection does lead to renal damage it must be sufficiently rare so as not to affect the management of the individual patient. This conclusion allows us to reassure the numerous women who present with urinary tract infection and at the same time make it unnecessary to treat asymptomatic episodes of infection in the non-pregnant woman. There are exceptions to this. For instance, urinary tract infection should be searched for and treated in patients whose defensive mechanisms are impaired as a result of steroid therapy or treatment with immuno-suppressive drugs or as a consequence of bone marrow or kidney failure. In these subjects urinary tract infection represents an important source of gram-negative septicaemia (McCabe & Jackson, 1962).

The problems which arise when attempting to treat urinary tract infection in the presence of end-stage kidney failure are particularly intriguing. They are summarized in Table 2. It seems that in these patients the most useful drugs are the penicillins, co-trimoxazole and gentamicin because adequate urinary concentrations of these drugs can be obtained without systemic toxicity. Thus in the case of co-trimoxazole, the sulphonamide moiety is well excreted despite the presence of advanced kidney failure (Williams *et al.*, 1968; Sharpstone, 1970). Although trimethoprim is retained in patients with end-stage kidney failure, its urinary concentration still exceeds the M.I.C. for most urinary pathogens (Sharpstone, 1969). A limited trial of co-trimoxazole in patients with glomerular filtration rates of less than 30 ml per minute and urinary tract infection due to *Esch. coli* and *Proteus spp*. yielded a cure rate of

70 per cent in 16 patients with *Esch. coli* infection, cure being defined as a sterile urine 6 weeks after stopping treatment. In a further group of 14 patients with infection due to *Proteus spp.* the cure rate was 50 per cent. In 12 patients with *Pseudomonas aeruginosa* urinary tract infection, treated with gentamicin using the regime described by Gingell and Waterworth (1968), 60 per cent were cured.

TABLE 2

PROBLEMS IN TREATMENT OF URINARY TRACT INFECTION IN THE PRESENCE OF CHRONIC KIDNEY FAILURE

1. Infections are usually acquired in hospital and thus more likely to be due to resistant organisms.
2. Therapeutic urinary concentrations of antibacterial agents may be difficult to attain without systemic toxicity.
3. Therapeutic urinary concentrations of antibacterial agents are more slowly established and drug resistance may therefore develop more readily during treatment.
4. Urinary acidification is not possible.
5. Disparity of functional impairment of the kidneys may lead to unequal excretion of antibacterial agents and persistence of infection in the kidney with the poorer function.

CONCLUSIONS

The management of non-obstructive infections of the urinary tract in adult women is concerned solely with the relief of symptoms since these infections in the absence of obstruction do not lead to progressive impairment of kidney function. Except in pregnancy, and in patients in whom defensive mechanisms are impaired, no benefit results from treating asymptomatic infection in the adult.

REFERENCES

ALTEMEIR, W. A., TODD, J. C. & WELLFORD, W. I. (1967). Gram-negative septicaemia: A growing threat. *Annals of Surgery*, **145,** 530.

ASSCHER, A. W., SUSSMAN, M., WATERS, W. E., EVANS, J. A. S., CAMPBELL, H., EVANS, K. T. & WILLIAMS, J. (1969). Asymptomatic significant bacteriuria in the non-pregnant woman. II. Response to treatment and follow-up. *British Medical Journal*, **1,** 804.

ASSCHER, A. W. & WATERS, W. E. (1971). Significant bacteriuria in the non-pregnant woman. In *Renal Infection and Renal Scarring* (Eds., Kincaid-Smith, P. & Fairley, K. F.), p. 25. Mercedes Publishing Services, Melbourne, Australia.

FREID, M. A. & VOSTI, K. L. (1968). The importance of underlying disease in patients with gram-negative bacteriuria. *Archives of Internal Medicine*, **121,** 418.

GINGELL, J. C. & WATERWORTH, P. M. (1968). The dose of gentamicin in patients with normal renal function and with varying degrees of renal impairment. *British Medical Journal*, **2,** 19.

GRÜNEBERG, R. N., LEIGH, D. A. & BRUMFITT, W. (1968). *Escherichia coli* serotypes in urinary tract infection: Studies in domiciliary, ante-natal and hospital practice. In *Urinary Tract Infection* (Eds., O'Grady, F. & Brumfitt, W.), p. 68. Oxford University Press.

KASS, E. H. (1960). The role of asymptomatic bacteriuria in the pathogenesis of pyelonephritis. In *Biology of Pyelonephritis* (Eds., Quinn, E. L. & Kass, E. H.), p. 399. Little Brown and Co.

LOGAN, W. P. D. & CUSHION, A. A. (1958). Morbidity studies from general practice. *Studies on medical and population subject*, No. 14, H.M.S.O.

MCCABE, W. R. & JACKSON, G. G. (1962). Gram-negative bacteriuria. *Archives of Internal Medicine*, **110**, 847.

SHARPSTONE, P. (1969). The renal handling of trimethoprim and sulphamethoxazole in man. *Postgraduate Medical Journal*, November Supplement, **45**, 38.

STAMEY, T. A., TIMOTHY, M., MILLAR, M. & MIHARA, G. (1971). Recurrent urinary tract infections in adult women. The role of introital enterobacteria. *California Medicine*, **115**, 1.

WHALLEY, P. J. (1967). Bacteriuria of pregnancy. *American Journal of Obstetrics and Gynecology*, **97**, 723.

WILLIAMS, D. M., WIMPENNY, J. & ASSCHER, A. W. (1968). Renal clearance of sodium sulphadimidine in normal and uraemic subjects. *Lancet*, **2**, 1058.

10

CHEMOTHERAPY OF URINARY TRACT INFECTIONS

J. D. Williams, J. Kosmidis and A. M. Geddes

Urinary tract infections are very common and in most cases respond rapidly to antibiotic therapy. When considering the treatment of any infection, three factors must be taken into account: the patient, the infecting organism and the antibiotic of choice. In urinary tract infection, all the factors in the equation show marked variability. Firstly, almost all systemic antibiotics have at some time been recommended for treatment of urinary infections in addition to agents specifically designed for these infections. Secondly, the organisms causing infection include gram-negative and gram-positive bacteria with unpredictable sensitivity patterns as well as candida and other less common organisms. Thirdly, the patients are of all ages with infections of different severity, and often with anatomical or functional variations in the urinary tract.

The organisms isolated from even the most straightforward groups of patients, for example symptomatic infections arising in females in the general community, are unpredictable. Although 80 per cent of the organisms are *Escherichia coli*, the remainder are mainly *Proteus mirabilis* and *Staphylococcus albus* which have different sensitivity patterns. In hospital acquired infections the range of organisms is much wider and includes Klebsiella *spp.*, *Pseudomonas aeruginosa*, indole positive proteus strains and other less commonly isolated bacteria with a wider range of antimicrobial sensitivity.

The range of antibiotics available for treatment of urinary tract infections grows longer each year (Table 1). Such is the variety of patients with urinary tract infections that each of the agents listed has a useful place in therapy and, despite the extensive choice, it is not uncommon to encounter a patient for whom only one of these agents is indicated. Urinary infection is so prevalent

Table 1

POSSIBLE AGENTS FOR TREATMENT OF URINARY TRACT INFECTIONS

Sulphonamides	*Other oral agents*	*Parenteral antibiotics*
Short Acting	Ampicillin	Ampicillin
(8 tabs. a day)	Amoxycillin	Colistin
e.g. sulphadimidine	Cephalexin	Kanamycin
Medium Acting	Nalidixic Acid	Streptomycin
(1 tab. a day)	Nitrofurantoin	Gentamicin
e.g. sulphametopyrazine	Co-trimoxazole	Cephaloridine
Long acting	Mandelamine	Cephalothin
(1 tab. a week)	Cycloserine	
e.g. sulphamethoxydiazine		

that occasionally one needs to use an antibiotic, such as erythromycin, which is not usually regarded as a urinary tract antibiotic (Zinner *et al.*, 1971).

The patients who acquire urinary tract infections may be classified into many clinical categories (Table 2). The patients in these groups present different chemotherapeutic problems, and show variable responses to treatment. Even within a specific group of patients, for example pregnant women

TABLE 2

CLINICAL GROUPS OF PATIENTS WITH URINARY TRACT INFECTIONS SHOWN TOGETHER WITH ADDITIONAL FEATURES WHICH INFLUENCE THE MANAGEMENT AND TREATMENT OF THE PATIENT

Young children	Vesico-ureteric reflux
	Urethral valves
	Normal renal tracts
Schoolgirls	Occasional symptomatic episodes
	Repeated infections
	Asymptomatic bacteriuria
Females of childbearing age	Occasional symptomatic episodes
	Repeated infections
	Pyelonephritis of pregnancy
	Asymptomatic bacteriuria in pregnancy
	Urethral syndrome
Older females	Genital prolapse
	Asymptomatic bacteriuria
Males (excl. young children)	Acute prostatitis
	Prostatic hypertrophy
	Asymptomatic bacteriuria (elderly only)
All ages	Bladder catheter
	Renal failure
	Post-operative infection
	Calculus formation

with significant bacteriuria, the response to treatment varies; some patients in this group have additional factors present such as a congenital malformation of the renal tract or calculus formation in the kidneys, ureter or bladder, which influence the outcome of treatment.

ORGANISMS RESPONSIBLE FOR URINARY TRACT INFECTIONS

The sensitivity of urinary pathogens to antimicrobial drugs varies considerably and unpredictably. Even in domiciliary infections where greatest uniformity of pathogen and sensitivity occurs, culture of the urine is necessary to determine whether it is a sensitive strain of *Esch. coli* causing the infection or one of the less common pathogens. Most clinicians, however, are satisfied to treat the patient on the basis of the likely organisms and sensitivity, and use culture of the urine as a test of cure or for identifying organisms not amenable to the initial therapy.

The most likely pattern of antimicrobial sensitivity of isolates from four clinical groups of patients is shown in Table 3. These organisms, consecutively

TABLE 3

SENSITIVITY PATTERNS OF ORGANISMS ISOLATED FROM URINARY TRACT INFECTIONS OCCURRING IN FOUR GROUPS OF PATIENTS AT DUDLEY ROAD HOSPITAL

All strains were collected in the first 3 months of 1972 except for the strains from women with asymptomatic bacteriuria collected during 1971. The organisms represent consecutive isolates and are unselected

Source of patient	*No. of strains tested*	*Percentage of strains resistant to* Ampicillin	*Sulphonamide*	*Nitrofurantoin*	*Nalidixic acid*	*Co-trimoxazole*	*Cephalexin*
General practice[a]	99	12	23	15	14	3	9 per cent
Pregnant women[a]	100	25	29	6	2	1	1 per cent
Hospital inpatients	553	49	42	37	22	21	17 per cent
Urological patients	54	56	57	46	52	20	29 per cent

[a] The organisms from general practice contain some strains of *Staph. albus* and *Strep. faecalis*, but from the pregnant women only gram-negetive bacilli were tested.

isolated from patients with urinary infections during 1971 or in the first few months of 1972, were tested against six oral agents commonly used to treat urinary tract infections. Sulphonamide-resistance was found in 23 per cent of isolates from domiciliary cases, but with the other agents resistance was unusual. A rather higher incidence of resistance to ampicillin was seen in organisms isolated from pregnant women from the same population. This probably reflects previous antibiotic treatment as many of the patients were multiparous and had several hospital admissions. The sensitivity of the organisms from hospital in-patients shows much more variability as this group includes patients with infections acquired in hospital with a wide range of organisms, many of which display multiple antibiotic resistance. Urological patients were infected with the most resistant organisms.

In Table 4 are shown the sensitivities of selected hospital urinary tract pathogens against six other antibiotics. The organisms selected for testing were those showing resistance to three or more of the oral agents. Such survey data become less valuable the wider the range of organisms included because the sensitivity patterns of one organism can distort the results: for

TABLE 4

SENSITIVITY PATTERNS OF 78 STRAINS ISOLATED FROM URINE OF PATIENTS IN MEDICAL AND SURGICAL WARDS

The strains were selected on the basis of resistance to 3 or more of the oral agents (see previous table)

Antibiotic	*Per cent resistant strains*
Streptomycin	69
Tetracycline	76
Colistin	21
Kanamycin	14
Gentamicin	3
Carbenicillin	60

These strains comprised 14 *Esch. coli*, 14 Proteus species, 32 Klebsiella, 10 Pseudomonas, 6 other gram-negative bacilli and 2 *Strept. faecalis*.

example, the differences between the kanamycin and gentamicin results reflect the sensitivity of the pseudomonas strains. Similarly, the incidence of colistin resistance reported in this table occurs mainly in the proteus isolates. It will be seen that culture of the urine and determination of sensitivity is essential in selecting appropriate therapy in hospital patients.

Recognition of the organisms responsible for the infection sometimes precedes the results of sensitivity testing and this enables predictions to be made about therapy while awaiting confirmation or sensitivity. Table 5 shows the probable sensitivities to antimicrobial agents or organisms isolated from urinary tract infections. This information varies in different hospitals. For example, if a klebsiella is isolated in Dudley Road Hospital, it will be almost certainly sensitive to kanamycin, while in the neighbouring Accident Hospital, 80 per cent of klebsiella strains are resistant to kanamycin (Roe & Lowbury, 1972). However, many of the resistances shown in this table are fixed and the patterns are generally applicable.

TABLE 5

PROBABLE SENSITIVITY PATTERNS OF URINARY PATHOGENS

Organism	*Probably sensitive to*	*Probably resistant to*
Esch. coli (domiciliary)	Sulphonamide and other agents	—
Esch. coli (hospital)	Co-trimoxazole, cephalexin, nalidixic acid	Sulphonamide, ampicillin, nitrofurantoin
Proteus mirabilis	Ampicillin, kanamycin	Tetracycline, colistin
Other proteus species	Kanamycin	Many agents
Klebsiella	Cephaloridine, colistin, kanamycin	Ampicillin
Staph. albus	Ampicillin, nitrofurantoin	Nalidixic acid, colistin
Strep. faecalis	Ampicillin, nitrofurantoin	Many agents
Ps. aeruginosa	Gentamicin, carbenicillin, colistin	Many agents

ANTIBIOTICS AND URINARY TRACT INFECTION

The term antibiotic will be used to denote both conventional antibiotics and other chemotherapeutic agents such as sulphonamides and nitrofurantoin. Three broad groups can be defined: sulphonamides, other oral agents and parenteral antibiotics, and some of their properties are summarized in Table 6. The major route of excretion of these agents is by way of the kidney and as a result significant quantities appear in the urine. Cycloserine, nalidixic acid and nitrofurantoin, however, do not give therapeutic concentrations in the blood and are therefore contra-indicated when severe renal infection and possible septicaemia are suspected.

Controversy has existed for some time about the necessity for therapeutic blood levels of antibiotics in the treatment of renal infections. Ampicillin blood levels are only marginally higher than the minimum inhibitory concentration (M.I.C.) of *Esch. coli* when the antibiotic is given by mouth and in severe infections intravenous administration of ampicillin has been shown to give superior results to oral therapy (Brumfitt *et al.*, 1964). This suggests that adequate serum levels of an antibiotic may be important in the treatment of urinary tract infections, but it would be wrong to assume that agents producing negligible blood levels are ineffective in renal infections. Studies of serum antibody levels measured against infecting organisms have suggested that 30 per cent of pregnant women with bacteriuria have some degree of renal involvement as judged by an antibody titre of 1/320 or greater (Percival, Brumfitt & de Louvois, 1964). However, nitrofurantoin is widely and successfully used in bacteriuria in pregnancy. The relationship of renal involvement as estimated by serum antibody levels and response to nitrofurantoin therapy is shown in Table 7. The cure rate was the same whether or not the kidney was involved. The extent of renal infection in these patients was not sufficient to affect the response to treatment. In patients with renal abnormalities or

TABLE 6

FACTORS INFLUENCING CHOICE OF ANTIBIOTICS IN URINARY TRACT INFECTIONS

Agents	
Short-acting sulphonamides	Most domiciliary infections are sensitive; very cheap; low toxicity; safe in pregnancy and childhood.
Longer-acting sulphonamides	Simple dose regimens; single dose therapy possible with some; more expensive; doubts over Stevens-Johnson syndrome associations.
Ampicillin, amoxycillin	Low toxicity but skin rashes in 5–10 per cent of patients. Klebsiella and other hospital pathogens often resistant. Used parenterally for severe community acquired infections.
Cephalexin	Used as alternative in ampicillin-hypersensitive patients. Active against some ampicillin-resistant gram-negative bacilli. Not cheap.
Nitrofurantoin	Cheap; broad spectrum of activity but not effective in proteus infections; low toxicity; some vomiting when high doses used. Polyneuritis with long courses.
Nalidixic acid	Broad spectrum of activity but resistance can develop during treatment. Not cheap; many doses necessary; not indicated in pregnancy or neonates.
Co-trimoxazole	Very active combination with high cure rates. Many uses in different types of U.T.I. but doubts over teratogenic and haematological effects.
Tetracycline	Little used because of effect on dentition—not in pregnancy or in young children. Proteus strains resistant.
Mandelamine	Many variations available for treatment; urine must be acid. Broad activity but slow in acute phases of infection.
Cycloserine	Most *Esch. coli* strains sensitive; high blood levels lead to neurotoxicity.
Aminoglycosides	Increasing range of activity from streptomycin to kanamycin to gentamicin but increasing toxicity also. All highly bactericidal. Used mainly in severe hospital acquired infections with different degrees of resistance. Ototoxic—modify dose in renal failure.
Colistin	Neurotoxic in renal failure; used in chronic infections in urological patients; not against proteus or gram-positive infections.
Cephaloridine	Indication similar to parenteral ampicillin but spectrum somewhat broader; avoided where possible in renal failure.
Carbenicillin	Usually reserved for pseudomonas infections; large doses necessary; expensive.

other complicating factors, high serum levels of antibiotic may be necessary but are probably not essential for eradicating less severe infections.

The levels of antibiotics in prostatic fluid are also of interest. In dogs, the only antibiotics found to attain therapeutic concentrations in prostatic fluid were oleandomycin and erythromycin (Stamey *et al.*, 1970). These agents are primarily active against gram-positive organisms, although they are effective against gram-negative bacilli in high concentration and at an alkaline pH (*British Medical Journal*, 1972). The prostatic fluid is normally acid, although it has been found to be alkaline in up to 75 per cent of patients with prostatitis

TABLE 7

RELATION OF ANTIBODY TITRE TO RESPONSE TO TREATMENT WITH NITROFURANTOIN

Antibody titre	*Number treated*	*Number cured at 6 weeks*
1/320 and above	18	14 (74 per cent)
Less than 1/320	35	24 (70 per cent)

(Ludvik, 1964). Trimethoprim is a weak base with a pK_a of 7·3, is very diffusable and may prove useful in the treatment of prostatitis when given in combination with a sulphonamide.

Newer agents

During the past 5 years, three new agents have become available for the treatment of urinary tract infection. Two of these, cephalexin and amoxycillin, are antibiotics, while trimethoprim is a chemotherapeutic compound given in combination with a sulphonamide as co-trimoxazole.

Cephalexin

Cephalexin is a cephalosporin antibiotic which has a side-chain similar to that of ampicillin and, like ampicillin, is excreted in the urine in high concentration. The spectrum of activity of cephalexin is wider than that of ampicillin particularly in klebsiella infections and those due to ampicillin resistant proteus species. Smith and Williams (1970) found that cephalexin produced similar cure rates to those obtained with ampicillin and nitrofurantoin when treating refractory urinary infections (i.e. low) and similar to that with sulphonamide (i.e. high) in uncomplicated infections in domiciliary patients. Cephalexin is particularly useful for the treatment of infections caused by sulphonamide-resistant organisms in patients who are hypersensitive to the penicillins (and therefore to ampicillin).

Amoxycillin

Amoxycillin (alpha-amino-*p*-hydroxybenzylpenicillin) is a semi-synthetic penicillin which has an antibacterial spectrum similar to that of ampicillin against urinary pathogens (Kosmidis *et al.*, 1972). Absorption from the gastrointestinal tract is, however, better than that of ampicillin and blood levels are therefore almost twice as high (Geddes *et al.*, 1971). Urine concentrations of amoxycillin are also significantly greater than those obtained with ampicillin Whereas urinary recovery of ampicillin varies from 30 to 40 per cent of an oral dose, up to 50 per cent of amoxycillin is excreted in the urine (Geddes *et al.*, 1971). The main advantage of amoxycillin over ampicillin in the treatment of urinary tract infections might be the less frequent dosage required as a result of the superior absorption. Ampicillin urine levels already greatly exceed the M.I.C. for *Esch. coli.* We treated 21 patients with bacteriuria in pregnancy with amoxycillin in a dose of 1000 mg twice a day for 7 days. All the patients had amoxycillin-sensitive organisms in the urine and radiologically normal renal tracts. Eradication of bacteriuria was achieved in all 21 women. A total of 69 patients suffering from various infections have been treated with amoxycillin with satisfactory results (Kosmidis *et al.*, 1972). Apart from skin rashes in 3 patients, there have been no serious untoward reactions to the antibiotic.

Co-trimoxazole

Trimethoprim and sulphamethoxazole, the components of co-trimoxazole, both produce therapeutic blood levels following oral administration. The ratio of sulphamethoxazole serum levels to those of trimethoprim is approximately 20:1 as compared with a 5:1 ratio in pharmaceutical preparations of co-trimoxazole (Table 8). Co-trimoxazole is well excreted in the urine, the

TABLE 8

CO-TRIMOXAZOLE SERUM LEVELS (μg/ml)

Two tablets every 12 hours (each tablet containing 80 mg of TMP and 400 mg of SMX)

Time after dose (hours)	*Trimethoprim (TMP)*	*Sulphamethoxazole (SMX)*
1	2·7	68
2	2·3	72
4	2·3	61
6	2·3	54
11	1·4	37

renal clearance of sulphamethoxazole increasing with rising urine flow rates and with alkalinization, while trimethoprim clearance is not affected by change in urine flow and increases with urinary acidification. Co-trimoxazole is well tolerated in childhood, giving satisfactory blood and urine levels (Table 9). The blood levels in children produce the same 20:1 ratio of sulphonamide to trimethoprim, but in urine the ratio is nearer 2:1.

TABLE 9

CO-TRIMOXAZOLE SERUM AND URINE LEVELS IN CHILDREN (μg/ml) FOLLOWING 40 mg TMP AND 200 mg SMX

	Trimethoprim (TMP)		*Sulphamethoxazole (SMX)*	
Age (months)	*Blood*	*Urine*	*Blood*	*Urine*
24	0·74	36	37	66
24	2·40	130	42	360
9	1·20	100	50	240

At the present time most hospital and domiciliary pathogens causing urinary infections remain sensitive to co-trimoxazole. However, while most domiciliary organisms remain sensitive to sulphonamide and to other simple agents, there is no necessity to change prescribing habits to co-trimoxazole. In hospital, a valuable agent such as co-trimoxazole should be used only when specifically indicated and not prescribed indiscriminately. It is disappointing, but not entirely unexpected, to see trimethoprim-resistant *Esch. coli* strains beginning to appear in hospital. These can be associated with resistance-transfer factors (Fleming *et al.*, 1972), and dissemination may be rapid. It would be unfortunate if this agent were to diminish in effectiveness because of colonization of the hospital environment by trimethoprim-resistant organisms.

Co-trimoxazole is an effective antibiotic for the treatment of urinary tract infections (Cox & Montgomery, 1968; Reeves *et al.*, 1969) and has been used successfully for long-term prophylaxis (Cattell *et al.*, 1971). If trimethoprim and sulphamethoxazole are mixed in solution, precipitation may occur and preparations of co-trimoxazole for parenteral administration are therefore not available. This is a serious disadvantage in that parenteral therapy is preferable to the oral route for the treatment of serious infections, especially in patients who are vomiting. We have recently successfully treated a small number of septicaemic patients with a combination of trimethoprim and sulphadiazine (there is no parenteral preparation of sulphamethoxazole) both given intravenously by bolus injection from separate syringes.

Trimethoprim is a folic acid antagonist and doubts have been expressed about the desirability of prescribing it during pregnancy because of the possibility of teratogenicity. There was, however, no increased incidence of abnormality in a series of babies born to women treated during pregnancy with co-trimoxazole (Williams *et al.*, 1969) and follow-up studies on these children showed normal development (E. K. Smith and J. D. Williams—unpublished data).

CHEMOTHERAPY PROBLEMS IN DIFFERENT GROUPS OF PATIENTS

Patients suffering from urinary tract infections are not a homogeneous group. Table 2 shows the clinically important categories of patients presenting with urinary tract infection. Some of the specific problems presented by these groups will now be outlined.

Young children

Pyelonephritis in childhood may lead to destruction of renal tissue at a time when growth is occurring and, as a result, the child may reach adult life with scarred contracted kidneys. Reflux of urine from bladder to ureter during micturition is an important factor in the aetiology of urinary tract infection in this age group and may lead to persistent or recurrent infection. Children with reflux should be instructed to practise 'double micturition' during and after antibiotic treatment of infection. As in adults, urinary infections are significantly more common in female children than in males after the first year of life. However, the presence of congenital urethral valves may underlie recurrent urinary tract infection in male children and antibiotic treatment will usually fail to eradicate infection until the valves have been surgically removed. All children with urinary tract infection should be given a 10-day course of an appropriate antimicrobial agent. Drugs such as tetracycline which are contra-indicated in childhood should not be used in this age group.

In adults, simple infections which do not lead to renal damage frequently occur in patients with normal urinary tracts; similar infections occur in childhood and respond to short courses of therapy, tend not to recur and do not produce continuing renal damage. These children should not be over-treated or excessively investigated. However, careful follow-up with regular urine cultures must be undertaken in *all* children treated for urinary tract infection, even when the renal tract is normal. If, after a 6-month period, infection has not recurred, follow-up can bé discontinued (MacGregor & Freeman, 1968). Two or more recurrences of symptoms with positive urine cultures are an indication for long-term suppressive therapy. Children with urinary tract infection associated with reflux and also those with non-correctible lesions of the renal tract such as horseshoe or cystic kidneys should also be given prophylactic chemotherapy (Smellie, 1970). Low-dose sulphonamide and nitrofurantoin have been recommended for this purpose. (Smallpiece, 1968; Normand & Smellie, 1965). The emergence of organisms resistant to these agents necessitates change of treatment to ampicillin, cycloserine (Murdoch *et al.*, 1968) or co-trimoxazole (Cattell *et al.*, 1971). The dose of an antibacterial drug for long-term prophylaxis depends on the agent selected but is usually one-quarter to one-third of the daily therapeutic dose. Duration of long-term therapy varies according to the presence or absence of reflux or other abnormality in the renal tract but should normally not be less than 6 months. Children with reflux should be maintained on low-dose therapy as long as reflux persists (Smellie, 1970).

Schoolgirls

Most interest in this age-group has focused on the 1 to 2 per cent of schoolgirls who have asymptomatic bacteriuria often associated with structural defects in the renal tract. These children are sometimes of smaller stature than non-bacteriuric classmates (Kunin *et al.*, 1960; 1970; Savage *et al.*, 1969). In schoolgirls with asymptomatic bacteriuria, the urine should be sterilized with a 10-day course of an appropriate antibiotic. Several recurrences of bacteriuria are an indication for long-term therapy. Occasional symptomatic episodes of infection or repeated infection in this group of patients should be managed as in women of child-bearing age.

Females of child-bearing age

Urinary tract infections occur more commonly in this age-group than in any other and certain sub-groups can be identified:

Occasional symptomatic episodes

These may take the form of either acute cystitis or of acute pyelonephritis. The latter condition may be associated with septicaemia and should be treated with an injectable bactericidal drug such as kanamycin (Geddes *et al.*, 1967). Less fulminating episodes of infection usually respond to a 7-day course of an oral agent to which the infecting organism is sensitive such as sulphonamide, nitrofurantoin or ampicillin.

Recurrent urinary tract infection

Frequent recurrences of urinary tract infection are a common cause of morbidity in women of child-bearing age and may be precipitated by known factors such as sexual intercourse (p. 94). In many women, however, there is no obvious triggering factor. Urine culture may yield an organism which is resistant to standard drugs, such as sulphonamides, nitrofurantoin and ampicillin, but sensitive to newer agents, such as cephalexin or co-trimoxazole, which is particularly effective in patients who have failed to respond to 'primary' treatment. Repeated episodes of urinary tract infection in women of child-bearing age are an indication for long-term chemotherapy. Cycloserine (Murdoch *et al.*, 1968), co-trimoxazole (Cattell *et al.*, 1971) and nitrofurantoin (Bailey *et al.*, 1971) have all proved satisfactory for this purpose. Mandelamine is also effective for long-term prophylaxis but the urine pH must be kept below 5 with an acidifying agent such as methionine.

Asymptomatic bacteriuria and pyelonephritis of pregnancy

These conditions are dealt with elsewhere (pp. 78, 95).

The urethral syndrome

Up to 50 per cent of the women consulting general practitioners because of frequency of micturition and dysuria are found to have sterile urine (Gallagher *et al.*, 1965; Mond *et al.*, 1965). This has been referred to as the urethral syndrome and is probably associated with low-grade infection in periurethral tissues. In one study, 58 per cent of females with this syndrome subsequently developed urinary infection (O'Grady *et al.*, 1970). Antibiotic therapy must be empirical in the urethral syndrome in the absence of bacteriological confirmation of diagnosis but co-trimoxazole given for 7 days produces relief in a proportion of women with this distressing condition (A. M. Geddes—unpublished data).

The middle-aged and elderly

Urinary tract infection in females in this age-group may be associated with gynaecological disorders such as genital prolapse, which should be corrected (Williams *et al.*, 1969a). Antibiotic therapy will then usually eradicate the infection. Asymptomatic bacteriuria is common in elderly women (Dontas *et al.*, 1966) and in most instances is probably not an indication for chemotherapy.

Acute prostatitis may occur in middle-aged males (and also sometimes in young men). Even after prostatic massage, positive cultures are only obtained in about one-third of these patients (Garland, 1967) and chemotherapy must therefore be 'blind' in the majority of cases. Co-trimoxazole appears to be effective in this condition (D. S. Reeves—personal communication). If relapse occurs following treatment, long-term chemotherapy is indicated.

Benign prostatic hypertrophy causing urethral obstruction and residual urine is the commonest cause of urinary tract infection in middle-aged and elderly males. Antibiotic therapy will usually fail in these patients until prostatectomy has been performed.

Catheterization and urinary tract infection

The insertion of a bladder catheter frequently leads to infection of the urine in spite of prophylactic antibiotics. Antibiotics should not be given to patients with indwelling bladder catheters and positive urine cultures unless there is evidence of systemic disturbance or blood stream invasion such as high fever and toxicity, as they are usually unsuccessful in eradicating the infection. These clinical features arise more frequently in patients who have been catheterized after operations on the urinary tract than in patients who are catheterized for medical reasons. In the former case, there is often an extensive operation site allowing access to the blood stream. If significant bacteriuria develops in catheterized medical patients, 100 ml of 1/5000 chlorhexidine solution or framycetin (500 mg in 50–100 ml of sterile water) can be instilled into the bladder once or twice a day and left there for 30 minutes. Following removal of a catheter residual urinary infection should be eradicated according to the sensitivity of the infecting organism.

Renal failure and urinary tract infection

The selection of an antibiotic for the treatment of urinary tract infection associated with renal failure requires particular care, as certain antibiotics are contra-indicated in renal failure and others must be used with caution. Tetracyclines should not be given to patients with renal failure, as they may cause further deterioration in renal function (Stott *et al.*, 1971) and, as nitrofurantoin cumulates in the blood of uraemic patients leading to peripheral neuropathy (p. 235), it is also contra-indicated. The dose of any drug which is principally excreted by the kidney should be modified in renal failure. Kunin (1967) provides guide-lines for the use of antibiotics in renal failure and recommends increasing the intervals between individual doses, depending on the degree of azotaemia. Particular care should be taken with drugs such as the aminohexoses, whose side-effects are related to blood levels, and serum concentrations of these antibiotics should be measured frequently during the treatment of urinary tract infections complicating renal failure. A formula has recently been recommended for calculating the dose of gentamicin in renal failure (Chan *et al.*, 1972). In renal insufficiency, the clearance of trimethoprim but not of sulphamethoxazole is impaired (Sharpstone, 1969). The clinical significance of this observation with regard to co-trimoxazole administration is as yet unknown.

CONCLUSIONS

The accurate identification of the infecting organism and careful determination of its sensitivity to antibiotics is a very important part of the management of urinary tract infection. This information is all that is required for the treatment of a first attack of urinary infection and in the majority of 'uncomplicated' cases clinical cure will be effected irrespective of the drug selected provided that it is excreted in therapeutic concentrations in the urine. The medical literature contains numerous reports of the treatment of urinary tract infections with new antibacterial agents with 'cure rates' of between 80 and 85 per cent in virtually every series. The 15 to 20 per cent of patients who failed to respond to treatment were usually found to have some abnormality in the renal tract or other complicating factor such as a bladder catheter or pregnancy. It is this latter group which must be identified and each patient managed individually.

REFERENCES

BAILEY, R. R., ROBERTS, A. P., GOWER, P. E. & DE WARDENER, H. E. (1971). Prevention of urinary tract infection with low dose nitrofurantoin. *Lancet*, **2**, 1112.

British Medical Journal (1972). Leading article—Chronic prostatitis, **3**, 1.

BRUMFITT, W., LEIGH, D. A., PERCIVAL, A. & WILLIAMS, J. D. (1964). An assessment of ampicillin in the treatment of urinary tract infection. *Postgraduate Medical Journal*, supplement to vol. **40**, 55.

CATTELL, W. R., CHAMBERLAIN, D. A., FRY, I. K., MCSHERRY, M. A., BROUGHTON, C. & O'GRADY, F. (1971). Long-term control of bacteriuria with trimethoprim-sulphonamide. *British Medical Journal*, **1**, 377.

CHAN, R. A., BENNER, E. J. & HOEPRICH, P. D. (1972). Gentamicin therapy in renal failure: a nomogram for dosage. *Annals of Internal Medicine*, **76**, 773.

COX, C. E. & MONTGOMERY, W. G. (1968). Combined trimethoprim sulphisoxazole therapy of urinary infections. *Postgraduate Medical Journal*, supplement to vol. **45**, 65.

DONTAS, A. S., PAPANAYIOTOU, P., PAPANICOLAOU, N., MARKETOS, S. & ECONOMOU, P. (1966). Bacteriuria in old age. *Lancet*, **2**, 305.

FLEMING, M. P., DATTA, N. & GRUNEBERG, R. N. (1972). Trimethoprim resistance determined by R factor. *British Medical Journal*, **1**, 726.

GALLAGHER, D. J. A., MONTGOMERIE, J. Z. & NORTH, J. D. K. (1965). Acute infections of the urinary tract and the urethral syndrome in general practice. *British Medical Journal*, **1**, 622.

GARLAND, J. B. (1967). Dissertation on the clinical condition of prostatitis, M.D. thesis, University of Manchester.

GEDDES, A. M., WILLIAMS, J. D., KOSMIDIS, J., GOODALL, J. A. D. & ANDREWS, J. (1972). Clinical pharmacological studies with a new semi-synthetic penicillin, Alpha-amino-*p*-hydroxybenzylpenicillin. In *Proceedings of 7th International Congress of Chemotherapy*, Prague. (In press.)

GEDDES, A. M., GRAY, J. A., MURDOCH, J. MCC. & WALLACE, E. T. (1967). The treatment of serious gram-negative infections with kanamycin. *Postgraduate Medical Journal*, May supplement, p. 44.

KOSMIDIS, J., WILLIAMS, J. D., ANDREWS, J., GOODALL, J. A. D. & GEDDES, A. M. (1972). Amoxycillin—pharmacology, bacteriology and toxicology. *British Journal of Clinical Practice*, **26**, 341.

KUNIN, C. M., SOUTHALL, I. & PAQUIN, A. J. (1960). Epidemiology of urinary tract infections. A pilot study of 3057 school children. *New England Journal of Medicine*, **263**, 817.

KUNIN, C. M. (1967). A guide to use of antibiotics in patients with renal disease. *Annals of Internal Medicine*, **67**, 151.

KUNIN, C. M. (1970). A ten year study of bacteriuria in schoolgirls: final report of bacteriologic, urologic and epidemiologic findings. *The Journal of Infectious Diseases*, **122**, 382.

LUDVIK, W. VON (1964). Zur diagnostik der chronischen prostatitis. *Deutsche Medizinische Wochenschrift*, **89**, 2366.

MACGREGOR, M. & FREEMAN, P. (1968). Sub-classification of childhood urinary tract infections as an aid to prognosis. In *Urinary Tract Infection* (Eds., O'Grady, F. & Brumfitt, W.), p. 95. Oxford University Press.

MOND, N. C., PERCIVAL, A., WILLIAMS, J. D. & BRUMFITT, W. (1965). Presentation, diagnosis and treatment of urinary tract infections in general practice. *Lancet*, **1**, 514.

MURDOCH, J. MC.C., SPEIRS, C. F., GEDDES, A. M., WRIGHT, N. & WALLACE, E. T. (1968). Treatment of recurrent urinary tract infection. In *Urinary Tract Infection* (Eds., O'Grady, F. & Brumfitt, W.), p. 227. Oxford University Press.

NORMAND, I. C. S. & SMELLIE, J. M. (1965). Prolonged maintenance chemotherapy in the management of urinary infection in childhood. *British Medical Journal*, **1**, 1023.

O'GRADY, F. W., RICHARDS, B., MCSHERRY, M. A., O'FARRELL, S. M. & CATTELL, W. R. (1970). Introital enterobacteria, urinary infection and the urethral syndrome. *Lancet*, **2**, 1208.

PERCIVAL, A., BRUMFITT, W. & DE LOUVOIS, J. (1964). Serum antibody levels as an indication of clinically inapparent pyelonephritis. *Lancet*, **2**, 1027.

REEVES, D. S., FAIERS, M. C., PURSELL, R. E. & BRUMFITT, W. (1969). Trimethoprim-sulphamethoxazole: Comparative study in urinary infection in hospital. *British Medical Journal*, **1**, 541.

ROE, E. & LOWBURY, E. J. L. (1972). Changes in antibiotic sensitivity patterns of Gram-negative bacilli in burns. *Journal of Clinical Pathology*, **25**, 176.

SAVAGE, D. C. L., WILSON, M., ROSS, E. M. & FEE, W. M. (1969). Asymptomatic bacteriuria in girl entrants to Dundee primary schools. *British Medical Journal*, **3**, 75.

SHARPSTONE, P., (1969). The renal handling of trimethoprim and sulphamethoxazole in man. *Postgraduate Medical Journal*, November supplement, **45**, 38.

SMALLPIECE, V. (1968). *Urinary tract infection in childhood and its relevance to disease in adult life*. Heinemann, London.

SMELLIE, J. M. (1970). Acute urinary tract infection in children. *British Medical Journal*, **4**, 97.

SMITH, E. K. & WILLIAMS, J. D. (1970). The use of Cephalexin monohydrate in chronic bacteriuria and acute urinary tract infection. *British Journal of Urology*, **42**, 522.

STAMEY, T. A., MEARES, E. M. & WINNINGHAM, D. G. (1970). Chronic bacterial prostatitis and the diffusion of drugs into prostatic fluid. *Journal of Urology*, **103**, 187.

STOTT, R. B., CAMERON, J. S., OGG, C. S. & TOSELAND, P. (1971). Tetracyclines and impaired renal function. *Lancet*, **2**, 1378.

WILLIAMS, J. D., BRUMFITT, W., CONDIE, A. P. & REEVES, D. S. (1969). The treatment of bacteriuria in pregnant women with sulphamethoxazole and trimethoprim. *Postgraduate Medical Journal*, supplement to vol. **45**, 71.

WILLIAMS, J. D., THOMLINSON, J. L., COLE, J. G. L. & COPE, E. (1969a). Asymptomatic urinary tract infection in gynaecological outpatients. *British Medical Journal*, **1**, 29.

ZINNER, S. H., SABATH, L. D., CASEY, J. I. & FINLAND, M. (1971). Erythromycin and alkalinisation of the urine in the treatment of urinary tract infections due to gram-negative bacilli. *Lancet*, **1**, 1267.

11

BACTERIAL ENDOCARDITIS FOLLOWING CARDIAC SURGERY

I. PHILLIPS AND SUSANNAH EYKYN

BACTERIAL endocarditis is an uncommon but serious complication of cardiac surgery. Intracardiac prostheses, in particular, appear to predispose the patient to infection, and potential sources of micro-organisms are legion. When a patient does develop endocarditis, the clinical signs are often atypical, making diagnosis difficult, and the combination of foreign material and often resistant organisms makes treatment too very difficult. It is the purpose of this paper to examine the role of antibiotics in the prevention and treatment of this type of endocarditis, in the light of experience at St. Thomas's Hospital.

PREVENTION OF INFECTION IN CARDIAC SURGERY

Type of surgery and incidence of infection

It has been appreciated for many years that the insertion of a prosthesis increases the risk of intracardiac infection after cardiac surgery. Table 1 shows that the incidence of endocarditis in 4570 cardiac operations performed before prostheses were in general use, was about 1 per cent (Taussig *et al.*, 1951; Scott, 1952; Koiwai & Nahas, 1956; Denton *et al.*, 1957). With the introduction of prosthetic surgery, the incidence in 1594 operations in seven different centres, averaged 3·6 per cent (Nelson *et al.*, 1965; Amoury *et al.*, 1966; Cohn *et al.*, 1966; Yeh *et al.*, 1967; Windsor *et al.*, 1968; Clarkson & Barrat-Boyes, 1970; Okies *et al.*, 1971).

Prophylactic antibiotics

Experience of the use of prophylactic antibiotics in general surgery originally led to the suggestion that they should not be used in cardiac surgery. Lord, Imparato, Hackel and Doyle (1961) collected information from many centres on patients treated by open-heart surgery but before valve prostheses were in common use, and found that the incidence of endocarditis in 315 patients given *pre-operative* prophylaxis only, was 2·2 per cent, while it was only 0·5 per cent among 2170 patients not given such prophylaxis. True prophylaxis of this kind, involving the administration of antibiotics only for a period before surgery, is not now generally practised. However, Linde and Heins in 1960 questioned the advisability of *post-operative* prophylaxis with the agents then available, and Kittle and Reed (1961) found, in a small series of 108 patients who had surgery under bypass, an incidence of endocarditis of 8·7 per cent among patients given a variety of antibiotics for varying times following operation, compared with only 3·2 per cent in those not given antibiotics.

TABLE 1

ENDOCARDITIS IN CARDIAC SURGERY. INFLUENCE OF PROPHYLACTIC ANTIBIOTICS

Type of surgery	Prophylaxis	Number of patients	Incidence of endocarditis		Organisms			
				Per cent	Staph. aureus	Staph. albus	Other	Per cent staph.
Other than valve prosthesis[a]	Inadequate	4570	50	1·1	6	18	8	75
Valve prosthesis[b]	Inadequate	1594	58	3·6	15	21	21	63
Valve prosthesis[c]	Adequate[d]	2700	22	0·8	1	4	16	24

[a] Taussig *et al.*, 1951.
Scott, 1952.
Koiwai & Nahas, 1956.
Denton *et al.*, 1957.

[b] Nelson *et al.*, 1965.
Amoury *et al.*, 1966.
Cohn *et al.*, 1966.
Yeh *et al.*, 1967.
Windsor *et al.*, 1968.
Clarkson & Barrat–Boyes, 1970.
Okies *et al.*, 1971.

[c] Nelson *et al.*, 1965.
Amoury *et al.*, 1966.
Windsor *et al.*, 1968.
Herr *et al.*, 1965.
Shafer & Hall, 1970.

[d] Adequate—prophylaxis that includes penicillinase-resistant penicillin.

Whether we call this post-operative administration of antibiotics prophylaxis or treatment, there now seems ample evidence to show that these early conclusions, made at a time when penicillinase-resistant penicillins were not generally available, were probably incorrect.

Table 1 shows that the incidence of endocarditis among 2700 patients from seven centres, given adequate prophylaxis, was only 0·8 per cent (Nelson *et al.*, 1965; Herr *et al.*, 1965; Amoury *et al.*, 1966; Stein *et al.*, 1966; Windsor *et al.*, 1968; Block *et al.*, 1970; Shafer & Hall, 1970). The poor results of Goodman, Shaffner, Collins, Battersby and Koenig (1968) suggest that adequate prophylaxis must be defined in terms of duration as well as antibiotic. In their small series, the incidence of endocarditis was not affected by the administration of oxacillin for only 3 days postoperatively. Firor (1967) attributed his high infection rate to the fact that prophylaxis was started *after* surgery rather than immediately before it. Nelson said in 1965 that 'the time has come when cardiac surgeons need not apologise for using prophylactic antibiotics' and it seems reasonable, after five more years of experience, for even a microbiologist to agree.

'Effective' prophylaxis

In order to explain the meaning of 'effective prophylaxis' it is necessary to look at the types of organism that cause endocarditis after cardiac surgery. Table 1 gives this information in simplified form, for the three groups already discussed. In the first group of cases, who did not have prostheses, and in whom prophylaxis was either not used or was inadequate, 75 per cent of 32 organisms isolated were staphylococci, usually coagulase negative (Koiwai & Nahas, 1956; Denton *et al.*, 1957). In the early days of valve prostheses, about the same proportion of staphylococci was found—63 per cent. However, when the importance of staphylococci was appreciated (Resnekov, 1959), and penicillinase-resistant penicillins came into use (Effler *et al.*, 1965), not only did the incidence of endocarditis fall as we have already noted, but the proportion of staphylococci also fell markedly—to 23 per cent in the series collected in Table 1. We can add to this our own experience at St. Thomas's Hospital where in 320 patients with valve prostheses given 4 g methicillin and 2 g ampicillin every 24 hours, starting the night before the operation and continuing for 3 weeks, we have not seen a single case of staphylococcal endocarditis.

Organisms from environmental sources

So far, we have considered organisms, such as staphylococci, that often come from the patient himself, or, when the ungloved finger was used to open a valve, from the surgeon, at the time of operation. However, there is another possible source of infection at the time of operation or soon after, and that is the apparatus used on the patient. These organisms are usually Gram-negative, with an unpredictable antibiotic sensitivity pattern, and in this context prevention by sterilization and good aseptic technique is more effective than antibiotic prophylaxis (Editorial, 1968).

The importance of proper sterilization of the heart-lung machine has been underlined by the experience of Keown, Gilman and Bailey (1957) and of Geraci, Dale and McGoon (1963) who attributed a number of cases of *Pseudomonas aeruginosa* endocarditis to a failure of a quaternary ammonium compound, and of Linde and Heins (1960) who failed to eradicate an Achromobacter with ethylene oxide.

The apparatus used in the immediate post-operative period has also been found responsible for infection. We reported three cases of *Pseudomonas cepacia* bacteraemia during the week following cardiac surgery, caused by contaminated pressure-monitoring apparatus (Phillips *et al.*, 1971). These patients were treated as for endocarditis and appear to have escaped cardiac lesions in spite of their bacteraemia, perhaps supporting the suggestion of Yeh and his colleagues (1967) that even patients who have just had cardiac surgery have some defences, particularly against small numbers of organisms in the blood stream. The only two patients with endocarditis in our series of 320 with valve prostheses, acquired their infections from contaminated intravenous infusions, a problem brought to prominence by the recent paper by Duma, Warner and Dalton (1971). The organisms were again pseudomonads, related to *Ps. cepacia*, and their main reservoir was the hospital's supply of softened and deionized water, used in a rapid-cooling autoclave. Sterilized bottled fluids inside the autoclave were cooled by a mist of contaminated water, which lodged under the foil cap. When bottles of the fluids were used, the needles of drip sets were pushed through this water into the bottles, thereby contaminating their contents.

Other sepsis

A further important source of cardiac infection in these patients has been clearly identified as post-operative sepsis elsewhere. Many groups have identified wound infection, respiratory tract infection, and urinary tract infection as important foci of infection that can seed the bare areas around a prosthesis, and all emphasize the importance of early, energetic treatment of such infections. An increased incidence of infections other than intracardiac, often due to resistant organisms, is one of the clear disadvantages of prophylactic antibiotics (Fekety *et al.*, 1969; Sallam *et al.*, 1971).

Late infection

The potential sources of infection are still not exhausted. In many series it has been noted that cases of endocarditis fall into one of two groups, either occurring within a few weeks of surgery, or after an interval of several months. We have so far considered only the first group. Late endocarditis, which may account for half of the cases, seems more to resemble endocarditis in patients with cardiac lesions who have not had cardiac surgery. It often follows such events as dental manipulations, labour, or cardiac catheterization, and although the causative organisms do include familiar streptococci, they also include a large proportion of staphylococci and other bacteria. For this reason broad-spectrum antibiotic prophylaxis is probably indicated whenever patients with intracardiac prostheses undergo operations that might give rise to a bacteraemia (Cohn *et al.*, 1966; Firor, 1967; Walker *et al.*, 1969). There is little published experience to judge the validity of this advice.

Emergence of Gram-negative bacilli and fungi

It has been suggested that the price of effective anti-staphylococcal prophylaxis would be their replacement by Gram-negative bacilli and fungi (Cumie & Rachmaninoff, 1965). There is no doubt that increasing numbers of cases, particularly of fungal endocarditis, are being reported, usually as single cases or as confusing collections of cases from the literature (Cumie & Rachmaninoff, 1965; Leffert & Hackett, 1967; Conway *et al.*, 1968; Jones *et al.*, 1969; Chaudhury, 1970). There has also recently been a report of a case of Q-fever endocarditis complicating cardiac surgery (Morgans & Cartwright, 1969). However, there seems little evidence from reports of endocarditis in large series of cases of cardiac surgery, that there is a true increase in incidence.

On the other hand, the reports of an increased incidence of Gram-negative infections of other sites by Sallam, Sammon, McGeachie and Bain (1971), who studied closed heart surgery, and by Fekety, Cluff, Sabiston, Seidl, Smith and Thoburn (1969), who studied prosthetic cardiac surgery, are supported by our own experience. This contributes little to the solution of the central problem of endocarditis however, and one cannot agree with a general conclusion (Sallam *et al.*, 1971) that prophylaxis does more harm than good.

DIAGNOSIS OF ENDOCARDITIS

If, in spite of careful prophylaxis, a patient does develop endocarditis, there arise the problems of diagnosis already mentioned (Linde & Heins, 1960). Among the more important is the fact that not all patients with bacteraemia following cardiac surgery have endocarditis, although one is often forced to treat them as if they had. Table 2 lists, in three groups, the patients with bacteraemia in our series. The first group includes patients with persistently positive blood cultures, and clinical signs suggestive of endocarditis. There were only two in our series. The second group, of 8 patients, includes those with transient bacteraemia with no signs of either continued infection or of endocarditis. Finally there is a group, again of 8 patients, who have terminal disease, such as hepatic, renal or severe cardiac failure, or uncontrolled infection elsewhere, but no definite signs of endocarditis, and who were found at autopsy to have no good evidence of intracardiac infection. Table 2 also shows that the organisms in each group are much the same, showing the results of occasional failures of asepsis, and of effective anti-staphylococcal prophylaxis, with only three staphylococci isolated. All the organisms were resistant to ampicillin, one of the drugs used in prophylaxis, and all but three were resistant to methicillin, the second drug.

TABLE 2

BACTERAEMIA FOLLOWING VALVE REPLACEMENT AT ST. THOMAS'S HOSPITAL. 18 OUT OF 320 PATIENTS. AMPICILLIN AND METHICILLIN PROPHYLAXIS

Category	*Number of patients*	*Incidence (per cent)*	*Staph. aureus*	*Staph. albus*	*Gram-neg. bacilli*	*Pseudomonas species*	*Fungi*
Proven endocarditis[a]	2	0·6	—	—	—	2	—
Bacteraemia[b]	8	2·5	—	2	2	4	—
Associated with terminal disease[c]	8	2·5	1	—	2	4	1

[a] Persistent positive blood cultures with appropriate clinical or autopsy findings.
[b] Single positive blood culture followed by one or more negative cultures before definitive treatment.
[c] Patients with usually single positive blood cultures, with terminal disease but no clinical or autopsy evidence of endocarditis.

TREATMENT OF ENDOCARDITIS

Antibiotics

It is generally stated that a bactericidal antibiotic or combination of antibiotics should be used to treat endocarditis following cardiac surgery, as in any other context. I would like to suggest that the facts at our disposal do not entirely support this. A significant number of patients reported in the literature have recovered on therapy that would seem designed to be as non-specific as possible, as well as non-bactericidal, while most of the patients who have had sound bactericidal treatment have died. It is difficult, under these circumstances to be certain of any principles.

Our experiences with two cases of post-operative endocarditis at St. Thomas's Hospital illustrate some of the problems of choosing the right antibiotics. Both patients were infected with an organism related to *Ps. cepacia*. Results of some *in vitro* tests of antimicrobial susceptibility are shown in Table 3. The organism was highly resistant to the usual anti-pseudomonas drugs polymyxin, gentamicin and carbenicillin, but was sensitive in terms of Minimal Inhibitory Concentration (M.I.C.) results, to cephalexin, sulphamethoxazole and trimethoprim and moderately sensitive to tetracycline, erythromycin and rifampicin. Minimal Bactericidal Concentrations (M.B.C.) were considerably higher for all agents, with a marked inoculum effect. No useful syngergism was demonstrated with any of the combinations examined.

One patient was treated at St. George's Hospital with oral rifampicin, cotrimoxazole and cephalexin. This successfully suppressed the infection, but as she is still receiving treatment 4 months later, it is not yet possible to say whether she is cured. (Maddocks, personal communication.) The other

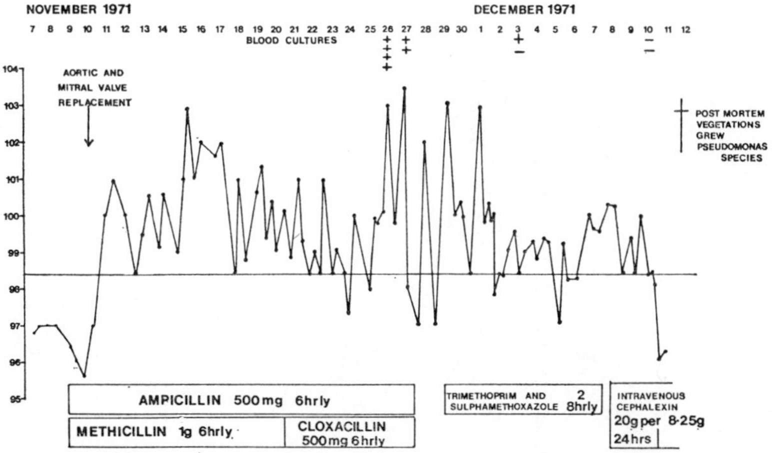

FIG. 1. Pseudomonas species endocarditis following aortic and mitral valve replacement in a 32-year-old man.

TABLE 3

ANTIMICROBIAL SENSITIVITY OF PSEUDOMONAS SPECIES ISOLATED FROM TWO PATIENTS WITH ENDOCARDITIS AT ST. THOMAS'S HOSPITAL

	Inoculum	*Carbenicillin*	*Ampicillin*	*Gentamicin*	*Kanamycin*	*Erythromycin*	*Cephalexin*	*Rifampicin*	*Sulphamethoxazole*	*Trimethoprim*
M.I.C.	10^6	1000	500	100	100	12·5	1·56	12·5	6·25	3·12
	10^2						0·02	0·8	0·4	0·4
							indifferent		indifferent	
M.B.C.	10^6				>100	100	250	50	>12·5	>12·5
	10^2				>100	50	0·9	12·5	1·56	3·12
							indifferent		slight synergism	

Cephalexin + Rifampicin and Sulphamethoxazole + Trimethoprim: various combinations in serum in therapeutic range—NO KILL 10^6, ALL KILLED 10^2

patient had a more rapid onset and fulminating course. Cotrimoxazole did not suppress the infection, and intravenous cephalexin in high dosage was substituted. Unfortunately a leak developed around the valve and before treatment could have any effect, the patient died. The pseudomonad was isolated from cultures of the necrotic tissue round the valve removed at autopsy (Fig. 1).

Removal of prosthesis

The importance of having foreign material in the heart is relatively clear. Koiwai and Nahas (1956) cured 77 per cent, and Denton (1957) 56 per cent of patients who had endocarditis complicating commissurotomies, but once a prosthesis is introduced, the mortality rate of endocarditis rises to about 70 per cent (Braimbridge, 1969). Should one therefore remove the prosthesis or first try to cure the infection with antibiotics? In many cases the question does not arise because the infection results in life-threatening haemodynamic consequences that need immediate surgical correction if the patient is to have any chance of survival. The question does arise however in patients whose valves continue to function (Fraser *et al.*, 1967). There is no doubt that patients have recovered as a result of energetic antibiotic treatment alone (Geraci *et al.*, 1963; Littlefield *et al.*, 1965; Amoury *et al.*, 1966; Stein *et al.*, 1966; Yeh *et al.*, 1967; Conway *et al.*, 1968; Block *et al.*, 1970; Okies *et al.*, 1971), and many surgeons feel that it is correct under these circumstances, to try antibiotics and undertake further surgery only if bacteraemia persists or there is haemodynamic deterioration (Stanton *et al.*, 1968; Walker *et al.*, 1969; Block *et al.*, 1970; Weinstein, 1972). There must always be an uncomfortable feeling that a patient who responds to antibiotics alone may not have endocarditis at all!

Assessment of effects

The report of Watanakunakorn and Hamburger (1970) on the management of a case of *Staph. albus* endocarditis, highlights the problem of assessment of cure. Their patient was treated with a semi-synthetic penicillin for 13 months and then relapsed on cessation of treatment. After an initial response to further treatment with the same antibiotic, the patient relapsed again, to be cured finally by removal of the infected valve. Others have commented on similar suppression of infection (Fraser *et al.*, 1967; Speller *et al.*, 1971). Another report from these same workers (Watanakunakorn *et al.*, 1968) draws attention to a further problem—the persistence of organisms as L-forms.

It may be said in conclusion that although we have made significant strides in the prevention of endocarditis following cardiac surgery by using effective chemoprophylaxis and more efficient asepsis, we appear to have made little progress in devising effective therapy when our preventive efforts fail.

REFERENCES

AMOURY, R. A., BOWMAN, F. O. & MALM, J. R. (1966). Endocarditis associated with intracardiac prosthesis. *Journal of Thoracic and Cardiovascular Surgery*, **51**, 36.

BLOCK, P. C., DESANCTIS, R. W., WEINBERG, A. N. & AUSTEN, W. G. (1970). Prosthetic valve endocarditis. *Journal of Thoracic and Cardiovascular Surgery*, **60,** 540.

BRAIMBRIDGE, M. V. (1969). Cardiac surgery and bacterial endocarditis. *Lancet*, **i,** 1307.

CHAUDHURY, M. R. (1970). Fungal endocarditis after valve replacements. *Journal of Thoracic and Cardiovascular Surgery*, **60,** 207.

CLARKSON, P. M. & BARRAT-BOYES, B. G. (1970). Bacterial endocarditis following homograft replacement of the aortic valve. *Circulation*, **42,** 987.

COHN, L. H., ROBERTS, W. C., ROCKOFF, S. D. & MORROW, A. G. (1966). Bacterial endocarditis following aortic valve replacement. *Circulation*, **33,** 209.

CONWAY, N., KOTHARI, M. L., LOCKEY, E. & YACOUB, M. H. (1968). Candida endocarditis after heart surgery. *Thorax*, **23,** 353.

CUMIE, A. R. W. & RACHMANINOFF, N. (1965). Fungal (Candida) endocarditis following open-heart surgery. *Journal of Thoracic and Cardiovascular Surgery*, **50,** 431.

DENTON, C., PAPPAS, E. G., URICCHIO, J. F., GOLDBERG, H. & LIKOFF, W. (1957). Bacterial endocarditis following cardiac surgery. *Circulation*, **15,** 525.

DUMA, R. J., WARNER, J. F. & DALTON, H. P. (1971). Septicaemia from intravenous infusions. *New England Journal of Medicine*, **284,** 257.

EDITORIAL (1968). Prophylactic antibiotics and heart surgery. *New England Journal of Medicine*, **278,** 162.

EFFLER, D. B., FAVALORO, R. & GROVES, L. K. (1965). Heart valve replacement. *Annals of Thoracic Surgery*, **1,** 4.

FEKETY, F. R., CLUFF, L. E., SABISTON, D. C., SEIDL, L. G., SMITH, J. W. & THOBORN, R. (1969). A study of antibiotic prophylaxis in cardiac surgery. *Journal of Thoracic and Cardiovascular Surgery*, **57,** 757.

FIROR, W. B. (1967). Infection following open-heart surgery, with special reference to the role of prophylactic antibiotics. *Journal of Thoracic and Cardiovascular Surgery*, **53,** 371.

FRASER, R. S., ROSSALL, R. E. & DVORKIN, J. (1967). Bacterial endocarditis occurring after open-heart surgery. *Canadian Medical Association Journal*, **96,** 1551.

GERACI, J. E., DALE, A. J. D. & MCGOON, D. C. (1963). Bacterial endocarditis and endarteritis following cardiac operations. *Wisconsin Medical Journal*, **62,** 302.

GOODMAN, J. S., SCHAFFNER, W., COLLINS, H. A., BATTERSBY, E. J. & KOENIG, M. G. (1968). Infection after cardiac surgery. *New England Journal of Medicine*, **278,** 117.

HERR, R., STARR, A., MCCORD, C. W. & WOOD, J. A. (1965). Special problems following valve replacement. *Annals of Thoracic Surgery*, **1,** 403.

JONES, T., MESHEL, L. & RUBIN, I. L. (1969). Aspergillus endocarditis superimposed on aortic valve prosthesis. *New York State Journal of Medicine*, **69,** 1923.

KEOWN, K. K., GILMAN, R. A. & BAILEY, C. P. (1957). Open heart surgery. *Journal of the American Medical Association*, **165,** 781.

KITTLE, C. F. & REED, W. A. (1961). Antibiotics and extracorporeal circulation. *Journal of Thoracic and Cardiovascular Surgery*, **41,** 34.

KOIWAI, E. K. & NAHAS, H. C. (1956). Subacute bacterial endocarditis following cardiac surgery. *Archives of Surgery*, **73,** 272.

LEFFERT, R. L. & HACKETT, R. L. (1967). Aspergillus aortitis following replacement of aortic valve. *Journal of Thoracic and Cardiovascular Surgery*, **53,** 866.

LINDE, L. M. & HEINS, H. L. (1960). Bacterial endocarditis following surgery for congenital heart disease. *New England Journal of Medicine*, **263,** 65.

LITTLEFIELD, J. B., MULLER, W. H. & DAMMANN, J. F. (1965). Successful treatment of *Pseudomonas aeruginosa* septicaemia following total aortic valve replacement. *Circulation*, **32** (Supplement 1), 103.

LORD, J. W., IMPARATO, A. M., HACKEL, A. & DOYLE, E. F. (1961). Endocarditis complicating open-heart surgery. *Circulation*, **23**, 489.

MORGANS, C. M. & CARTWRIGHT, R. Y. (1969). Case of Q-fever endocarditis at site of aortic valve prosthesis. *British Heart Journal*, **31**, 520.

NELSON, R. M., JENSON, C. B., PETERSON, C. A. & SANDERS, B. C. (1965). Effective use of prophylactic antibiotics in open heart surgery. *Archives of Surgery*, **90**, 731.

OKIES, J. E., VIROSLAV, J. & WILLIAMS, T. W. (1971). Endocarditis after cardiac valve replacement. *Chest*, **59**, 198.

PHILLIPS, I., EYKYN, S., CURTIS, M. A. & SNELL, J. J. S. (1971). *Pseudomonas cepacia* septicaemia in an intensive care unit. *Lancet*, **i**, 375.

RESNEKOV, L. (1959). Staphylococcal endocarditis following mitral valvotomy with special reference to coagulase-negative *Staphylococcus albus*. *Lancet*, **ii**, 597.

SALLAM, I. A., SAMMON, A., MCGEACHIE, J. & BAIN, W. H. (1971). Prophylactic antibiotics in closed heart surgery. *Chest*, **60**, 252.

SCOTT, H. W. (1952). Surgical treatment of patent ductus arteriosis in childhood. *Surgical Clinics of North America*, **32**, 1299.

SHAFER, R. B. & HALL, W. H. (1970). Bacterial endocarditis following open heart surgery. *American Journal of Cardiology*, **25**, 602.

SPELLER, D. C. E., STEPHENS, M. E. & VIANT, A. C. (1971). Hospital infection by *Pseudomonas cepacia*. *Lancet*, **i**, 798.

STANTON, R. E., LINDESMITH, G. G. & MAYER, B. W. (1968). *Escherichia coli* endocarditis after repair of ventricular septal defects. *New England Journal of Medicine*, **279**, 737.

STEIN, P. D., HARKEN, D. E. & DEXTER, L. (1966). The nature and prevention of prosthetic valve endocarditis. *American Heart Journal*, **71**, 393.

TAUSSIG, H. G., KING, J. T., BAUERSFIELD, R. & SWARAMAKRISHNE, P. (1951). Results of operation for pulmonary stenosis and atresia. *Transactions of the Academy of American Physicians*, **64**, 67.

WALKER, S. R., SHUMWAY, N. E. & MERIGAN, T. C. (1969). Management of infected cardiac valve prostheses. *Journal of the American Medical Association*, **208**, 531.

WATANAKUNAKORN, C., CARLETON, J., GOLDBERG, L. M. & HAMBURGER, M. (1968). Candida endocarditis surrounding a Starr-Edwards prosthetic valve. *Archives of Internal Medicine*, **121**, 243.

WATANAKUNAKORN, C. & HAMBURGER, M. (1970). *Staphylococcus epidermidis* endocarditis complicating a Starr-Edwards prosthesis. *Archives of Internal Medicine*, **126**, 1014.

WEINSTEIN, L. (1972). Infective endocarditis: past, present and future. *Journal of the Royal College of Physicians of London*, **6**, 161.

WINDSOR, H. M., FAGAN, P. & SHANAHAN, M. X. (1968). Bacterial endocarditis, mitral regurgitation, and intra-atrial thrombosis following mitral valve replacement. *Thorax*, **23**, 11.

YEH, T. J., ANABTAWI, I. N., CORNETT, V. E., WHITE, A., STERN, W. H. & ELLISON, R. G. (1967). Bacterial endocarditis following open-heart surgery. *Annals of Thoracic Surgery*, **3**, 29.

12

SURGERY FOR BACTERIAL ENDOCARDITIS OF HEART VALVES

M. V. Braimbridge

Bacterial endocarditis is a not uncommon incident in the history of patients who require valve surgery. For instance at St. Thomas's Hospital 14 of 140 aortic valve replacements had previously had bacterial endocarditis and in almost all it was the cause of the cardiac deterioration that had necessitated surgical intervention. An even higher percentage of patients requiring aortic and mitral valve replacement had had bacterial endocarditis, 7 of 55 (13 per cent). Bacterial endocarditis of the mitral valve alone, causing damage severe enough to warrant surgery, was less common. Only 2 of 116 mitral valve replacements (2 per cent) and 1 of 200 mitral valvotomies (0·5 per cent) had a previous history of endocarditis. This contrasts markedly with the overall incidence of bacterial endocarditis which affects primarily the mitral rather than the aortic valve (86 per cent compared with 55 per cent) (Lepeschkin, 1952), and reflects the more marked destruction caused to the flimsier aortic valve and the greater intolerance of the left ventricle to acute aortic regurgitation.

INDICATIONS FOR OPERATIVE TREATMENT

The necessity for surgery in the management of bacterial endocarditis implies that medical treatment has been unable to arrest the course of the disease, either because too much destruction of cusp tissue had occurred before the infection was brought under control or because the microbiologist had been unable to kill the organism.

For ideal operating conditions, the patient should be out of heart failure with the valve area affected clear of infection. To achieve this in practice, 6 weeks at least—preferably 3 months, should have elapsed since the last positive blood culture so that the operative area becomes fibrotic and free of vegetations and oedema. Stitches placed in the valve ring will then hold well. Of 14 aortic valve replacements performed at St. Thomas's Hospital for bacterial endocarditis, 10 were carried out under these conditions. One of these 10 patients died from a sudden and unexpected rise of serum potassium in the immediate post-operative period, causing irreversible ventricular fibrillation. The remainder left hospital. There was 1 late death, a man who developed a subarachnoid haemorrhage and had to have his anticoagulants stopped. His aortic valve thrombosed.

None of the surviving 8 patients has developed a leak around the prosthesis. The usual incidence of such leakage after operations on healed bacterial endocarditis is due to the fibrous tissue in the aortic valve ring being particularly tough and holding the fixing sutures well.

The results of surgery for healed bacterial endocarditis in patients who are not in frank cardiac failure at the time of surgery are satisfactory. However, there are patients whose degree of valve destruction produces catastrophic cardiac failure or whose organisms are resistant to available therapy. These patients will inevitably die if the infection cannot be cured and the regurgitation through the destroyed valve alleviated. Surgery, therefore, has to be carried out in an infected, oedematous operative field in a patient who is in severe cardiac failure and often in pulmonary oedema. The problems of surgery are then entirely different (Braimbridge, 1969).

REVIEW OF THE LITERATURE

Eighty-three patients who had undergone urgent valve surgery for acute cardiac failure secondary to bacterial endocarditis or who had active infections resistant to therapy have been abstracted from the literature (Acar *et al.*, 1966; Kennedy *et al.*, 1966; Braniff *et al.*, 1967; Ehrenhaft, 1967; Gahagan, 1967; Hurley *et al.*, 1967; Kaiser *et al.*, 1967; Kristinsson & Bentall, 1967; Robiczek *et al.*, 1967; Scott *et al.*, 1967; Wilcox *et al.*, 1967; Windsor & Shanahan, 1967; Kay *et al.*, 1968; Stason *et al.*, 1968; Kretschmer & Lawrence, 1969; Wallace *et al.*, 1969; Manhas *et al.*, 1970; Neville *et al.*, 1971; Ribot *et al.*, 1971; Wise *et al.*, 1971). The paper by Hutter *et al.* (1970) has not been used as the patient with SBE appears to have been included in Stason's paper from the same institution (Stason *et al.*, 1968). Two patients with Coxiella infection in the paper by Wise *et al.* (1971) are not included as they form part of the communication by Kristinsson and Bentall (1967). Only the personal cases of Kretschmer and Lawrence (1969) are used. Hatcher does not mention the organisms involved in the acute cases which have not therefore been incuded (Hatcher *et al.*, 1971).

St. Thomas's Hospital

Included among the 83 patients are 4 patients with bacterial endocarditis of the aortic valve operated on urgently for cardiac failure at St. Thomas's Hospital. The responsible organisms were *Streptococcus viridans*, *Streptococcus faecalis*, a non-haemolytic streptococcus and an unidentifiable coccobacillus. Two patients died. One of these was admitted moribund with a 100 cm^3 sized sinus of Valsalva aneurysm encircling the coronary artery and right atrium, and the other had a large myocardial infarct 2 days before surgery. The remaining 2 are well.

Causative organisms

The causative organisms were of the usual distribution (Table 1). 51 per cent were streptococci, usually viridans, but with a fair percentage of others.

Staphylococci accounted for 20 per cent, usually *Staphylococcus aureus*, with coagulase negative staphylococci being relatively uncommon. Coxiella, fungi

TABLE 1

VALVE REPLACEMENT IN 83 PATIENTS. CARDIAC FAILURE AND ACTIVE ENDOCARDITIS—ORGANISMS RESPONSIBLE

Streptococcus			42	51 per cent
viridans 26)	B. haemolytic (3)			
pneumoniae (4)	Other (4)			
faecalis (5)				
Staphylococcus			17	20 per cent
aureus (11)				
albus and coagulase negative (6)				
Coxiella			4	
Fungus			2	
Candida (2)				
Other organisms			7	
Klebsiella (2)	Neisseria (1)	Brucella (1)		
Serratia (1)	Corynebacterium (1)	Coccobacillus (1)		
Unknown			11	
			83	

and other organisms were also uncommon and there were a fair percentage where organisms were seen in the valves removed at surgery but could not be cultured. The type of organism, therefore, is no different in the acute case from the less urgent one.

Valve replacements

In the 83 patients, 70 required aortic valve replacements, supporting the view that it is infection of the aortic valve that produces the greatest haemodynamic disturbance. One patient required replacement of both aortic and mitral valves; 6 the mitral valve alone and 1 the tricuspid valve. Four patients had valvoplasties, 3 mitral and 1 tricuspid. One patient died on induction of anaesthesia.

Operative mortality

Twenty-three of the patients died in hospital, an operative mortality of 30 per cent. This mortality is some three times the mortality of surgery carried out on the aortic valve under less acute conditions but is a marked improvement on the 100 per cent mortality that would otherwise have occurred. The increased operative mortality was due mainly to the poor pre-operative condition of the patients. Several patients, including one of ours, developed cardiac arrest before surgery and one died on induction of anaesthesia before any surgery could be performed. Sinus of Valsalva sinuses were also frequent, one of ours being 100 cm^3 in size, and the friable nature of the necks of the sinuses increase the difficulties of closing them. The infected valve ring is oedematous and holds stitches poorly so that recurrent regurgitation past the prosthesis may occur if stitches pull through which prejudices post-operative recovery.

Post-operative progress

Once the patient has survived surgery, however, his prognosis appears to be no different from an elective valve replacement. There were only 3 late deaths reported, a late mortality of 4 per cent, though admittedly the length of follow-up was not reported in every case so that proper comparison was not possible. One of the late deaths was due to candida infection of the implanted valve and 2 to myocardial disease.

The incidence of valve dehiscence varied markedly. Manhas *et al.* (1970) reported that all their 12 patients had leaks following acute aortic valve replacement. Stason *et al.* (1968) reported a 31 per cent incidence in 13 patients. Neville *et al.* (1971) however stated that none of their valves had developed a leak, a striking difference from the other series, and perhaps due to the fact that their sutures were carried through the aortic valve wall and tied over Teflon felt buttresses.

Reinfection of the implanted prosthetic valve with the organism responsible for the original bacterial endocarditis was not a major problem. Only one patient become so infected, the organism being brucella. Five other patients, however, developed post-operative bacterial endocarditis with other organisms, staphylococci and candida, and one of these subsequently died.

SUMMARY

Surgery for bacterial endocarditis affecting heart valves is safe and satisfactory if sufficient time can be allowed to elapse between eradication of infection and surgery. Nevertheless, when this is impossible due to active resistant endocarditis or intractable cardiac failure, valve replacement is still advised, though the operative mortality is trebled. Once the patient has left hospital however, his prognosis is no different from any other valve replacement patient.

REFERENCES

ACAR, A. G., CABROL, C., CARTIER, F. & FOUCHARD, A. (1966). Cure chirurgicale d'une endocardite bacterienne avec insuffisance aortique. *Archives des Maladies due Coeur et des Vaisseaux*, **5**, 757.

BRAIMBRIDGE, M. V. (1969). Cardiac surgery and bacterial endocarditis. *Lancet*, **i**, 1307.

BRANIFF, B. A., SHUMWAY, N. E. & HARRISON, D. C. (1967). Valve replacement in active bacterial endocarditis. *New England Journal of Medicine*, **276**, 1464.

ENRENHAFT, J. L. (1967). Discussion of paper by Kaiser *et al.*

GAHAGAN, T. (1967). Discussion of paper by Kaiser *et al.*

HATCHER, C. R., SYMBAS, P. N., LOGAN, W. D., MANSOUR, K. A. & ABBOTT, C. A. (1971). Surgical management of complications of bacterial endocarditis. *Annals of Surgery*, **173**, 1045.

HURLEY, E. J., ELDRIDGE, F. L. & HULTGREN, H. N. (1967). Emergency replacement of valves in endocarditis. *American Heart Journal*, **73**, 798.

HUTTER, A. M., DESANCTIS, R. W., NATHAN, M. J., BUCKLEY, M. J., MUNDTH, E. D., DAGGETT, W. M. & AUSTEN, W. G. (1970). Aortic valve surgery as an emergency procedure. *Circulation*, **41**, 623.

KAISER, G. C., WILLMAN, V. L., THURMANN, M. & HANLON, C. R. (1967). Valve replacement in cases of aortic insufficiency due to active endocarditis. *Journal of Thoracic and Cardivascular Surgery*, **54**, 491.

KAY, J. H., BERNSTEIN, S., TSUJI, H. K., REDINGTON, J. V., MILGRAM, M. & BREM, T. (1968). Surgical treatment of candida endocarditis. *Journal of the American Medical Association*, **203**, 105.

KENNEDY, J. H., SABGA, G. A., FIST, A. A. & SANCETTA, S. M. (1966). Isolated tricuspid valcular insufficiency due to subacute bacterial endocarditis. *Journal of Thoracic and Cardiovascular Surgery*, **51**, 498.

KRETSCHMER, K. D. & LAWRENCE, G. H. (1969). Valve replacement in patients with bacterial endocarditis. *American Journal of Surgery*, **118**, 273.

KRISTINSSON, A. & BENTALL, H. H. (1967). Medical and surgical treatment of Q fever endocarditis. *Lancet*, **ii**, 693.

LEPESCHKIN, E. (1952). On the relation of the site of valvular involvement in endocarditis and the blood pressure resting on the valve. *American Journal of Medical Science*, **224**, 318.

MANHAS, D. R., HESSEL, E. A., WINTERSCHEID, L. C., DILLARD, D. H. & MERENDINO, A. K. (1970). Open heart surgery in infective endocarditis. *Circulation*, **41**, 841.

NEVILLE, W. E., MAGNO, M., FOXWORTHY, D. T. & MOFFAT, J. E. (1971). Emergency aortic valve replacement in bacterial endocarditis. *Journal of Thoracic and Cardiovascular Surgery*, **61**, 916.

RIBOT, S., GILBERT, L., ROTHFELD, E. L., PARSONNET, V. & JACOBS, M. G. (1971) Bacterial endocarditis with pulmonary oedema necessitating mitral valve replacement in a hemo-dialysis dependent patient. *Journal of Thoracic and Cardiovascular Surgery*, **62**, 59.

ROBICZEK, F., PAYNE, R. B., DAUGHERTY, H. K. & SANGER, P. W. (1967). Bacterial endocarditis of the mitral valve treated by excision and replacement. *Collected Works on Cardiopulmonary Disease*, **13**, 36.

SCOTT, S. M., FISH, R. G. & CRUTCHER, J. C. (1967). Early surgical intervention for aortic insufficiency due to bacterial endocarditis. *Annals of Thoracic Surgery*, **3**, 158.

STASON, W. B., DESANCTIS, R. W., WEINBERG, A. N. & AUSTEN, W. G. (1968). Cardiac surgery in bacterial endocarditis. *Circulation*, **38**, 514 (cases 5, 7, 10, 12, 13).

WALLACE, A. G., YOUNG, W. G. & OSTERHOUT, S. (1969). Treatment of acute bacterial endocarditis by valve excision and replacement. *Circulation*, **31**, 450.

WILCOX, B. R., PROCTOR, H. J., RACKLEY, C. E. & PETERS, R. M. (1967). Early surgical treatment of valvular endocarditis. *Journal of the American Medical Association*, **200**, 116.

WINDSOR, H. M. & SHANAHAN, M. X. (1967). Emergency valve replacement in bacterial endocarditis. *Thorax*, **22**, 25 (cases 1–5).

WISE, J. R., BENTALL, H. H., CLELAND, W. P., GOODWIN, J. F., HALLIDIE-SMITH, K. A. & OAKLEY, C. M. (1971). Urgent aortic valve replacement for acute aortic regurgitation due to infective endocarditis. *Lancet*, **ii**, 115.

5

13

ANTIBIOTIC USE IN HOSPITAL

Round Table Discussion
Chairman: E. J. L. LOWBURY

Dr. E. J. L. Lowbury

A major dilemma in the use of antibiotics arises from the emergence of antibiotic resistance, which is to some extent a peculiar hazard of hospital infection, although it is obviously not restricted to that sphere, as we may hear later in the discussions on the emergence of resistant gonococci. The dilemma might be expressed as an aphorism: 'If we use an antibiotic, we may lose it to-morrow; if we don't use an antibiotic, we may lose our patient to-day'. This, of course, is an over-simplification, and we have seen a number of examples which give us a more optimistic outlook on the possibility of keeping ahead of the resistant organisms. We have, for example, the case of *Streptococcus pyogenes*; even if this organism has not lost virulence to the extent that is sometimes imagined, infection caused by it has certainly become a very small problem compared with what it used to be. The problem which persists is not associated with penicillin resistance, even after 30 years, although we must not rule out the possibility that penicillin-resistant *Strept. pyogenes* may emerge one day; after all, we waited 12 years from the introduction of neomycin before neomycin-resistant staphylococci appeared.

In this session I think we should consider the ways in which we can attempt to preserve the antibiotics for use in hospitals as effectively as possible. We have a team of distinguished experts, and I will call on them to speak and tell us something about their experiences which are relevant to this problem. Their experience covers a wide range of clinical situations. The first speaker whom I will call upon is Dr. M. T. Parker of the Central Public Health Laboratory, one of whose interests has been the emergence of methicillin-resistant staphylococci. Dr. Parker, would you tell us something about this disturbing problem, and the studies on it which you have made?

ANTIBIOTICS AND RESISTANCE OF STAPHYLOCOCCI

Dr. M. T. Parker

I should prefer to be a little more general, and to make some observations on the resistance of staphylococci to antibiotics with particular reference to the situation in hospitals. I shall take as my starting point what I like to call Barber's law. You will remember that, over 25 years ago, Mary Barber showed that two factors were concerned in the increasing frequency of penicillin-resistant staphylococci among patients. First, exposure to antibiotics led to the disappearance of sensitive organisms from the flora, and second, organisms which were already antibiotic resistant were acquired by cross-infection (Barber 1947a, b). The prevalence of resistant organisms in the hospital population will therefore be influenced, on the one hand, by the proportion of the population receiving antibiotics, and on the other, by the extent to which each treated patient is isolated from other patients. This subsequently proved to be true for other staphylococcal resistances.

Changes in sensitivity pattern of staphylococci

Now, *Staphylococcus aureus* leads a blameless sexual life, and is apparently incapable of transferring genetic material by conjugation. Its resistance determinants appear to be transferred only by transduction by phage, and, with a few exceptions, to be acquired and transferred singly. Despite these apparent disadvantages, however, problems with multiple-antibiotic resistance in *Staph. aureus* appeared in hospitals early in the 1950s, long before we had similar trouble with transferable drug resistance in the enterobacteria, although both groups of organisms were similarly exposed to antibiotics in hospital.

It is clear, therefore, that multiple resistance can arise, and resistant strains can become widely distributed in the hospital population, without genetic linkage between resistance determinants, or transferability by conjugation. In *Staph. aureus* the resistance determinants, though in the main unlinked,

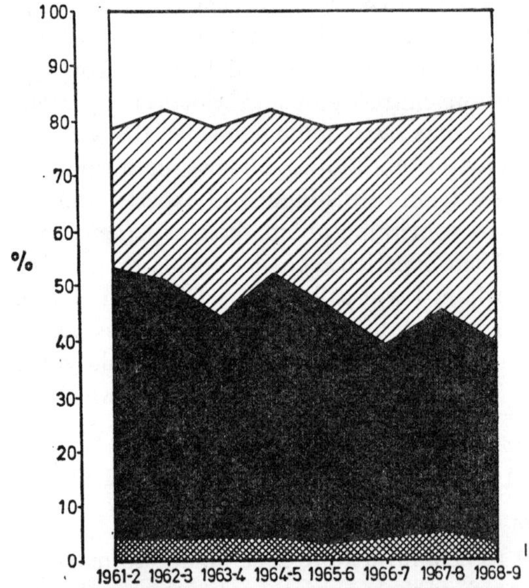

FIG. 1. *Staphylococcus* strains isolated from lesions of patients in eight London hospitals. Percentages: □, sensitive to all antibiotics; ▨, resistant only to penicillin; ■, resistant to penicillin and one or more other antibiotics; ▩, resistant to one or more antibiotics (not penicillin).

are ecologically associated. The advantage conferred by a wide spectrum of resistance ensures that the strains that persist endemically in hospital will acquire fresh resistances as further antibiotics are brought into use (Richmond *et al.*, 1964). The epidemiological evidence suggests that transfer of resistance between different staphylococcal strains is a slow process. For example, the 83A and 84/85 strains of *Staph. aureus* each took over 2 years to acquire methicillin resistance (Parker & Hewitt, 1970), and neomycin resistance was confined to the 84/85 strains for several years (Jevons *et al.*, 1966). But the restriction of a resistance to a single strain, or to a small number of strains, does not prevent trouble if the strains themselves spread widely through the population.

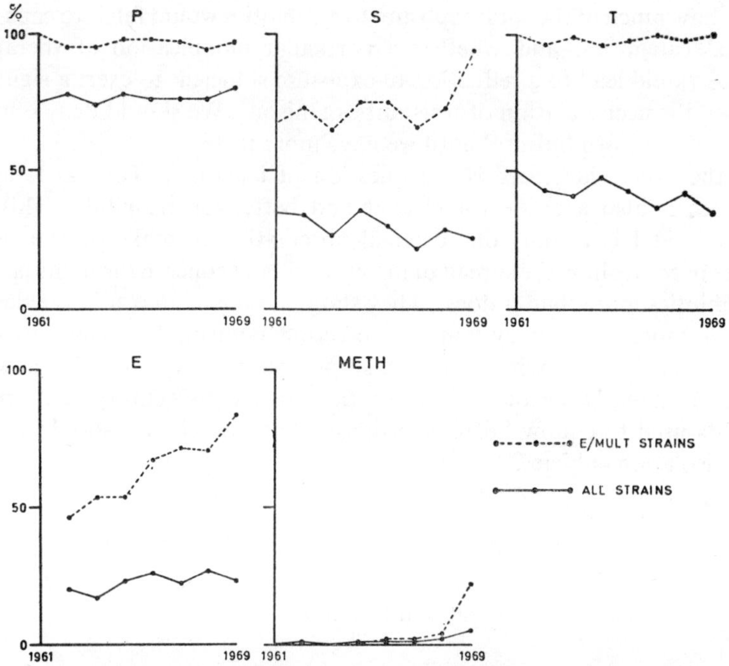

FIG. 2. Resistance of strains of *Staph. aureus* from lesions of patients in eight London hospitals to individual antibiotics. E/MULT = multiple-antibiotic resistant strains that were endemic in the hospitals (i.e. made up ⩾ 3 per cent of a series of consecutive isolates). P = penicillin; S = streptomycin; T = tetracycline; E = erythromycin; METH = methicillin.

What is the present position with regard to multiple-antibiotic resistance in staphylococci in hospital? Our survey of resistance in the *Staph. aureus* strains isolated from lesions in eight London hospitals suggests the following. Between 1961 and 1969 there was a slow fall in the proportion of strains resistant to two or more antibiotics from about one-half to a little more than one-third (Fig. 1). On the other hand, the endemic, multiple-antibiotic resistant strains increased the number of their resistances (Fig. 2). Here we may have been seeing Mary Barber's law at work; a great deal of effort has gone into infection control in the last 10 years, and our hygienic measures may have been responsible for limiting the spread of the endemic strains.

RESTRICTION OF ANTIBIOTICS OR ISOLATION OF PATIENTS

What can we do in the future? We can reduce the exposure of the hospital population to antibiotics or we can increase the degree of isolation of the patients from each other. Obviously we must try to do both. There has been a good deal of talk in this symposium about the 'misuse' of antibiotics, but it was clear that one man's misuse is another man's antibiotic policy! None of us knows how much of the total exposure to antibiotics would fall into each of the 'misuse' categories, and whether a particular modification of therapeutic practice would lead to a reduction of exposure sufficient to exert a significant effect on the accumulation of resistant organisms. We should deny ourselves the use of the word 'misuse' until we have more facts.

On the other side there is the question of isolation. The battle against resistance is also a battle for cleaner and better-run hospitals. This is so obvious that I have only one original observation to make on the subject. Success in controlling the spread of infection should concern the manufacturers of antibiotics more than it does. They should take an interest in the development of more efficient systems of infection control, both by supporting research and by improving facilities, so protecting their expensive new antibiotics from early obsolescence. In the nineteenth century, rich philanthropists used to endow hospital beds; perhaps Beecham's should begin to endow isolation cubicles.

Dr. E. J. L. Lowbury

I think that leads logically to Dr. Mark Ridley's topic; I have asked him to tell us something about the application of an antibiotics policy which he studied at St. Thomas's Hospital in London.

HOSPITAL ANTIBIOTIC POLICIES

Dr. M. Ridley

We started our antibiotic policy at St. Thomas's Hospital in the dark days of 1958 when 18 per cent of coagulase-positive staphylococci isolated from patients, and sometimes causing life-threatening infections, were resistant to penicillin, streptomycin, tetracyclines, erythromycin and novobiocin. This left us only toxic drugs such as vancomycin and ristocetin with which to treat those with serious infections.

Like Dr. Parker I ended up listening to some of the contributions on resistance with gloomy feelings which I am sure are false at this moment in time.

In the dark days I mentioned we had to follow the second of Mary Barber's Laws; that is to say we had to withhold the use of certain antibiotics throughout the hospital. Fortunately it was the clinicians who asked for advice and accepted this tactical manoeuvre when it was suggested. All prescribing of erythromycin and novobiocin was forbidden. In a matter of a few months these truly multiple-resistant strains disappeared and we re-introduced the use of erythromycin and novobiocin but only in combination for strains resistant to penicillin, streptomycin and tetracycline.

Then we were saved by the bell. Beecham's brought out Celbenin (methicillin) the first of the penicillinase-stable penicillins.

We were able, therefore, to alter the policy slightly. The policy then became benzyl penicillin for penicillin-sensitive staphylococci, erythromycin combined with novobiocin for penicillin-resistant staphylococci and methicillin to be used only for penicillin and erythromycin and/or novobiocin-resistant staphylococci. We kept this policy in operation for about a year. As we used the drugs we again saw a rise in the percentage of erythromycin and novobiocin-resistant strains but these were no longer a worry because we had methicillin.

As methicillin resistance did not seem to be common we simplified the policy by recommending benzylpenicillin for penicillin-sensitive staphylococci and methicillin or cloxacillin for all other staphylococci.

We have had no great problem with methicillin-resistant staphylococci although we have been looking for these routinely since 1964 using a high concentration of salt in our medium and a 10 microgram methicillin disc, which is one of the essential special methods for detecting methicillin resistance.

METHICILLIN RESISTANCE

Although we use a vast amount of methicillin and cloxacillin, amounting to over £15,000 worth per annum, we do not see the fairly high percentage of methicillin resistance that has been reported elsewhere. Since October 1964 when we began to use the special type of sensitivity test that is required to detect methicillin resistance our figures show that the percentage of methicillin-resistant strains has increased from about 0·1 per cent to about 1·3 per cent during 1971. Although all these methicillin-resistant strains are also resistant to penicillin, streptomycin and tetracycline there has always been another antibiotic that we could use. We have been fairly careful to avoid cross infection with these rare methicillin-resistant strains by treating the patient whether treatment is clinically indicated or not, and if possible by isolation of the patient.

I think that with these drugs and stratagems I feel much more confident about the future than earlier speakers.

PERSISTENCE OF ANTIBIOTIC RESISTANT BACTERIA

Dr. E. J. L. Lowbury

How do you feel, in the light of your experience, about the emergence of multi-resistant strains in which there is a genetically-linked resistance to several antibiotics? With such strains, the use of one antibiotic may select resistance to several others, and the deliberate avoidance of an antibiotic to which many strains are resistant will not necessarily lead to the elimination of these resistant strains. I see Dr. Parker shaking his head, so perhaps you can both comment on that.

Dr. M. T. Parker

I shouldn't think the patient would worry whether the resistance was linked when he was infected with the organism! In effect there has been an ecological linkage between the major resistances of staphylococci for the last 20 years. Staphylococci are resistant to a number of antibiotics because it is, from a Darwinian point of view, of advantage to them to be resistant to many different antibiotics that they may encounter within a short period of time in a hospital and so the patient doesn't mind which staphylococcus he gets infected with. OK—there is a resistant staphylococcus—patients get infected with it when their sensitive organisms get cleared out. That's the story as far as I can see.

Dr. E. J. L. Lowbury

I can remember the time (in the 1950s) when we were using only tetracycline for treatment of infection with *Strept. pyogenes* in our Burns Unit, and found a high incidence of tetracycline-resistant *Staph. aureus* in the burns. Then we stopped using tetracycline for streptococcal infection and switched to erythromycin. The incidence of tetracycline resistance in *Staph. aureus* came down after this change, but the incidence of erythromycin-resistant staphylococci rose steeply. Today there seems to be much more linked resistance to two, three or more antibiotics, and I wonder if we would have the same experience if we made such an experiment today?

Dr. M. T. Parker

Yes, a few instances of two linked resistances have been described in *Staph. aureus* (e.g. penicillin and erythromycin, penicillin and kanamycin), but they appear to be uncommon so far. We carried out a fairly extensive search for them some time ago but found none.

Dr. E. J. L. Lowbury

Would you like to comment on that, Dr. Ridley?

Dr. M. Ridley

The only comment that I have to make is that since we stopped using erythromycin and novobiocin (currently we spend less than £30 per annum on these drugs), strains resistant to them have remained rare.

The one worry that I have, although I am not a biochemist and may not have understood everything said yesterday by Professor Mark Richmond, is that if there was ever a slight change in the type of penicillinase produced by staphylococci then perhaps methicillin and cloxacillin might be hydrolysed by such 'new' enzymes.

Dr. E. J. L. Lowbury

So far we have talked only about staphylococci, apart from an occasional glance at the gram-negative bacilli; I think we might now consider the problems of gram-negative bacilli and the use of antibiotics for treatment of infection with these organisms. I'd like to ask Dr. Asscher if he could take up the threads —he's had a great deal of experience in the treatment of urinary tract infections in patients with renal insufficiency.

RENAL IMPAIRMENT AND ANTIBIOTIC USE

Dr. A. W. Asscher

Dr. Parker mentioned the value of cubicles, in relation to the problem of hospital infections. We do have a cubicle but unfortunately all our bacteria are concentrated in it. In fact it is our dialysis unit, which is a veritable culture medium. One of the commonest causes of death in a dialysis unit is gram-negative septicaemia. Fifty per cent of all deaths in dialysis units are associated with gram-negative infections, and the commonest source of these infections is the urinary tract. For this reason I would like to consider the problem of treating urinary tract infection in the presence of impaired kidney function. There are many difficulties in the way of treating these infections successfully. Firstly, the organisms which cause the infections are usually acquired in hospital and are, therefore, more likely to be resistant to the commonly used antibacterial agents. Secondly, it is difficult to achieve an adequate urinary concentration of an antibacterial agent whilst avoiding systemic accumulation of toxicity. Thirdly, antibacterial agents reach an adequate urinary concentration more slowly than normal, thus giving greater opportunity for the organisms to develop resistance during treatment. In addition, urinary acidification cannot be achieved and finally, where kidney function is unequally impaired most of the antibacterial drug will be excreted by the better functioning kidney, thus by-passing the poorly functioning kidney where infection may persist.

Renal handling of antibacterials

A few years ago we set out to try and solve the problem. In the first instance we had a look at the excretion of sulphadimidine in patients with end-stage kidney failure, with creatinine clearances of less than 30 ml/min. We were surprised to find that in patients with kidney failure sulphadimidine clearance was not impaired; presumably because although less of the drug is filtered, tubular reabsorption is equally diminished. At first this observation appeared to be only of academic interest because the majority of organisms isolated from the urinary tract of patients with kidney failure were resistant to sulphonamides, but our observations became of more than theoretical interest when co-trimoxazole became available. Sharpstone showed that the sulphonamide component of co-trimoxazole (sulphamethoxazole) behaved like sulphadimidine and was well excreted in the urine of patients with end-stage kidney failure. The trimethoprim component, however, was retained even though enough of the drug appeared in the urine to be effective. We have used co-trimoxazole in the treatment of patients with non-oliguric kidney failure whose urinary tract was infected with coliforms and proteus spp. Six weeks after a 7-day course of co-trimoxazole tabs. 2 b.d., a 60 per cent cure rate was observed in 42 patients in whom glomerular filtration rate was less than 30 ml/min. This is very satisfactory considering the extreme difficulty in treating these infections. One interesting point which emerges from the use of co-trimoxazole in patients with impaired kidney function is that the ratios of sulphonamide to trimethoprim in the urine vary widely because the sulphonamide is rapidly cleared whereas the trimethoprim is retained, thus very high sulphonamide/trimethoprim ratios are observed. Despite this the synergism between the two drugs is retained. Could it be that most of the 'goodness' of co-trimoxazole is attributable to the trimethoprim?

Components of co-trimoxazole

Dr. E. J. L. Lowbury

Can you give these two drugs separately to a patient, with different periods of administration?

Dr. A. W. Asscher

Yes, you may well have to adjust the dose of sulphonamide and trimethoprim individually when you are using this combination of drugs in patients with kidney failure. By doing so it might be possible to achieve the ideal 20 to 1 sulphonamide/trimethoprim ratio in the urine. It is not certain, however, how critical this ratio is. As you know, Dr. Reeves and Professor Brumfitt showed in 1968 that sulphonamide/trimethoprim ratios ranging between 2 to 1 and 10 to 1 were all equally effective against the common gram negative urinary pathogens.

Dr. M. Ridley

I think the thing with trimethoprim and sulphamethoxazole is that the ratio has been chosen using subjects with normal kidneys producing the same type of curve with both compounds. Dr. Lennox-Smith is in the audience and he ought to know.

Dr. I. Lennox-Smith

The original work on blood and urine levels was indeed undertaken using healthy volunteers but those of us who were in Prague last year heard Professor

Rieder's results and recommendations concerning dosage with different degrees of renal failure (Rieder & Fernex, 1971). A copy of the manuscript of this paper is available to anyone who is particularly interested. Summarized very briefly, the recommendations are that normal doses may be used with creatinine clearances above 25 ml/min: one tablet twice daily is sufficient for values between 15 to 25 ml/min: one tablet daily is recommended for those with creatinine clearance below 15 ml/min. Blood levels of total sulphamethoxazole should be monitored. These recommendations need to be confirmed in larger series of patients.

The excretion of *active* sulphamethoxazole is little affected by decreasing renal function but metabolites accumulate. The elimination of trimethoprim is retarded by a factor of 2–3 in severe renal failure.

There are many things that I could add about the fixed 1:5 ratio and how and why it was chosen but I cannot go into this now; discussion on the subject is often more philosophical than practical. Suffice it to say that there were good grounds for the choice: it is desirable to have only one rather than a plethora of combinations; and we know by very wide experience that this one works.

Dr. A. W. Asscher

The amounts of trimethoprim and sulphonamide in co-trimoxazole were chosen so as to give a 20 to 1 ratio in the blood since this is the most effective ratio for synergism for the majority of pathogens with the exception of gonococcus, for which the ratio of 1 to 1 has been found to be the most successful.

INFECTIONS IN SUSCEPTIBLE PATIENTS

Dr. E. J. L. Lowbury

One of the hospital departments which deals with susceptible patients and uses sophisticated apparatus is the renal dialysis unit. I would like to ask Sister Harris who is in charge of the nursing aspects of such a unit how antibiotics are used there.

Renal dialysis unit

Sister M. E. Harris

We have been more fortunate than Dr. Asscher and are concerned mainly with shunt infections. The commonest organism in our dialysis unit is *Staph. pyogenes* which is usually discovered through routine monthly nasal swabs of each patient. The staphylococci are usually sensitive to neomycin used as a topical application twice daily in the form of Naseptin cream. We continue the treatment for 3 weeks and leave 1 week clear and then re-swab. It is rarely necessary to repeat this treatment.

Shunts and arterio-venous fistulae infections usually occur with *Staph. pyogenes* sensitive to cloxacillin and other antibiotics and our usual choice of antibiotic is cloxacillin. Some shunts have become infected with *Pseudomonas aeruginosa* and this can eventually result in septicaemia. On each occasion that this has happened it has occurred with a patient who has his machine at home and dialyses himself. They have failed to report the primary infections either to their G.P. or the Renal Unit until they feel unwell. Shunt swabs and blood cultures then reveal pseudomonas. The treatment in these patients has been 5 grams of carbenicillin given three times weekly via the venous line during the post-dialysis washing. Sometimes this has been combined with gentamicin 80 mg. These infections are usually discovered by the nurse who can alert the physician so that the appropriate action can be taken. I feel that the nurse is in close contact with the patient 24 hours a day and is therefore able to observe these reactions more closely than the physician. The prompt treatment of infection in our unit is due to our close liaison with the medical team.

Dr. E. J. L. Lowbury

It is interesting that the pseudomonas infections developed in patients having home dialysis. Have you any idea about the possible source of the organisms, and whether these infections were caused by the patients' flora or acquired from an external source? We regard *Ps. aeruginosa* as an organism common in hospital but rare in the home.

Renal transplant patients

Mr. H. J. O. White

May I say a few words about infection in the context of kidney transplantation. Of the two methods of preventing infection, antibiotic therapy or isolation of the patient, we rely mainly on avoidance of contact between organisms and the patient. We are dealing with a very special group of patients. Because of uraemia and immunosuppression, they are more liable to infection than the general population. Such infections may be caused by the usual pathogens and also by organisms which are not normally pathogenic to the otherwise healthy individual, and this type of infection includes organisms for which antibiotics have limited effect such as fungi, viruses and *Pneumocystis carinae*. I think that the most important point and the one that Sister Harris has made, is that every aseptic precaution should be taken. There must be absolutely scrupulous asepsis both in the theatre and outside, particularly in the care of these patients' arteriovenous shunts and fistulae.

Problem of the donor

Considering the cadaveric donor, it is easy to 'transplant' infection with the kidneys. Each donor must therefore be carefully assessed with this in mind. In this context there are two groups of cadaveric donors. Firstly, the cadaver donor who is already dead when the transplant surgeon is informed and so it is too late to take steps to prevent infection. However, this is usually a sudden death and the donor is not normally infected. The second group is the potential cadaver donor on a ventilator and this group is particularly liable to infection, especially if they have been on a ventilator for 2 or more days. Many of them develop a bacteraemia and the majority of transplant surgeons would avoid using kidneys from such a source when the ventilator has been in use for 48 hours or more. There is a place for prophylactic antibiotics in the prevention of infection when kidneys are to be used from donors on a ventilator if the medical team looking after the donor agree, and it is hard to think of a circumstance in which this might be against the potential donor's interest. I can quote one case in which a pair of kidneys were transplanted from a donor in Cambridge who had been on a respirator for 2½ days. Ten days later *Escherichia coli* was cultured from the arterial anastomosis following a secondary haemorrhage in one of the recipients. In the other, the same organism was cultured from an abscess which had developed at the junction of the donor ureter and the recipient bladder.

Infection in the recipient

Turning to the recipient, can we do anything to prevent infection before the transplant operation itself? Certainly, if you can't eradicate infection from the kidneys of patients on maintenance dialysis, then possibly you should take them out. This is our policy with polycystic kidneys as it is thought that even though the fluid in those cysts may be initially sterile in the non-immunosuppressed patient, they are a potential source of infection after immunosuppression is started. Following re-anastomosis of the donor kidney in the recipient, it is the policy in some units to give a single prophylactic injection of one or more antibiotics at this time. We do not adopt this policy unless the kidney has come from a ventilator death.

Following transplantation again two groups may be considered. Firstly, in the minority of cases the donor kidney may immediately function satisfactorily and in such cases there is usually very little problem in keeping their lower urinary tract sterile. However, in the other group which constitutes the majority, the renal transplant undergoes acute tubular necrosis, so that from a few days to a month little urine is produced. During part of this time there will be an indwelling urethral catheter and possibly also a catheter splinting the donor ureter. It is certainly our practice to use neomycin bladder washouts two or three times a day until either the urethral catheter is removed or urine is being produced in quantity. In all cases we practice reverse barrier nursing but somebody has already argued that this may be unnecessary.

Antibiotic use

With regard to the use of antibiotics for established infection following transplantation, we prefer to know the bacteriology and sensitivities and then treat each infection specifically with a narrow-spectrum drug. Particular care has to be exercised in the use of antibiotics because of the dangers of accumulation in the presence of poor renal function or nephrotoxicity or even under-excretion as was previously mentioned by Dr. Asscher with respect to sulphonamides. The other point that has been made is that a patient may require dialysis in the immediate post-transplant period. Antibiotic may be rapidly dialysed out of the patient so that immediately after dialysis has ceased, a further booster dose is required; gentamicin is such an example.

The last point I make is that it has become a kidney transplant surgeon's philosophy that we must, if need be, lose transplants and save patients and place them back on dialysis. On occasion it is impossible to eradicate infection from the immunosuppressed transplanted patient and it is preferable to remove a poorly-functioning graft, particularly when there have been a number of episodes of threatened rejection, and place the patient back on dialysis in the hope that one day that patient may again be fit for a second or third transplant.

PROPHYLACTIC USE OF ANTIBIOTICS IN SURGERY

Dr. E. J. L. Lowbury

Thank you very much, Mr. White. You referred to the use of chemotherapeutic agents for prophylaxis in this special field, and also emphasized that special methods are needed for high risk patients. I'd like now to ask Mr. Williams, who is a general surgeon, to give us his views on the prophylactic use of antibiotics in surgery, both in the high risk and in the general surgical field.

Wound infection rates

Mr. J. Alexander Williams

Thank you Dr. Lowbury. I am not sure why I have been included on this panel but I think I am here to represent the common man. I am officially a representative of general and abdominal surgery and, Heaven knows, we in general surgery need all the help possible from bacteriologists as our record is not good and our rate of wound infection is still high. I am diffident about quoting the figures from papers when the author also happens to be sitting on the panel. Perhaps I have read your paper more recently than you have, Professor Williams, but if I make any mistakes when quoting you I hope that you will correct me. In 1966 there was published a comprehensive report on wound infection in a book by you and your colleagues (Williams *et al.*, 1966). The infection rate that you then reported for such simple operations as a hernia was 6 per cent. For varicose veins it was 9 per cent, for cholecystectomy 15 per cent and for bowel surgery it was something like 25 per cent—an appalling rate of suppurative wound infection. You will have realized that surgeons are a grubby group but we are not quite as bad as that!

There may be surgeons in the audience who will say 'My infection rate is not as high as that'. To them I say review your own results critically or have someone else do so. We checked our own figures recently and today's *British Journal of Surgery* contains a report from our own unit on a study of wound infection while we were engaged in a trial of plastic wound guards (Williams *et al.*, 1972). In this trial the bacteriologist examined the patients after operation and inspected their wounds. He found that our rate was almost as high as that reported in Professor Williams' survey. After cholecystectomy it was 13 per cent, after gastric operations 6 per cent, after colon operations 18 per cent—still a very high infection rate. This infection rate is dependent on a number of factors, not only on the scruffiness of the surgeon but also on the length of time he takes to operate and particularly on the type of operation. If he is operating on a patient with acute cholecystitis or on the large bowel then he will have a high rate of infection.

Prevention of abdominal wound infection

Naturally the surgeon who is aware that some of his wounds are becoming infected wishes to do something to try to reduce the incidence. It is very tempting for the surgeon to try to prevent or minimize infection by achieving a sufficient level of the appropriate antibiotic in the wound. I have been interested in trying to reduce the incidence of infection in our patients and after looking at the available evidence have come to the following conclusions.

We are trying to achieve a high level of antibiotic in the wound in order to improve the chances of destroying any organisms that may reach the wound before they can produce infection. We can do it in two ways either by instilling topical antibiotics (Nash, 1967), or by giving a high dose of parenteral antibiotic so that it will enter the wound (Polk & Lopez-Mayor, 1969). In the published reports there is great enthusiasm expressed by a number of authors who claim that since using a certain antibiotic wound infections have disappeared. There have been a number of reports on the use of topical ampicillin in wound infection which are quite convincing. There has not been an absolutely impeccable controlled trial with ampicillin but there have been extremely good controlled trials using multiple topical antibiotic sprays. Jackson, Pollock and Tindall (1971) reported an elegant controlled trial using topical antibiotics and found the wound infection rate was exactly the same in the treated and the control groups. Like Ellis (1969) I have tried to weigh up the evidence from those reports that claim benefit from topical antibiotics and those that do not and I can find just as many and as convincing reports on one side as on the other. I personally, and perhaps irrationally do use topical antibiotics.

Operations using foreign body implants

I have been performing one operation in which I was particularly anxious to avoid infection; this was a method of hernia repair using a prosthesis. I used this method in order to send the patients out of hospital on the day of operation. A very atraumatic hernia repair without tension was needed and therefore I used a patch of nylon to repair the posterior inguinal wall; this makes a comfortable hernia repair, and the patients get out of bed on the same day and walk about the following day. However, if you are placing foreign material in a wound it is very important to prevent infection because if there is infection plus a foreign body the infection will persist. We have used the topical (polymyxin-bacitracin) antibiotic spray in this group of patients and have just surveyed the results in 160 patients. We have encountered only one persistent wound infection and three of minor untreated superficial sepsis, which is better than the reported infection rate of 6 per cent. We have not conducted a control trial but with such good results I am loath to do so. There may be a number of other factors contributing to the good result and possibly a major factor is that we send the patient home on the same day. It may also be that we are extra careful in securing haemostasis in a patient we are intending to send home.

Systemic antibiotics

There is no unequivocal published evidence that topical antibiotics in the wound make any difference to the incidence of infection. There have been reports on the effects on wound healing of systemic ampicillin and cephaloridine. In a controlled trial, ampicillin given at the beginning of the operation was shown not to have the slightest effect on wound infection rates (Pollock & Tindal, 1972) while cephaloridine lowered the infection rate (Polk & Lopez-Mayor, 1969). I always tend to believe a report in which the results come out showing no benefit for a drug. Almost every report that comes out saying that this or that antibiotic is the answer to the problem of wound infection is followed by one that shows that it produces no effect.

Pre-operative bowel preparation

Finally I would like to discuss pre-operative bowel preparation. Because of the high risk of wound infection in patients with operations on the bowel, surgeons have attempted to 'sterilize' the gut before bowel surgery. A former Birmingham gastroenterologist Dr. Jack French had a saying, which is very true; he said 'if you wish to sterilize the bowel, the only way to do so is to take it out and boil it'. There is a great deal of published work on antibiotic bowel preparation and the evidence so far from controlled trials is that there is no difference between patients who have had pre-operative antibiotics and those who have had no antibiotics, providing that the patients have had equally thorough mechanical bowel preparation. If you thoroughly wash out the bowel by enemata and purgation, it seems that it makes not the slightest difference whether you give the patient antibiotics by mouth before or after operation (Ellis, 1969). There is some evidence to suggest that the risk of infection is greater if you give a patient pre-operative bowel antibiotics (Altemeier *et al.*, 1968; Polacek & San Felippo, 1968). My own survey of the available evidence in the literature leads me to believe there is no proof that there is a place for routine antibiotic prophylaxis in any form of general surgery.

Dr. E. J. L. Lowbury

I wonder if Mr. White would like to make any observations on that?

Mr. H. J. O. White

It was refreshing to hear another general surgeon cleansing the large bowel because I am quite convinced that this is the most important thing. May I ask Mr. Williams if he does not give long-acting sulphonamides prophylactically prior to large bowel surgery?

Mr. J. Alexander Williams

I do not.

Mr. H. J. O. White

I admire your courage. Most surgeons still give long-acting sulphonamides. If you ask a hundred surgeons you would still get 90 per cent hoping for benefit from long-acting sulphonamides and perhaps 50 per cent using neomycin, again without very much belief in it.

Dr. E. J. L. Lowbury

I think it is very important that we should have as much material from controlled studies as possible. Prophylactic use of antibiotics is one of the controversial questions on which emotion rather than knowledge tends to determine people's opinion; there is clearly a need for more knowledge.

We are fortunate to have Professor Petersdorf with us, and I would like to ask him if he would give us his views on this problem in the general context of his experience in the United States.

EXPERIENCE IN THE UNITED STATES

Staphylococcal infections

Professor R. G. Petersdorf

Some very challenging statements have been made and pearls of wisdom have been dropped. In the United States we seem to have the general impression that we are on top of the staphylococcal resistance problem. This may be a false hope but in a very carefully controlled study in our hospital, Drs.

Bulger and Sherris (1968) showed that staphylococci in 1968 were far less resistant than in 1959. I think this is a favourable trend and may reflect in part more careful usage of antibiotic drugs. However, there is more to the story than this. As one of the speakers pointed out, we have used kilograms of methicillin and have encountered few methicillin-resistant organisms. As a matter of fact, the only real epidemic we have seen, was carried in from outside the hospital by a patient who was in a nursing home and who had not been in contact with the general hospital setting (O'Toole *et al.*, 1970).

Gram-negative infections

With gram-negative organisms the problem is more complicated. While it is true that antibiotic usage is related in some way to the emergence of resistant strains, we don't know the mechanism of resistance in many cases. Simply restricting antibiotics does not seem to be handling this problem. An example is the Infectious Disease Service at the Boston City Hospital on which antibiotic usage is controlled quite rigidly. However, it was from this very service that the first major report on overwhelming gram-negative bacteremia during the last decade appeared (Finland *et al.*, 1959). There are probably many factors accounting for the emergence of resistant gram-negatives; one is that we seem to be working on a weaker substrate. By that I mean patients with transplants receiving immunosuppressive drugs or undergoing cardiac surgery are being kept alive by heroic measures only to be parasitized by a variety of organisms. The ones with which we seem to be having the most trouble in the U.S., as well as in the U.K., are klebsiella-enterobacter, pseudomonas, and serratia.

Antibiotic use

There have also been some striking changes in the use of antibiotics in the last 10 years. It is my distinct impression that we are using fewer drugs now than we ever did before. We use virtually no chloramphenicol and much less tetracycline. Novobiocin is off many formularies and oleandomycin was never on most. So we are dealing with comparatively few bacteriostatic drugs. Even among the bactericidal agents, a number are falling by the wayside. In our institution, it is now rare for a patient to have a prescription for kanamycin; almost all receive gentamicin. Because the regulatory agency in the United States, the Food and Drug Administration, has not yet released co-trimoxazole for clinical use, we cannot, of course, employ it. We still use a good deal of ampicillin and although our patterns of *Esch. coli* resistance to this drug have not been as dramatic as in this country, we are seeing more refractory *Esch. coli* strains. We use cephalothin a good deal, much less cephaloridine than in the U.K. and very little polymyxin. Hence, if the number of antibiotics that are circulating about the hospital are counted it becomes apparent that there are many fewer than there were 10 years ago. This is probably a wholesome development which may herald a plateau indicating that we may not have to confront new waves of resistant bacteria. However, I have the uncomfortable feeling that this is a false hope and will not turn out to be the case. It is my distinct impression that our usage of antibiotics, just like yours, has become a great deal more sophisticated. Unfortunately, this statement does not apply to most surgeons who are still using penicillin and streptomycin for every operation.

Effects of antibiotic restriction

Dr. E. J. L. Lowbury

I wonder about the possible benefits or disadvantages of restricting the range of available antibiotics. You said that novobiocin has fallen out, and that certain other antibiotics have not become available in the United States. Many of us feel that having a large range of available antibiotics, some of which are kept in reserve while others are being used, gives flexibility to ring the changes in an antibiotics policy which can help to keep us 'ahead of resistance'. How does this concept apply in the successful antibiotic policy which you have used in Seattle?

Professor R. G. Petersdorf

We make no formal attempt to impose a policy but there are a fair number of people on our faculty who have worked in the field of antimicrobial therapy. Dr. William M. M. Kirby and Dr. Marvin Turck, in addition to myself, are examples. As a result, many of the younger men on the faculty, the practicing physicians in the community, and the housestaff have been exposed to a good deal of practical teaching. In a sense, then, we set the policy by example. We usually agree on drug usage and in the case of novobiocin, an agent which is accompanied by a good deal of gastrointestinal distress, and which has been replaced by other alternative drugs, we simply don't use it. When a pharmacist sees that an agent has not been used for 6 months, he quits buying it so that it falls by the way by natural attrition and not by decree.

Dr. E. J. L. Lowbury

Thank you very much. Professor Williams, would you like to make some observations on these problems?

HOSPITAL ACQUIRED INFECTION

Prophylactic antibiotics

Professor R. E. O. Williams

There are one or two points that emerged from what has been said that are worth comment.

On the question of antibiotic prophylaxis, I would certainly agree with what has been said about the published evidence in this field, that there is very little evidence that you can effectively prevent post-operative infections by antibiotic prophylaxis. There is, however, one situation where it really does seem to be mandatory to use antibiotic prophylaxis and that is for thigh amputation to prevent gas gangrene. We heard from Dr. Phillips that the literature suggests that there is a marginal value for antibiotic prophylaxis in cardiac surgery and I suppose that is one situation where the emotion will sustain the practice simply because of the appalling problem of infection if it does develop in a valve prosthesis that has been locked up in the heart.

In relation to antibiotic prophylaxis in the gut I am sure that the statement is right that there is at the moment virtually no good evidence that you can prevent post-operative infection in colon surgery by antibiotic prophylaxis. However, the sort of antibiotics that have generally been used do not by any means affect a very large proportion of the bacteria in the gut. In order to reduce the bacteroides in the gut, for example, you have to use antibiotics other than neomycin. It is possible that if you could be really sufficiently sophisticated in the kind of antibiotic prophylaxis that you use, some benefit might be derived. Then we get to the dilemma which Dr. Parker posed at the beginning that the greater the load of antibiotics used in the hospital the more certainty there will be of a greater population of resistant strains of bacteria. So that although you may be doing good for this patient today you may be putting yourself in a situation where you are going to be much worse off for a large number of patients in the future.

Isolation of patients

In looking at what Dr. Parker said about the maintenance of antibiotic sensitivity among the bacteria in hospitals by hygiene as well as by abstinence from antibiotic usage, one must remember that the pool of resistant strains in the hospital is in general not a pool of overt infections—it is a pool in carrier sites of one sort and another. The more one looks at the behaviour of bacteria around the hospital, the more you see that patients entering hospital change their flora very very rapidly. They change their gut flora, they change their nose flora, they change their skin flora. It is the endemic resistant strains going around from one carrier to another that maintain the pool from which the odd patient becomes infected. So the sort of hygiene that we have to consider is not simply the hygiene of preventing the bacteria from a wound infection which has got pus in it from being transferred to another patient; it is a much more complicated problem of preventing patients spreading their organisms from one person to another.

Hospital hygiene

There are some general measures we can take which are effective and are practicable. A large part of the transfer of gut organisms probably relates to food and drink, and kitchen hygiene in the broadest sense is a practical way of making some effect on this—though in fact we don't yet know that. All the work we have done in the last few years indicates how difficult it is to prevent spread of staphylococci to the nose and to the skin, and that there comes a time when one may have to consider that the acquisition of some resistant strains may be inevitable for many patients. There are some patients, however such as those to be subjected to transplantation, or whose diseases make them particularly susceptible, for whom one really may have to take very much more stringent precautions against the acquisition of resistant strains.

Variations in micro-organisms

We have heard several times of the change in the pattern of resistance in staphylococci, and there has been reference also to changes in the streptococcal situation. We tend to attribute these changes either to what we do or what we don't do. A point that hasn't been mentioned is that there has been a very substantial change in the distribution of the staphylococci as recognized by phage type in the last 20 years, and I think that you could make a good case for arguing that one of the reasons why the staphylococcal situation looks as though it is under control at the moment is because we don't happen to have, in the late sixties and early seventies, so many of the particularly virulent communicable staphylococci as we had in the early fifties. I am sure we should look more at this possibility of long-term changes in the behaviour of the organisms to explain some of the differences in the epidemiological pattern. Perhaps this is the explanation of the sudden upsurge of infections with serratia, which has occurred on the other side of the Atlantic but which does not seem yet to have struck this country. I wonder whether there may not be an element of change in the character of the gonococcus that accounts for some of the changes in the epidemiological pattern, rather than simply all the things that people are alleged to do nowadays which it is said they used not to do.

Sensitive or resistant

Dr. E. J. L. Lowbury

The emergence of serratia as a hospital pathogen reminds me of the emergence of the carbenicillin-resistant pseudomonas which we discussed yesterday, and which presented us with a new pattern of Gram-negative bacillary infection in certain hospitals. It also poses a new problem of definition. What is 'sensitivity' and what is 'resistance' to carbenicillin when the main pathogen (e.g. *Ps. aeruginosa*) is present in a mixed culture? We found, for example, that when proteus or klebsiella carrying a particular R factor was growing in the same burn as a sensitive pseudomonas, within two or three days of starting the use of carbenicillin the pseudomonas became highly resistant to carbenicillin. The laboratory correctly reported the original *Ps. aeruginosa* as sensitive but are we now required to report on the sensitivity of other organisms which might potentially infect the pseudomonas and make it resistant. After all, the word 'sensitive' in a laboratory report means 'you may expect successful therapy with this antibiotic'. I am just throwing this out as a rather awful last thought!

REFERENCES

ALTEMEIER, W. A., CULBERTSON, W. R. & HUMMEL, R. P. (1968). Surgical considerations of endogenous infections—sources, types and methods of control *Surgical Clinics of North America*, **48,** 227.

BARBER, M. (1947a). Coagulase-positive staphylococci resistant to penicillins. *Journal of Pathology and Bacteriology*, **59,** 373.

BARBER, M. (1947b). Staphylococcal infection due to penicillin-resistant strains. *British Medical Journal*, **2,** 863.

BULGER, R. J. & SHERRIS, J. C. (1968). Decreased incidence of antibiotic resistance among *Staphylococcus aureus*. *Annals of Internal Medicine*, **69,** 1099.

ELLIS, H. (1969). The place of antibiotics in surgical practice to-day. *Annals of the Royal College of Surgeons of England*, **45,** 162.

FINLAND, M., JONES, W. E. & BARNES, M. W. (1959). Occurrences of serious bacterial infections since introduction of antibacterial agents. *Journal of the American Medical Association*, **170,** 2188.

JACKSON, D. W., POLLOCK, A. V. & TINDALL, D. S. (1971). The value of plastic adhesive drape in the prevention of wound infection. A controlled trial. *British Journal of Surgery*, **58,** 340.

JEVONS, P. M., JOHN, M. & PARKER, M. T. (1966). Cultural characteristics of a newly recognised group of hospital staphylococci. *Journal of Clinical Pathology*, **19,** 305.

NASH, A. G. (1967). Topical ampicillin and wound infection in colon surgery. *British Medical Journal*, **1,** 471.

O'TOOLE, R. D., DREW, W. L., DAHLGREN, B. J. & BEATY, H. N. (1970). An outbreak of methicillin-resistant *Staphylococcus aureus* infection. Observations in hospital and nursing home. *Journal of the American Medical Association*, **213,** 257.

PARKER, M. T. & HEWITT, J. H. (1970). Methicillin resistance in *Staphylococcus aureus*. *Lancet*, **i,** 800.

POLACEK, M. A. & SANFELIPPO, P. (1968). Oral antibiotic bowel preparation and complications in colon surgery. *Archives of Surgery*, **97,** 412.

POLK, H. & LOPEZ-MAYOR, J. F. (1969). Post-operative wound infection: A prospective study of determinant factors and prevention. *Surgery*, **66,** 97.

POLLOCK, A. V. & TINDAL, D. S. (1972). The effect of a single-dose antibiotic in the prevention of wound infection. *British Journal of Surgery*, **59,** 98.

RICHMOND, M. H., PARKER, M. T., JEVONS, P. M. & JOHN, M. (1964). High penicillinase production correlated with multiple antibiotic resistance in *Staphylococcus aureus*. *Lancet*, **i,** 293.

RIEDER, J. & FERNEX, M. (1971). Pharmacokinetic data of the combination sulphamethoxazole plus trimethoprim in patients with renal involvement. *Proceedings of the VIIth International Congress of Chemotherapy, Prague* (In press).

SHARPSTONE, P. (1969). The renal handling of trimethoprim and sulphamethoxazole in man. *Post-graduate Medical Journal Supplement*, **49,** 38.

WILLIAMS, J. A., OATES, G. D., BROWN, P. P., BURDEN, D. W., MCCALL, J., HUTCHINSON, A. G. & LEES, L. J. (1972). Abdominal wound infections and plastic wound guards. *British Journal of Surgery*, **59,** 142.

WILLIAMS, R. E. O., BLOWERS, R., GARROD, L. P. & SHOOTER, R. A. (1966). *Hospital Infection—Causes and Prevention*, p. 272. Lloyd-Luke, London.

14

TREATMENT OF RESPIRATORY TRACT INFECTION: A BACTERIOLOGIST'S VIEWPOINT

A. PERCIVAL

THE view is very common among clinicians that the usual type of laboratory report on specimens from the respiratory tract is not of much value. Certainly, little attention to detail appears to be expended on diagnostic specimens. Most general practitioners treat sore throat and exacerbations of chronic bronchitis without taking specimens and, in hospital, a frequent occurrence is for stale saliva or sputum to be collected by night nurses, left to stew on the ward for a period and then sent to the laboratory, without clinical data on the request form informing the laboratory, for example, that the patient has been receiving antibiotics for several days. The confusion is further compounded by those laboratories which merely culture a loopful of material and report sensitivities to antibiotics of any potential pathogen and often unlikely ones also. Little attempt is made to assess the possible clinical significance of the organisms isolated and it would be unreasonable to expect even a highly skilled technician to have sufficient medical knowledge to make such judgement. Another contributory factor during 30 years of antibiotic therapy has been the view that the commonest infecting bacteria, *Haemophilus influenzae* and pneumococci, are predictably sensitive to antibiotics and, therefore, treatment need not be based on bacteriological investigations. As a result microbiological advice is only sought after failure of 'blind' therapy, when it is difficult to identify the reasons for failure to respond. Therefore, many of the problems seem to be due to lack of communication and care in obtaining and processing specimens. The purpose of this communication is to review the procedures available for assessing bacterial infections of the respiratory tract and to discuss difficulties encountered in treatment.

SIGNIFICANCE OF BACTERIAL ISOLATIONS FROM SPUTUM

Many respiratory tract infections are probably initiated by viruses or mycoplasma, although in exacerbations of chronic bronchitis *H. influenzae* and pneumococci appeared to be more often responsible (Fisher *et al.*, 1969). The initial infection may then impair local defence mechanisms and allow secondary bacterial invasion by the more pathogenic bacteria present in the upper respiratory tract at the time. Of these, *H. influenzae* and pneumococci are the commonest infecting organisms. *H. influenzae* can be isolated from the upper respiratory tract of between 60 and 80 per cent of young children and a somewhat lower percentage of adults (Turk & May, 1967). Only 3 to 4 per cent are capsulated strains, but these are more pathogenic than non-capsulated strains, being frequently associated with severe infections in adults as well as children (Holdaway & Turk, 1967). The carrier rate for pneumococci in the upper respiratory tract in normal adults is approximately 40 per cent and is higher in children and in adults with chronic chest disease (Clifton *et al.*, 1955). Again certain sero-types are of relatively greater pathogenicity and communicability, being associated with more severe disease and with outbreaks of infection. In lobar pneumonia, approximately half the infections used to be caused by sero-types 1 and 2 (Grist *et al.*, 1952) but more recently type 3 has become predominant and types 1 and 2 relatively uncommon (Calder *et al.*, 1970).

Because the commonest infecting bacteria may be present in sputum merely as contaminants from the normal flora, laboratory assessment can not be based on a qualitative difference in the bacterial content. Indirect evidence for the pathogenicity of particular bacteria in respiratory infections (May, 1968) is a greater frequency of isolation from purulent than from non-purulent material, the response to chemotherapy, re-appearance of particular organisms during relapse and the association of high levels of serum antibodies to different organisms in chronic respiratory infections. This provides a rational basis for determining probabilities, but is not of specific help to a clinician confronted by a seriously ill patient and is no substitute for diagnostic investigation in the individual case. Bacteria from the upper respiratory tract are equally likely to contaminate purulent and non-purulent sputum and a serological response to an acute infection takes at least a week to develop.

In chronic bronchitis, the difficulty in bacteriological interpretation is accentuated since direct culture of the bronchi usually reveals bacterial colonization, whereas the bronchi are normally sterile in health (Brumfitt *et al.*, 1957; Lees & McNaught, 1959). In these studies, *H. influenzae* was most frequently isolated from the bronchi. Comparison with sputum culture showed that pneumococci were commonly recovered from sputum when this organism was not present in bronchial cultures. These findings suggest that, in chronic mucopurulent bronchitis, the damaged lower respiratory tract may be permanently colonized and that an episode of virus infection or of atmospheric irritation (smoke, fog, anaesthetic gases) could be sufficient to precipitate an acute exacerbation caused by more extensive invasion of tissues by bacteria already present in the bronchial tree. The therapeutic implications of such a concept are that antibacterial therapy should be designed to kill the bacteria in the bronchi of chronic bronchitics and this requires penetration of the antibacterial agent into bronchial secretions in sufficient amounts for a bactericidal level to be reached (May, 1968).

The clinical significance of bacteria other than *H. influenzae* and pneumococci has been much less clearly defined. In particular, a consequence of the widespread use of broad spectrum antibiotics has been the tendency for the normal upper respiratory tract flora to be replaced during treatment by more resistant organisms such as *Escherichia coli*, Klebsiella, Proteus or *Pseudomonas aeruginosa*. These organisms may be present in varying numbers in foods prepared in hospitals and canteens (Shooter *et al.*, 1971), but apparently have difficulty in establishing themselves in the upper respiratory tract unless the normal flora is suppressed by antibiotics. Table 1 shows

TABLE 1

THE EFFECT OF ANTIBIOTICS ON THE OCCURRENCE OF 'COLIFORMS' IN SALIVA

Subjects	*Number tested*	*'Coliforms' per ml of saliva* below 10	$10–10^2$	$10^2–10^3$	*above* 10^3	*Per cent positive*
Normal adults						
No hospital food	20	20	0	0	0	0
Hospital canteen	20	14	5[a]	1	0	30
Hospital patients						
No antibiotics	27	22	4	1	0	19
Antibiotics given	28	10	4[a]	6	8	64

[a] In each group, 3 contained 'coliforms' after but not before lunch.

salivary counts of these organisms related to source of food and antibiotic treatment. In the hospital patients studied, Enterobacteria were isolated in greater numbers and from a greater proportion of those receiving antibiotics. In 6 subjects, the organisms appeared in the saliva after eating. Therefore, the same problem of interpretation arises in patients receiving antimicrobial therapy; to assess the clinical significance of organisms which may be only secondary throat flora. Correct evaluation can be more crucial because Enterobacteria are usually isolated from patients with severe illness; for example those in intensive care units and particularly when a tracheostomy has been performed. A mortality rate of 49 per cent was observed in one group of patients thought to have pneumonia caused by *Esch. coli* (Tillotson & Lerner, 1967) and treatment of infection by such organisms will often require toxic antibiotics to be given in high dosage.

In an attempt to determine the significance of Enterobacteria and Pseudomonas in sputum (Percival & Roberts, 1972) we found 20 per cent of sputa contained these organisms but in only 4·4 per cent of sputa were they isolated in profuse growth. Nevertheless, they were thought to be responsible for 11 per cent of infections and in half the infections, there was clinical and radiological evidence of severe lower respiratory tract disease. It is impossible to know if these findings suggest an increasing incidence of pulmonary infection by 'coliforms', particularly when compared with earlier studies such as that by Brumfitt *et al.* (1957), who found 'coliforms' in the bronchi of 4 (18 per cent) of 22 chronic bronchitics yielding a positive culture. The infecting organisms in sputa received during 1970 and 1971 in the Liverpool Royal Infirmary laboratory, are shown in Table 2. These figures, which include all types of infection, do not reveal any notable differences in frequency of infecting organisms from those given in papers written 20 years ago.

TABLE 2

INFECTING ORGANISMS IN SPUTUM FROM PATIENTS IN THE ROYAL INFIRMARY, LIVERPOOL

Organism	*Percentage of those infected*[a]
H. influenzae	48
Pneumococci	19
H. influenzae and pneumococci	12
'Coliforms'	10
Neisseria	4
Others (mainly *Staph. aureus*)	3
Other mixed infections	4

[a] 975 (25 per cent) of 3900 sputa were infected.

Probably infection by coliforms will present an increasing problem in specialized units, where the infection may be introduced from contaminated nebulizers (Reinarz *et al.*, 1965) or ventilators, especially in those with tracheostomies. Such infections also occur in patients with severe chronic diseases, for example Pseudomonas infections in chronic bronchitics with bronchiectasis and in cystic fibrosis. This results from continued antibiotic treatment and even in more acute infections in susceptible patients the use of broad spectrum antibiotics appears to increase the incidence of infection by coliforms. For example, Price and Sleigh (1970) described an outbreak of infection by Klebsiella in an intensive care unit, which followed greatly increased usage of ampicillin and was not controlled until prophylactic and therapeutic use of antibiotics was discontinued.

EXAMINATION OF SPUTUM IN THE LABORATORY

First, sputum should be examined visually and classified according to its consistency and purulence. Specimens consisting only of saliva are rejected and a further specimen requested. We prefer to record only 3 types; mucoid, mucopurulent and purulent, because degrees of purulence are difficult to assess.

Microscopy

The importance of examining a gram-stained film appears to be undervalued in many laboratories. In a recent final examination for the I.M.L.T., only 5 of 30 technicians noticed *H. influenzae* in a film containing very large numbers of this organism together with pneumococci. In particular, a search should be made for bacteria associated in large numbers with polymorphs and only when this is seen should a potential pathogen be regarded as being of probable significance clinically. Unfortunately, this criterion has its limitations because when organisms are added to the sputum, they may infiltrate into purulent areas within as little as 2 hours. Microscopy will also show whether a specimen is stale and can be valuable in diagnosis of staphylococcal pneumonia, when patients can die within 24 hrs before the results of culture are known. Unfortunately, this condition is commonly unsuspected clinically and treated inadequately with either ampicillin or tetracycline. When an allergic condition is a possibility a special stain for eosinophils should be carried out.

Culture

The bacterial content of sputum is unevenly distributed (May, 1953) and random culture using a single loopful taken from a purulent area may miss pathogenic bacteria present in another part of the same specimen. Selective culture of purulent 'flakes', after washing 3 times in buffered saline, has been recommended (Mulder, 1938), but is time consuming and, in the author's experience, often fails to remove the salivary organisms. A more representative culture can be obtained by homogenizing the specimen. Shaking with glass beads and the original technique of Rawlins (1953) using 1 per cent buffered pancreatin incubated at 37°C for 1 hr or more fail to homogenize an appreciable number of specimens. More recently much better methods have been described which liquefy almost all specimens within 10 min at room temperature. In the author's experience a 2 per cent solution of *N*-acetyl-1-cysteine (B.D.H. Ltd.), prepared as described by Mead and Woodhams (1964), has proved satisfactory. However, in a comparative trial, Rawlins (1968) found a mixture of trypsin and 1 per cent pancreatin to be more effective than *N*-acetyl-1-cysteine as a liquefying agent and to give a higher yield of pathogenic organisms from muco-purulent specimens.

Pathogenic bacteria may be isolated from a higher percentage of patients with purulent sputum if multiple specimens are examined (May & Delves, 1964), but in ill patients, this could lead to unnecessary delay in beginning treatment. Unfortunately, no satisfactory method has been described for transporting sputum by post without a considerable loss in the rate of isolation of pathogenic bacteria and overgrowth by contaminants.

Quantitative culture

Quantitative techniques have greatly simplified the interpretation of the results of culturing urine and provided a rational basis for the diagnosis of urinary infection, but have been much less used in sputum culture. The finding of bacteria in the lower bronchi was observed to be invariably associated with numbers exceeding 10^6 per ml of exudate (Laurenzi *et al.*, 1961) and homogenates of purulent sputum to contain very large numbers of potential pathogens (Cooper *et al.*, 1961; Louria, 1962). Dixon and Miller (1965) found that when homogenized specimens were diluted 1 in 10,000, 70 per cent yielded either no growth or a pure growth of a single organism and recommended this as a routine procedure in sputum culture.

We carried out quantitative counts of coliforms in 190 sputa (Percival & Roberts, 1972). In purulent specimens, where gram-negative rods could be seen to be associated with polymorphs in the gram film, the counts always exceeded 10^5 per ml of homogenized sputum. However, counts of this order were also obtained in fresh non-purulent specimens and the overall distribution of counts for all specimens containing coliforms was not bi-modal. Thus, although quantitative enumeration of bacteria in sputum provides a guide to possible clinical significance, it will not differentiate infection from contamination as reliably as it does in urinary infections. This is not unexpected, because lower respiratory tract secretions, unlike bladder urine, are contaminated by passage through a vestibule containing very large numbers of organisms.

RESISTANCE OF RESPIRATORY PATHOGENS TO ANTIBIOTICS

Fortunately, changes in the sensitivity to antibiotics of the commonest infecting organisms have only occurred to a limited extent. Pneumococci have remained fully sensitive to the penicillins except recently in New Guinea (Hansman *et al.*, 1971) where a single sero-type 25 times less sensitive to benzyl penicillin was isolated from 15 different subjects. However, the circumstances were unusual in that penicillin had been given to large numbers of people once monthly at a low dosage for many years. Increase in resistance to penicillin can be induced *in vitro* but occurs in small steps and would only be expected to arise *in vivo* under circumstances such as those described or, of course, when a single dose regimen is used as in the treatment of gonorrhoea. Increased resistance of *Streptococcus pyogenes* to tetracycline had become common (approximately 40 per cent) among the general population by 1960 (Parker *et al.*, 1962) and more recently we found an increasing incidence of tetracycline-resistant pneumococci in the Liverpool area (Percival *et al.*, 1969). At the Royal Infirmary, Liverpool, tetracycline-resistant strains increased from 6 per cent in 1967 to 23 per cent in 1968 and included a variety of different sero-types. Table 3 shows the incidence of resistant strains throughout the years 1968 and 1969. There was a progressive rise to a maximum during the summer months. This suggests that the main reservoir of these strains was in patients with chronic disease, because infection in summer tends to occur mostly in them. However, resistant strains appeared also to be spreading in the community at home, since they were also found in children on admission to hospital. With a number of strains, the resistance of pneumococci to tetracycline would be missed in laboratories using too high a disc strength of the antibiotic, for example 50 micrograms as recommended in the Association of Clinical Pathologists Broadsheet on Antibiotic Sensitivity Tests (Barber & Stokes, 1966).

TABLE 3

INCIDENCE OF TETRACYCLINE-RESISTANT PNEUMOCOCCI IN SPUTUM FROM PATIENTS IN THE ROYAL INFIRMARY, LIVERPOOL

Period	*No. pneumococci isolated*		*Per cent tetracycline resistant*	
	1968	1969	1968	1969
Oct. to Jan.[a]	60	40	6	10
Feb. to Mar.	27	40	22	22
Apr. to May	44	26	23	20
Jun. to Sept.	24	45	33	32

[a] 1967–68 and 1968–69 respectively.

Resistance of *H. influenzae* to tetracycline (minimum inhibitory concentration 12·5 μg per ml or above) is less common, being only 7·6 per cent of the last 150 isolates in this laboratory. As yet, evidence of increasing resistance of *H. influenzae* to penicillins has not been described. However, of the last 150 isolates we have tested, the M.I.Cs. of ampicillin were 5 μg per ml for 6 strains (4 per cent) and 2·5 μg per ml for another 9 (6 per cent); the normal range being between 0·3 and 1·0 μg per ml by the method we use. Only sequential testing will show whether there is a trend toward an increasing proportion of strains showing diminished sensitivity, but the tendency for the organism to persist after treatment and the difficulty in attaining adequate levels of antibiotic in the bronchial secretions suggest that such a trend is a possibility.

When significant changes occur in the frequency of resistance of common infecting organisms, the choice of antibiotic for initial treatment on a best guess basis should be altered accordingly. In an area with 25 per cent or more strains resistant to tetracycline, this agent should no longer be used for lower respiratory infection unless and until the causative organism has been identified and found to be sensitive. Unfortunately, general practitioners continue to use tetracycline for the treatment of sore throat despite the high level of resistant *Strept. pyogenes* in the community and the damage this agent can cause to the teeth of young children.

ERADICATION OF BACTERIA FROM THE RESPIRATORY TRACT

The difficulty of eradicating *Strept. pyogenes* from the upper respiratory tract in order to prevent rheumatic fever is well known. For example, Brumfitt and Slater (1957) found that after a 4-day course of procaine penicillin 300,000 units and benzyl penicillin 100,000 units given intramuscularly twice daily, the convalescent carrier-rate was identical with that of an untreated group. Recently, Ross (1971) using the more sensitive method of salivary counting rather than throat swabs found failure rates of 23 and 13 per cent at 5 and 9 days respectively in children given oral penicillin 0·5 to 1 g orally daily.

Therapy for 10 days has previously been shown to be necessary for eradication (Wannamaker *et al.*, 1953). Pneumococci are also highly sensitive to antibiotics but with this organism, sero-typing has shown that they may persist in the upper respiratory tract of chronic bronchitics for many months despite antimicrobial treatment (Calder & Schonell, 1971).

If such sensitive organisms as pneumococci and *Strept. pyogenes* can persist in the upper respiratory tract despite antibacterial treatment, it is not surprising that *H. influenzae* which is 10 to 20 times less sensitive to penicillins will be even more difficult to eradicate. The type of regimen usually recommended for exacerbations of chronic bronchitis of tetracycline 250 mg or ampicillin 0·5 to 1 g four times daily for at least 5 days (McNicol, 1969) may well effect symptomatic improvement, but not infrequently can be expected to be insufficient to ensure eradication of the infecting organism to prevent the possibility of relapse. Therefore, a reappraisal of the amount and duration of antibiotic treatment to be given to patients with underlying chest disease appears to be overdue. Treatment should be designed to remove the pathogenic organism from the respiratory tract and should be given at a dosage and for a period more likely to achieve this than are the currently prescribed regimens.

PENETRATION OF ANTIBIOTICS INTO SPUTUM

Most antibiotics penetrate poorly into sputum, the concentrations being lower than those in the serum. Sputum concentrations are commonly below or at best only slightly higher than those required to inhibit common infecting organisms such as *H. influenzae*. The marginal relationship between sputum and inhibitory levels for some of the commonly used antibiotics is reviewed by May (1968). In addition, he showed that, for ampicillin, the sputum concentration tended to be lower in mucoid than purulent specimens, but irrespective of purulence was still not directly related to blood levels in different individuals. Furthermore, although increased sputum concentrations could be obtained by increasing the dose of ampicillin, apparently there was a limit for a particular subject beyond which further increase in sputum level could not be achieved by raising the dose. These observations have been confirmed for a variety of different antibiotics in patients with cystic fibrosis (Saggers & Lawson, 1968). In 40 patients receiving ampicillin, the author has also confirmed the relationship between dose and sputum concentration. Figure 1 shows the range of M.I.Cs. for *H. influenzae* related to sputum levels of ampicillin obtained with different dosage. It can be seen that 1 g of ampicillin is needed to inhibit most strains of *H. influenzae*, but that in some patients inhibitory levels are not attained even with this high dose. The clinical value of attention to detail in prescribing an adequate dose of antibiotic is suggested by May's experience that 1 g of ampicillin given 6 hourly for 7 days may be followed by relatively prolonged remissions whereas at a lower dose, relapse soon follows when treatment is stopped.

It should be remembered that some of the more recently developed antimicrobials, such as lincomycin, clindamycin, cephaloridine and cephalexin, are relatively much less active against *H. influenzae* than are antibiotics already much used in treatment of respiratory infection. The M.I.Cs. of these agents for *H. influenzae* are often higher than the blood levels obtained by conventional therapeutic dosage and, although data of sputum concentrations are unavailable, it is unlikely that these would be sufficiently high to justify the use of these antibiotics for chest infections caused by *H. influenzae*. On the other hand, trimethoprim is highly active against *H. influenzae* and is concentrated in lung tissue in animals (Bushby & Hitchings, 1968). Trimethoprim sputum concentrations exceeding those in the blood by a factor of

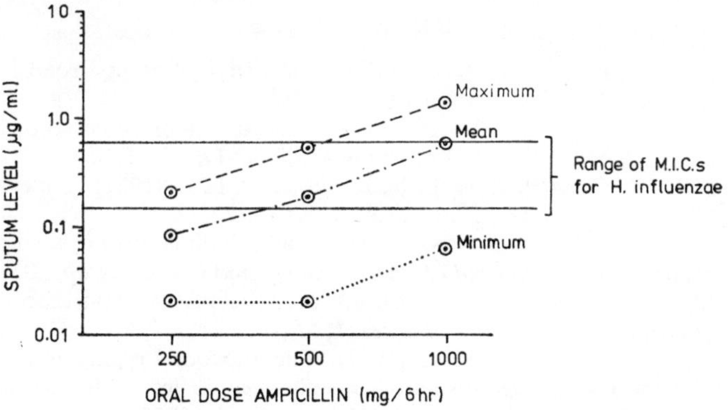

FIG. 1. Relationship between sensitivity of *H. Influenzae* and sputum levels of Ampicillin according to dose.

2·5 have been reported following oral administration (Pechere & Beck, 1969) and if these findings are confirmed, this would offer an explanation for the promising clinical results reported in a trial of co-trimoxazole in treatment of exacerbations of chronic bronchitis (Hughes, 1969).

CONCLUSIONS

Laboratory diagnosis of respiratory tract infection is difficult because the usual infecting organisms may occur in the normal flora. However, providing that fresh specimens of sputum are sent to the laboratory without delay before antimicrobial treatment is started, assessment by microscopy and culture after homogenization should enable the causative bacteria to be identified. Quantitative cultures are of value in judging the possible significance of organisms isolated, but will not differentiate between infection and upper respiratory tract contamination in every instance. Diagnosis becomes even more difficult when the normal flora is replaced by resistant organisms as a result of antimicrobial therapy and a profuse growth of an organism such as *Ps. aeruginosa* from a purulent specimen derived from a patient with a tracheostomy need not be an indication for treatment unless the clinical and radiological findings suggest pulmonary involvement. Because infection by such resistant organisms is very difficult to treat, more attention should be given to disinfection of the sources of these bacteria.

Eradication of even the more sensitive pathogenic bacteria from the respiratory tract often requires a longer course of antibiotics than is commonly given and at increased dosage. Effective therapy is limited by the poor penetration of many antimicrobials into sputum and relapse due to persistence of bacteria in the bronchial tree is the rule rather than the exception in subjects with chronic respiratory tract disease.

REFERENCES

BARBER, M. & STOKES, E. J. (1966). Antibiotic sensitivity testing, Broadsheet No. 55, Association of Clinical Pathologists.

BRUMFITT, W. & SLATER, J. D. H. (1957). Treatment of acute sore throat with penicillin. A controlled trial in young soldiers. *Lancet*, **1**, 8.

BRUMFITT, W., WILLOUGHBY, M. L. N. & BROMLEY, L. L. (1957). An evaluation of sputum examination in chronic bronchitis. *Lancet*, **2**, 1306.

BUSHBY, S. R. M. & HITCHINGS, G. H. (1968). Trimethoprim, a sulphonamide potentiator. *British Journal of Pharmacology and Chemotherapy*, **33**, 72.

CALDER, M. A., MCHARDY, V. U. & SCHONELL, M. E. (1970). Importance of pneumococcal typing in pneumonia. *Lancet*, **1**, 5.

CALDER, M. A. & SCHONELL, M. E. (1971). Pneumococcal typing and the problem of endogenous or exogenous re-infection in chronic bronchitis. *Lancet*, **1**, 1156.

CLIFTON, M., POWNALL, M. & STUART HARRIS, C. H. (1955). Observations on the carriage of pneumococci by patients with chronic bronchitis and their families. *Journal of Hygiene (Cambridge)*, **53**, 225.

COOPER, A. W., WILLIAMSON, G. M. & ZINNEMAN, K. (1961). Chronic bronchitis; changes in the bacterial flora of the sputum associated with exacerbations and long term antibacterial treatment. *British Journal of Diseases of the Chest*, **55**, 23.

DIXON, J. M. S. & MILLER, D. C. (1965). Value of dilute inocula in culture examination of sputum. *Lancet*, **2**, 1046.

FISHER, M., AKHTAR, A. J., CALDER, M. A., MOFFAT, M. A., STEWART, S. M., ZEALLEY, H. & CROFTON, J. W. (1969). Pilot study of factors associated with exacerbations in chronic bronchitis. *British Medical Journal*, **4**, 187.

GRIST, N. R., LANDSMAN, J. B., ANDERSON, T., ROWAN, G. & SMITH, A. (1952). Studies in the aetiology of pneumonia in Glasgow 1950–1951. *Lancet*, **1**, 640.

HANSMAN, D., GLASGOW, H., STURT, J., DEVITT, L. & DOUGLAS, R. (1971). Increased resistance to penicillin of pneumococci isolated from man. *New England Journal of Medicine*, **284**, 175.

HOLDAWAY, M. D. & TURK, D. C. (1967). Capsulated *Haemophilus influenzae* and respiratory tract disease. *Lancet*, **1**, 358.

HUGHES, D. T. D. (1969). Single blind comparative trial of trimethoprimsulphamethoxazole and ampicillin in the treatment of exacerbations of chronic bronchitis. *British Medical Journal*, **3**, 470.

LAURENZI, G. A., POTTER, R. T. & KASS, E. H. (1961). Bacteriologic flora of the lower respiratory tract. *New England Journal of Medicine*, **265**, 1273.

LEES, A. W. & MCNAUGHT, W. (1959). Non-tuberculous bacterial flora of sputum and of the upper and lower respiratory tract in pulmonary tuberculosis. *Lancet*, **2**, 1115.

LOURIA, D. B. (1962). Uses of quantitative analysis of bacterial populations in sputum. *Journal of the American Medical Association*, **182**, 1082.

MCNICOL, M. W. (1969). Chronic bronchitis. *Prescribers Journal*, **9**, 90.

MAY, J. R. (1953). The bacteriology of chronic bronchitis. *Lancet*, **2**, 534.

MAY, J. R. (1968). *Chemotherapy of Chronic Bronchitis.* English University Press, Ltd., London.

MAY, J. R. & DELVES, D. M. (1964). The survival of *H. influenzae* and pneumococci in specimens of sputum sent to the laboratory by post. *Journal of Clinical Pathology*, **17**, 254.

MEAD, G. R. & WOODHAMS, A. W. (1964). *N*-acetyl-1-cysteine as liquefying agent in the bacteriological examination of sputum. *Tubercle, London*, **45**, 370.

MULDER, J. (1938). *Haemophilus influenzae* (Pfeiffer) as an unbiquitous cause of common acute and chronic purulent bronchitis. *Acta Medica Scandinavica*, **94**, 98.

PARKER, M. T., MAXTED, W. R. & FRASER, C. A. (1962). Tetracycline-resistant haemolytic streptococci. *British Medical Journal*, **1**, 1550.

PECHERE, J. C. & BECK, H. (1969). Cited in Hughes (1969)—see above.

PERCIVAL, A., ARMSTRONG, E. C. & TURNER, G. C. (1969). Increased incidence of tetracycline-resistant pneumococci in Liverpool in 1968. *Lancet*, **1**, 998.

PERCIVAL, A. & ROBERTS, C. (1972). Significance of Enterobacteria and Pseudomonas in sputum. In *Microbiology of the Seventies* (Ed., Baker, F. J.), Butterworths, London.

PRICE, D. J. E. & SLEIGH, J. D. (1970). Control of infection due to *Klebsiella aerogenes* in a neurosurgical unit by withdrawal of all antibiotics. *Lancet*, **2**, 1213.

RAWLINS, G. A. (1953). Liquefaction of sputum for bacteriological examination. *Lancet*, **2**, 538.

RAWLINS, G. A. (1968). Use of pancreatin-trypsin solution for liquefaction of sputa for routine bacteriological examination. *Journal of Clinical Pathology*, **21**, 531.

REINARZ, J. A., PIERCE, A. K., MAYS, B. B. & SANFORD, J. P. (1965). The potential role of inhalation therapy equipment in nosocomial pulmonary infection. *Journal of Clinical Investigation*, **44**, 831.

ROSS, P. W. (1971). Bacteriological monitoring in penicillin treatment of streptococcal sore throat. *Journal of Hygiene* (*Cambridge*), **69**, 355.

SAGGERS, B. A. & LAWSON, D. N. (1968). *In vivo* penetration of antibiotics into sputum in cystic fibrosis. *Archives of Diseases of Childhood*, **43**, 404.

SHOOTER, R. A., FAIERS, M. C., COOKE, E. M., BREADEN, A. L. & O'FARRELL, S. M. (1971). Isolation of *Esch. coli, Pseudomonas aeruginosa* and Klebsiella from food in hospitals, canteens and schools. *Lancet*, **2**, 390.

TILLOTSON, J. R. & LERNER, A. M. (1967). Characteristics of pneumonias caused by *Escherichia coli. New England Journal of Medicine*, **277**, 115.

TURK, D. C. & MAY, J. R. (1967). Haemophilus influenzae; *its clinical importance.* English University Press, Ltd., London.

WANNAMAKER, L. W., DENNY, F. W., PERRY, W., RAMMELKAMP, C. H., ECKHARDT, G. C., HOUSER, H. B. & HAHN, E. O. (1953). The effect of penicillin prophylaxis on streptococcal disease rates and the carrier state. *New England Journal of Medicine*, **249**, 1.

15

TREATMENT OF RESPIRATORY TRACT INFECTION: A CLINICIAN'S VIEWPOINT

D. J. LANE

THERE is little doubt that 30 years of antibiotic therapy have transformed the picture presented by respiratory tract infections. This survey will glance back at our achievements, use them to point to present-day problems and attempt to peep briefly into the future.

ANTIBIOTICS AND DEATH RATES FROM RESPIRATORY DISEASES

As to achievement, it is evident that antibiotic therapy is, to a large extent, responsible for the dramatic decline in specific bacterial respiratory tract infections. The enormous changes in mortality from pneumonia are illustrated in Figure 1 which refers to male subjects of all ages in England and Wales

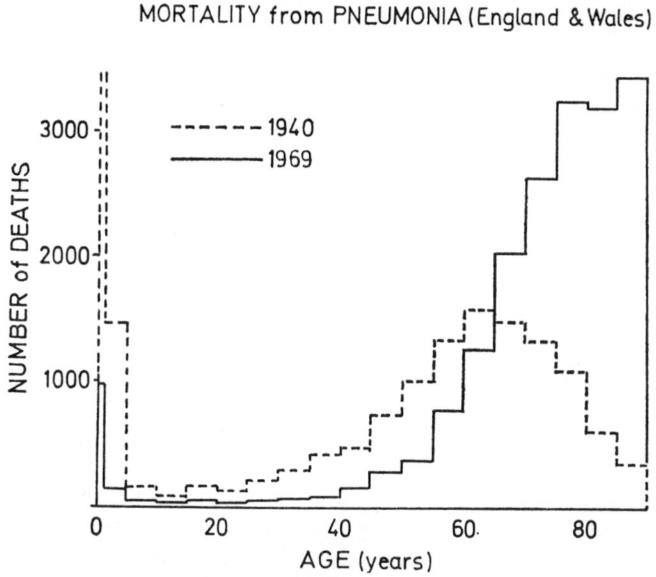

FIG. 1. Mortality from pneumonia (England and Wales) in 1940 and in 1969.

in the 2 years 1940 and 1969 which span the antibiotic era. The dramatic improvement in pneumonia deaths in children and young adults is very obvious. At the other end of the age scale, in the elderly, the peak incidence of death from pneumonia has receded from around 60 into the over 80s. But interestingly, the total number of deaths due to pneumonia in males of all ages in 1969 was greater by 15 per cent than pneumonia deaths in 1940 even though the total numbers dying from all causes were almost identical.

To illustrate from another specific infection, deaths from tuberculosis have been declining since the beginning of the century but this trend has certainly hastened since the introduction of specific chemotherapy in the 1950s as seen in Figure 2. On the other hand, this figure also shows that mortality from chronic bronchitis has remained obstinately static (Registrar General's Statistical Return, 1966).

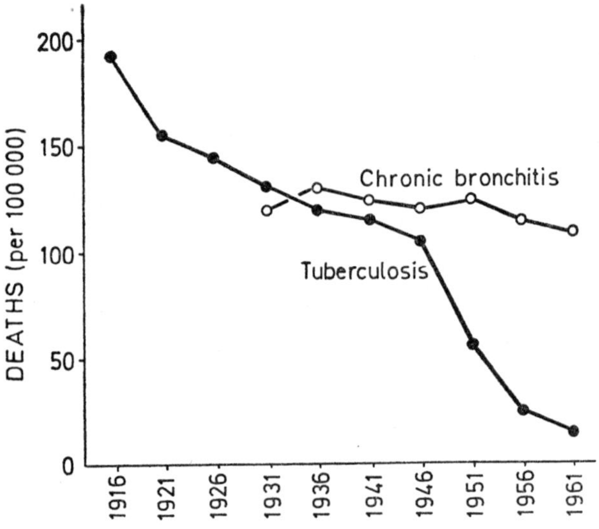

FIG. 2. Death rates from tuberculosis and chronic bronchitis by 5-year periods in males aged 45–64 from 1916 to 1965.

PERSISTENCE OF CHRONIC BRONCHITIS

The reasons for the persistence of chronic bronchitis and perhaps of pneumonia in the elderly, which is often secondary to bronchitis, are of course complex: an increasing incidence of chronic lung disease associated with cigarette smoking but a decreasing incidence due to control of air pollution: changes in the overall pattern of other diseases and in the reliability of death certification and so on. However, the fundamental problem is that chronic bronchitis is not basically an infective illness, but a chronic irritative lesion of the bronchi. Respiratory tract infections occur as clinically important, but pathologically incidental, events in a long drawn out process which starts with a smoker's cough and ends with ventilatory failure. Nonetheless, infection in chronic bronchitis represents the major demand for antibiotic therapy in respiratory disease today.

The decline in specific infections and the emergence of chronic bronchitis have been two factors contributing to the greatly altered pattern of respiratory tract infection over the last 30 years. In the pre-antibiotic era for example, infection with a pneumococcus appeared to cause a relatively clear cut picture of lobar pneumonia. Furthermore, it seemed that the pneumococcus did little else when invading the lung and that lobar pneumonia was seldom due to any other organisms. Similar, though not always as clear cut relationships, were thought to exist between staphylococci, streptococci, Friedlanders bacillus and other different clinical pictures, whereas *Haemophilus influenzae*, *Escherichia coli*, Pseudomonas *spp.* and their ilk were thought to play little part in respiratory tract infections.

RELATIONSHIP OF PATHOGENS TO DISEASE TODAY

In the 1970s following 30 years of the use of antibiotics, that perhaps all too neat pattern has been so altered that diagnostic correlations between microbiology and clinical features are no longer clearly defined. Although it is more than uncharitable to suggest that the use of antibiotics has anything directly to do with our present diagnostic confusion, it is perhaps worth reflecting that an effective therapy is sometimes an unfortunate damper to further investigation. The patho-physiology of pulmonary emphysema, about which we can do so little, has been exhaustively studied: respiratory tract infection for which we can do so much is far less well investigated.

DIFFICULTIES IN PRECISE DIAGNOSIS

The reasons for present-day diagnostic difficulties are threefold:

(1) A basic diagnostic dilemma.
(2) A clinical indifference.
(3) A genuine change in microbial flora.

There is a basic, somewhat fundamental, dilemma in relation to respiratory tract infection which it is very difficult to overcome, namely:

A particular clinical syndrome may be produced by a variety of infective agents.
The same infective agent may produce a variety of different syndromes.

Thus primary atypical pneumonia is often due to infection with *Mycoplasma pneumoniae* but may also be a result of rickettsial, bedsonia or various viral infections. Conversely, *M. pneumoniae* infection of the respiratory tract may be entirely symptomless or may cause a variety of syndromes apart from primary atypical pneumonia, ranging from a simple upper respiratory tract infection to a bullous myringitis or a tracheobronchitis.

Secondly, we appear to suffer from clinical lethargy. We fail to pick up important clues in the patient's history, examination or environmental circumstances which would lead us to suspect one organism rather than another and antibiotics are used with gay abandon, often without any attempt to make a proper bacterial diagnosis.

For example, in 1967, the position in relation to pneumonia in the Radcliffe Infirmary was assessed by Dr. D. C. Turk. In a group of 77 patients with pneumonia as diagnosed on clinical and radiological grounds, sputum was sent in only 44 per cent and of these, only just over one-third grew a respectable pathogen. Blood cultures were taken in 18 per cent and only one was positive. This survey of our bacteriological endeavour appeared rather dismal in scientific terms although there was insufficient evidence to decide whether the lack of bacteriological precision had had any adverse effect on the clinical outcome in individual cases.

The third factor causing diagnostic confusion is that there appears to have been a change in the microbial flora in relation to respiratory tract infections. It is of course difficult to decide how much of this is genuine, how much a consequence of changes in technique or interpretation. Certain organisms are more easily grown using modern culture media. Thus *H. influenzae*, formerly a 'commensal', is now more often a 'significant pathogen'. The last 30 years have also seen the development of effective techniques for the detection of viral infection. What part viruses played in respiratory tract infections in pre-antibiotic days, we shall never know. However, despite these factors, there do seem to have been genuine changes, particularly in relation to gram-negative organisms where the interpretation of sputum microbiology has become exceedingly complex as Dr. Percival's paper has so clearly pinpointed.

A LOGICAL APPROACH TO RESPIRATORY INFECTIONS

To circumvent these diagnostic difficulties, a three-pronged attack can be proposed:

(a) a detailed survey of the correlations between various clinical syndromes and microbiological studies.
(b) an exploration of different techniques for obtaining material for microbiological study.
(c) the evolution of a rational therapeutic approach based on the knowledge so gained and constantly revised in the light of new information.

Relating clinical and laboratory findings

Various centres have been reporting over recent years the results of clinical/microbiological associations. The patterns for the viral agents responsible for acute upper respiratory tract infections in various parts of the world are emerging (Evans, 1967). The aetiology of primary atypical pneumonia is now known to be much broader than mycoplasmal infection and clues leading the clinician to suspect mycoplasma, rickettsia or bedsonia organisms have been suggested. A detailed study of this type of correlation in pneumonia has come from Schonell *et al.* (1969) from Edinburgh. They divided 106 patients into 53 who showed serological evidence of viral or mycoplasmal infection and 53 who did not. Bacterial isolations were slightly more common in the latter group (52 per cent compared to 35 per cent) but there were no clear cut differences between the groups in terms of sputum purulence, clinical features, ESR, degree of leucocytosis or radiological findings. Despite these somewhat disappointing findings, it seems important to press ahead with this type of analysis and I have recently attempted to do so from the opposite angle, namely to make an analysis of the types of respiratory illness associated with infection with one particular organism namely *H. influenzae*.

As the organism responsible for human influenza, its star rose and fell equally precipitously and it was not until the 1950s that it was resurrected by May and others as of fundamental importance in infective episodes occurring in patients with chronic bronchitis. But it was only one organism amongst many. *H. influenzae* may occur in 15–50 per cent of cases but it shares the infective honours with *Streptococcus pneumoniae*, *Staphylococcus aureus* and several other organisms. This is an example of the association between one clinical state and several organisms.

The reverse of this, the clinical states associated with the isolation of one organism, has been less well documented for *H. influenzae*. At one end of the scale, it is well known that significant growths of this organism may be obtained from mucoid sputa in patients symptomless at least as far as infective features are concerned. However, at the other end of the scale, undoubted cases of cavitating pneumonia have been reported in which *H. influenzae* has been isolated from blood culture as well as from the sputum or lungs (Goldstein *et al.*, 1967).

To obtain a more balanced general picture, I recently used Dr. Turk's *H. influenzae* records to trace a series of patients from whose sputa *H. influenzae* had been isolated. These came from the general wards of the Radcliffe Infirmary and included both medical and surgical cases. The first surprise was to find so relatively few patients in this survey who presented with an acute infective exacerbation of chronic bronchitis. Table 1 details the findings. Half the patients developed a chest infection after some spell of unconsciousness, whether this was anaesthesia for surgery, head injury or some medical cause of coma. The slightly elevated WBCs and ESRs found in some patients gave mean values not significantly different in the two groups. The frequency of fever was unexpected as were the radiological findings. It certainly seemed that this organism could be quite frequently associated with parenchymal lung involvement. X-rays had been taken in 72 of the 83 patients and showed related abnormalities in 43 per cent. Collapse was common, not only in the loss of consciousness group, and in 10, there was consolidation, 2 of these presenting the picture of a cavitating pneumonia. *H. influenzae* thus appears to be a genuine pathogen quite often and not just a relatively innocent bystander in the bronchi.

TABLE 1

HAEMOPHILUS INFLUENZAE SPUTUM ISOLATIONS
RADCLIFFE INFIRMARY 1970–71

	No. of patients
Group I: Medical cases of primarily respiratory illness	
Acute infective exacerbations of chronic bronchitis, bronchiectasis or asthma	17
Pneumonia, carcinoma of bronchus	10
Miscellaneous	13
	40
Group II: Loss of consciousness cases	
Anaesthesia for surgery	31
Trauma	11
Medical (C.V.A., overdose, etc.)	6
	48

	Group I	*Group II*	*Significance of difference*
Smoker/Bronchitic	31/40	35/48	N.S.[a]
Mean temp. °C	37^3	37^8	$P < 0.005$
Mean WBC/mm^3	9310	10,960	N.S.
Mean ESR mm/h	43·9	33·6	N.S.
Chest X-ray—Pneumonia	6	7	N.S.
Collapse	7	7	
Other	13	22	
No lesion	12	14	

[a] N.S. = Not significant.

Collection of specimens for bacteriological examination

An alternative approach to better diagnosis is a more careful attention to technical detail. The clinician must ruefully accept the bacteriologists' sarcastic comments about sputum sample collection. This is all too often carried out in an unintelligent, slipshod fashion. The difficulties inherent in the examination of the expectorated secretions of the respiratory tract should perhaps encourage us to examine other techniques for obtaining material suitable for bacteriological examination. Blood culture is a neglected art and is more often positive in an early, untreated pneumococcal pneumonia than the scanty sputum. Most pneumonias extend to the pleura and cause sufficient reaction to provide a source of a few drops of bacteriologically precious fluid obtainable by simple pleural tap.

In infants, from whom sputum is seldom available, Mimica *et al.* (1971) have recently revived a technique for bacteriologic diagnosis in pneumonia first described in 1880—lung puncture. They obtained positive bacterial cultures, chiefly *Staph. aureus*, from 45 per cent of 505 infants less than 2 years of age. Their findings were used to establish a more rational 'blind' antibiotic regime for treating pneumonia in these children. In the same infants, positive cultures of the same organisms were obtained from the pharynx in only 11 per cent, from the anterior nares in 13 per cent and from the trachea in 20 per cent. Transtracheal aspiration of sputum is a technique applicable to other age groups (for few would be keen on lung puncture in adult bronchitics). Hahn and Beaty (1970) recently reported on the use of this technique in adults, finding it especially useful in the early stages of a pneumonia or in semi-conscious patients. Tracheal aspirates gave positive isolations in about two-thirds more instances than did expectorated sputum.

Rational approach to antibiotic therapy

But whilst further study and better techniques are undoubtedly going to be of importance, the clinician must face the situation as it presents itself here and now and work out a rational approach to antibiotic therapy accepting the diagnostic difficulties that exist and basing his recommendations on available knowledge. The treatment of sub-acute or chronic chest infections, when there is time to wait for a bacteriologic report, will be strongly influenced by that report and the antibiotic sensitivities reported as a result of *in vitro* testing. Leaving these cases aside, I would like to suggest an approach to the patient presenting with an acute respiratory tract infection either to the G.P.'s surgery or to the hospital emergency room. In both instances, the doctor will rely largely on clinical judgement. Although the houseman will have the doubtful advantage of the chest X-ray, no bacteriology will be available apart from a sputum gram stain which will be of value providing it is carried out by somebody with competence.

The first step is to place the patient in some workable diagnostic category such as that listed in Table 2. Even this relatively short list is too long for the

TABLE 2

SYNDROMES OF RESPIRATORY TRACT INFECTION

1. The common cold (coryza)
2. The sore throat (acute tonsilitis and pharyngitis)
3. Acute upper respiratory tract infection (influenza)
4. Croup—children only (acute laryngo-tracheo-bronchitis)
5. Acute lower respiratory tract infection (tracheo-bronchitis, bronchitis: also primary atypical pneumonia)
6. Acute bronchiolitis—children only
7. Pneumonia
8. Acute exacerbation of chronic bronchitis

circumstances being considered and I would like to confine my attention to syndromes 5, 7 and 8; acute lower respiratory tract infections, pneumonia and acute infective exacerbations of chronic bronchitis. These diagnostic categories must then be matched to the three therapeutic categories as outlined in Table 3.

TABLE 3

INDICATIONS FOR ANTIBIOTIC THERAPY IN RESPIRATORY TRACT INFECTIONS

1. Conditions in which bacterial infection is highly likely and therefore antibiotics are essential
2. Conditions in which a significant number of cases presenting with a given syndrome are likely to be due to bacteria and where antibiotics are indicated because of a reasonable chance that such bacteria will be present
3. Conditions in which bacteria may be responsible for super-infection in a primarily non-bacterial illness and for which the use of antibiotics is problematical, although they may afford an amelioration of certain symptoms

Conditions in which bacterial infection is highly likely and therefore antibiotics are essential.

Clinical or radiological evidence of consolidation will put the patient into this category because bacteria are very often implicated. If there are good grounds for suspecting a pneumococcus, then benzyl penicillin is adequate but in the presence of an influenza epidemic, the greatly increased likelihood of staphylococcal infection points to a need for an anti-staphylococcal antibiotic e.g. cloxacillin or flucloxacillin. In a dose capable of demolishing the resistant staphylococcus, these antibiotics will also kill off the pneumococci. Many series have emphasized the coccal nature of most pneumonias associated with influenza. A few other pneumonias are primarily viral but, at least in previously healthy subjects, very few are primarily of gram-negative origin, so that a broad spectrum antibiotic is not indicated.

Conditions in which a significant number of cases presenting with a given syndrome are likely to be due to bacteria.

When there is no evidence of consolidation and the patient is not a bronchitic, the diagnosis is that of a simple acute lower respiratory tract infection. Three in four cases would be due to a virus but from time to time, *M. pneumoniae* would be implicated and a tetracycline or erythromycin should be considered. Indeed, one might advocate this antibiotic in all such cases on this one in four chance, though most clinicians would prefer some hint based on clinical or laboratory data that an epidemic is around.

Conditions in which bacteria may be responsible for super-infection in a primarily non-bacterial illness and for which the use of antibiotics is problematical

Acute infective exacerbations of chronic bronchitis are placed in the problematic group to emphasize several aspects. Firstly, as previously stated, chronic bronchitis is not primarily an infective illness. The trachea and major bronchi of the bronchitic, unlike those of normal subjects which are sterile, are permanently colonized by bacteria. Various insults ranging from a change in atmospheric conditions to an acute viral infection will upset this relatively saprophytic arrangement and allow bacterial over-growth giving the clinical picture of an acute infective exacerbation of chronic bronchitis. Secondly, prophylactic antibiotics, once strongly advocated, have never been scientifically shown to be of any value in chronic bronchitis. Thirdly, some authors, notably Elmes *et al.* (1965), have suggested that antibiotics are not necessary in acute infective exacerbations of chronic bronchitis at least as seen in hospital practice. Several criticisms can be levelled at that paper but it serves as a reminder that many other factors besides antibiotics are important in chronic bronchitis; bronchodilators, diuretics, oxygen and physiotherapy to mention but a few.

Despite these reservations, antibiotics are generally both used and needed in the acute infective exacerbation in a chronic bronchitic. For the ambulant patient having one or perhaps two exacerbations per winter, any of several anti-microbials which will attack *H. influenzae* and *Strept. pneumoniae*, will suffice. Tetracyclines are still used by many but the increasing incidence of resistant strains of both of these organisms is causing concern. Ampicillin 250 mg q.d.s. is my first choice although others prefer cotrimoxazole 2 tablets b.d. In fact, it seems to matter little which agent is used since all are of similar efficacy. For the patient having more frequent exacerbations, the regime of ampicillin 1 g q.d.s. suggested by May (1968) is sometimes successful in prolonging the infection-free period after an exacerbation. For the serious exacerbation requiring hospitalization, systemic antibiotics are often mandatory, the broad spectrum agents again generally being favoured (e.g. ampicillin or cephaloridine).

Pneumonia in chronic bronchitis

The question of what antibiotic to use in the bronchitic who develops pneumonia especially during an influenza epidemic is a thorny one. Data on pneumonia during the 1957 epidemic collected from Sheffield showed clearly the fatal consequences of staphylococcal infection, overall mortality being 48 per cent compared with 16 per cent in non-staphylococcal pneumonias (Stuart-Harris, 1965). This tendency was more marked in patients with previous chronic chest disease, chiefly chronic bronchitis (staphylococcal pneumonia mortality 54 per cent compared with previously healthy subjects, mortality 42 per cent). During the 1969 epidemic, more cases were reported in whom gram-negative organisms were isolated. The reasons for this are undoubtedly complex. Two possibilities may be suggested. Firstly, the too liberal use of broad-spectrum antibiotics giving a free field for *Escherichia coli* and pseudomonas and secondly, a greater use of apparatus for ventilatory assistance. Humidifiers and ventilators readily harbour gram-negative organisms especially pseudomonas and although they are rarely true pathogens, they can become so in seriously debilitated bronchitic patients. So in general, the recommendations for pneumonia should perhaps be allowed to override the antibiotic recommendations for the straight acute infective exacerbation of chronic bronchitis and the choice be that of flucloxacillin for the chronic bronchitic with pneumonia. At the time therapy is initiated, sputum samples will be sent off. If a gram-negative organism is cultured consistently in association with clinical and radiological changes, then an appropriate antibiotic is required. For *H. influenzae*, the choice of ampicillin is easy and effective. For pseudomonas, the choice is more complex and controversial. Some of the available series are summarized in Table 4 and lead to the conclusion that a gentamicin/carbenicillin combination is about the most effective available at present. Each antibiotic is administered by the systemic and inhalation routes (20 G carbenicillin systemically; 4 G orally; 300 mg gentamicin systemically, 160 mg orally daily) (Pines *et al.*, 1970).

TABLE 4

ANTIBIOTICS IN PSEUDOMONAS PULMONARY INFECTIONS
A summary of some reported cases

Therapy	*Number*	*Recovered*	*Improved*	*Failed*
Gentamicin	38	10	7	21 (55 per cent)
Carbenicillin	64	31	12	21 (33 per cent)
Carbenicillin + Gentamicin	17	10	2	5 (29 per cent)

In conclusion, it is evident that these recommendations are somewhat empirical. A thorough reappraisal of the microbiology of respiratory tract infections and a re-definition of the clinical syndromes associated with the isolation of different organisms from the respiratory tract are required. Thirty years of antibiotics have bestowed great benefits, posed great problems and provided a constant challenge to clinical medicine.

REFERENCES

ELMES, P. C., KING, T. K. C., LANGLANDS, J. H. M., MACKAY, J. A., WALLACE, W. F. M., WADE, O. L. & WILSON, T. S. (1965). Value of ampicillin in the hospital treatment of exacerbations of chronic bronchitis. *British Medical Journal*, **2,** 904.

EVANS, A. S. (1967). Clinical syndromes in adults caused by respiratory infection. *Medical Clinics of North America*, **51,** 803.

GOLDSTEIN, E., DALY, A. K. & SEAMANS, C. (1967). Haemophilus influenzae as a cause of adult pneumonia. *Annals of Internal Medicine*, **66,** 35.

HAHN, H. H. & BEATY, H. N. (1970). Transtracheal aspiration in the evaluation of patients with pneumonia. *Annals of Internal Medicine*, **72,** 183.

MAY, J. R. (1968). *Chemotherapy of Chronic Bronchitis and Allied Conditions.* Published by English Universities Press Ltd., London.

MIMICA, I., DONOSO, E., HOWARD, J. E. & LEDERMANN, G. W. (1971). Lung puncture in the etiological diagnosis of pneumonia. *American Journal of Diseases of Children*, **122,** 278.

PINES, A., RAAFAT, H., SIDDIQUI, G. M. & GREENFIELD, J. S. B. (1970). Treatment of severe pseudomonas infections of the bronchi. *British Medical Journal*, **1,** 663.

Registrar General's Statistical Returns for England and Wales, 1966.

SCHONELL, M. E., GRAY, W., MOFFAT, M. A. S., CALDER, M. A. & STEWART, S. M. (1969). The relationship between the aetiology of pneumonia in adults and certain clinical and radiographic findings. *British Journal of Diseases of the Chest*, **63**, 140.

STUART-HARRIS, C. H. (1965). *Influenza and Other Virus Infections of the Respiratory Tract*. Published by Edward Arnold Ltd., London.

DISCUSSION

Chest infections in surgery

Question. Could Dr. Lane make some comments on the treatment of post-operative chest infections? These are a great problem in hospitals.

Dr. D. J. Lane. Physiotherapy is essential. I always think that this is something that is grossly neglected in certain hospitals, especially on the surgical wards. I was a little surprised by the number of patients with *Haemophilus influenzae* in the sputum in post-operative chest infections. I must of course go back and look at it from the clinical point of view and investigate post-operative chest infections and see which organisms are isolated. If *H. influenzae* turned out to be very common, and I suspect it is only common in smokers, then I would suggest that ampicillin was indicated but would stress the importance of physiotherapy.

Question. As an anaesthetist I find that I am invariably faced with a bronchitic patient who has been started on ampicillin immediately on admission. I can't help feeling that this is bad.

Dr. D. J. Lane. It is bad if the patient is merely a bronchitic without an acute exacerbation. If he has got an acute infective exacerbation then there is some reasonable evidence that giving a course of ampicillin will reduce the duration of that illness. If he has got mucoid sputum there is very little evidence, as Dr. Percival has said, that the ampicillin penetrates and we have no evidence that it is going to do much if it does. I agree.

Gram-negative organisms and respiratory tract infection

Professor W. Brumfitt. At St. Mary's Hospital Mr. Bromley and I studied bronchitic patients and normal subjects who were being bronchoscoped for reasons such as exclusion of a tumour (Brumfitt *et al.*, 1957). The interesting thing was that the chronic bronchitics, although well and asymptomatic at the time, had bronchi colonized by *H. influenzae*. If you take a throat swab *H. influenzae* is not present in my experience, unless it is also present in the lung. The pneumococcus, on the other hand, is very commonly present in the normal throat (Masters *et al.*, 1958) so that the finding of this organism in sputum is not of very great significance, unless you can exclude that it's from the throat (Brumfitt & Willoughby, 1958).

You also mentioned serotyping of *H. influenzae* in chronic bronchitis. I have never found a serotypable *H. influenzae* in chronic bronchitis. Thus, although capsulated, the striking thing is that they don't belong to any of the Pitman types. Perhaps Dr. Percival will comment on that.

The next organism that he mentioned was *Escherichia coli*. We had a very interesting paper from one of the veterinary investigators pointing out that pigs suffer from *Esch. coli* pneumonia. He said that this only occurs following mycoplasma infections and I wonder whether the same thing applies in humans. In other words, the mere presence of this organism in the throat is usually harmless and it only colonizes the bronchus when triggered by some viral or other infection, although of course, Tillotson & Lerner (1967) have shown that you can get *Esch. coli* infections embolically from the pelvis and so on, which is a different matter.

Finally, the question of lung puncture as a method of diagnosis. This should be done with a high speed drill and not by direct puncture. It can be a very dangerous procedure unless there are pleural adhesions (in the absence of which a pneumothorax occurs). Perhaps you would comment on these points.

Dr. A. Percival. Professor Brumfitt possibly missed the beginning of my paper, because I clearly mentioned his work in 1957 which established that in approximately 80 per cent of chronic bronchitics, the bronchi were colonized by bacteria even during remission. However, I do not agree that *H. influenzae* only occurs in the throat when it is also present in the bronchi or that the presence of pneumococci in the throat excludes the possibility that they may also be in the lower respiratory tract.

I quite agree with his second point that serotypable strains of *H. influenzae* are uncommonly isolated from sputum—only in approximately 5 per cent according to Turck.

His third question is an interesting and plausible suggestion. In chickens, a fulminating infection of the air sacs can be induced by introducing both a mycoplasma and an *Esch. coli* at the same time, but not with either alone. The *Esch. coli* serotype in this situation is O2, one of the common ones in human urinary infections and I agree that a primary infection by a virus or mycoplasma may frequently be needed to allow secondary bacterial infection in the human respiratory tract, and just possibly also in the human urinary tract. It is certainly not my experience that most Gram-negative pneumonias arise by haematogenous spread as described by Tillotson and Lerner in their essentially retrospective study of hospital records. We have observed prospectively patients found to have a consistently profuse growth of Gram-negative bacilli in purulent sputa. One half of them had clinical and radiological evidence of a severe pulmonary infection; abscess, empyema, pneumonia of bronchiectasis, and there was usually no evidence at all of its being caused by bacteraemic spread. The other half of this group of patients were either chronic bronchitics or had no radiological or clinical evidence of pulmonary infection. In them the 'coliforms' may just be superficial in the bronchi and in the absence of clinical or radiological evidence of pulmonary infection, I recommend that no antibiotic treatment be given merely because the sputum contains large numbers of 'coliforms'.

Now the last question—lung puncture. I would like to add another objection; it is analogous to the use of renal biopsy to diagnose chronic pyelonephritis. Pneumonia is a patchy condition and how many punctures have to be made? Can you imagine someone puncturing the lung of an adult smoker and seeing the patient expire from pneumothorax as a puff of smoke emerges—I think it is rather dangerous. Dr. Lane, however, was referring to children under the age of 2 where it is very difficult to obtain adequate specimens of sputum.

REFERENCES

BRUMFITT, W., WILLOUGHBY, M. L. N. & BROMLEY, L. L. (1957). An evaluation of sputum examination in chronic bronchitics. *Lancet*, **2**, 1306.

BRUMFITT, W. & WILLOUGHBY, M. L. N. (1958). Laboratory differentiation of chronic bronchial disease. An investigation of 117 cases. *Lancet*, **1**, 132.

MASTERS, P. L., BRUMFITT, W., MENDEZ, R. L. & LIKER, M. (1958). Bacterial flora of the upper respiratory tract in Paddington families, 1952–4. *British Medical Journal*, **1**, 1200.

TILLOTSON, J. R. & LERNER, A. M. (1967). Characteristics of pneumonia caused by *Escherichia coli*. *New England Journal of Medicine*, **277**, 115.

16

TREATMENT OF GASTRO-INTESTINAL INFECTION: A BACTERIOLOGIST'S VIEWPOINT

R. R. GILLIES

INFECTION of the gastro-intestinal tract can be caused by bacteria, viruses, protozoa or fungi but only in the case of those of bacterial origin are antimicrobial agents of possible use and it should be noted that the use of tetracyclines in treating amoebic dysentery probably has only an indirect effect by reducing the population of bowel bacteria which form part of the food supply for the causal amoebae. This brief communication therefore will be restricted to a consideration of the part played by antimicrobial agents in treating infections of the bowel.

BACILLARY DYSENTERY

Increasing incidence

A distinguished but ill-informed professor, whilst referring to the dramatic reduction in morbidity and mortality from communicable diseases in the first half of this century, commented that the introduction of antimicrobial agents, by providing bacteriologists with the need for *in vitro* sensitivity testing, saved them from mass redundancy.

One area in which there has probably been an increase in *morbidity* is from gastro-intestinal infections and of those bacillary dysentery has increased in incidence more dramatically than any other infection. This is reflected in Figure 1 which gives the average annual incidence of notification of dysentery in Scotland from 1920 and, as will be shown later, this represents only the tip of the dysentery iceberg. Some authorities argue that this increase is only relative and can be explained away by improved laboratory facilities coupled with the introduction of more sophisticated isolation techniques which allow the causal organisms to be harvested more readily; similarly an increasing awareness of the disease on the part of the general medical practitioner is suggested as an explanation for the increasing incidence. None of these suggestions are valid so far as Scotland is concerned. There has been virtually no provision of *additional* bacteriology laboratories in the last 20 years. The most recent advance in the isolation of dysentery bacilli was in 1942 with the introduction of desoxycholate citrate agar and, as can be seen from Figure 2, if there is an increasing awareness of the notification on the part of practitioners their awareness seems to wax and wane over periods of approximately 5 to 7 years!! Figure 2 also demonstrates the almost unrelenting increase in the notified incidence of the disease.

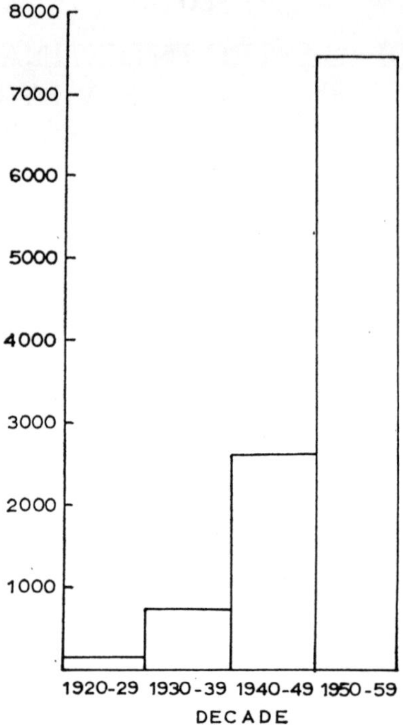

FIG. 1. Average annual incidence of notified bacillary dysentery in Scotland.

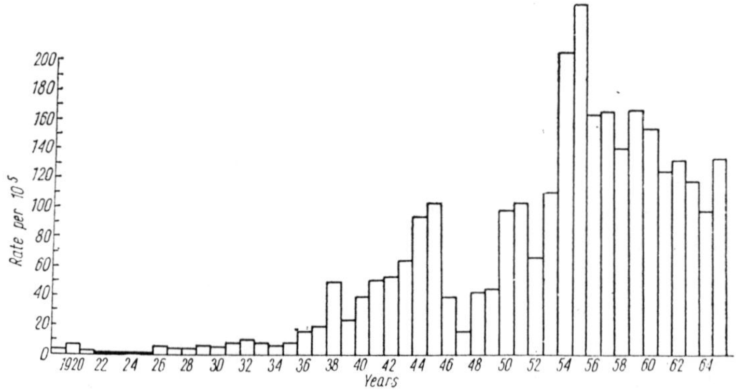

FIG. 2. Bacillary dysentery: Annual notification rates per 100,000 of Scottish population.

The Edinburgh survey

A few years ago, with the collaboration of a group of general practitioners, we undertook a prospective study over 4 years of diarrhoeal diseases in one part of the City of Edinburgh and Table 1 summarizes the laboratory findings in 1354 index cases of diarrhoea which were judged by the practitioner to be of infective origin. It will be noted that only 22·7 per cent proved to be bacterial in origin and in the latter part of the study when a search was almost

TABLE 1

RESULTS OF STOOL CULTURE IN 1354 INDEX CASES OF 'GASTRO-INTESTINAL INFECTION'

	Per cent
No pathogens isolated	77·3
Shigella sonnei	19·3
Pathogenic *Esch. coli*	1·9
Salmonellae	1·2
Shigella flexneri	0·3
	100

made for enteroviruses the proportion of cases shown to be caused by micro-organisms rose only to 30 per cent. The predominance of *Shigella sonnei* was to be expected but one of the important lessons from this survey was that highly competent physicians could not differentiate between cases which were infected and those patients from whom no acceptable pathogen could be isolated by sophisticated laboratory techniques. Similarly, in the laboratory, macroscopic and microscopic examination of stool specimens did not assist in differentiation of the infected from the uninfected patient. Further details of this survey have been published (Gillies, 1968). The larger part of this contribution will therefore concentrate on the part to be played by antibiotics in the management of the case and carrier of Sonne dysentery.

Sonne dysentery

The ease and speed with which *Sh. sonnei* made a successful takeover bid from other members of the genus as the causal organism of bacillary dysentery in Britain is, in retrospect, quite remarkable and apart from the milder course of the infection some notable changes also took place in the epidemiology of the disease. For example, a great increase in incidence even as judged by official notifications (Figure 2) and similarly there is evidence that gross undernotification occurs (Figure 3). Similarly the disparity in incidence between Counties and Burghs became even more evident when *Sh. sonnei* replaced other species and a periodicity in incidence of 5 to 7 years became even more marked.

Sonne dysentery has rightly been described as an enigmatic disease and we are no nearer solving most of the riddles which it presents than we were a decade or two ago and one unsolved problem concerns the use of antibiotics. Specific treatment is not required in the vast majority of cases since it is primarily a social inconvenience rather than a disease. Nor is there unequivocal evidence that the use of antimicrobial agents, even when exhibited on the basis of *in vitro* sensitivity tests, significantly shortens the duration of symptoms or reduces the period of time over which the clinically recovered patient continues to excrete the causal organism.

If it is agreed that part of the aim of treatment of such cases is to eliminate *Sh. sonnei* as rapidly as possible and thus protect from infection other individuals who have to share the same, often public, toilet accommodation as the patient, then the most efficient method of combining treatment of the patient with prophylaxis to others is to use an agent which controls rapidly the primary symptom—diarrhoea. Hutchinson (1956) has shown that the degree of contamination with shigellae in the toilet is dramatically reduced when the stool

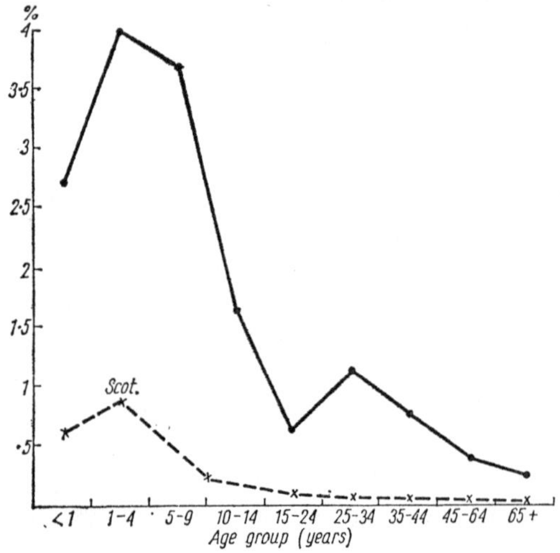

FIG. 3. Bacillary dysentery: Age specific incidence.
×---× cases notified (Scotland).
·——· cases proven by laboratory investigation.

is formed and remains thus until flushed from the toilet pedestal. Her experimental observations are backed up by epidemiological evidence which shows that the carrier with a formed stool plays a very much less significant part as a source of infection for other people than does the acute case with a soft stool which becomes fluid in the toilet water.

Use of antimicrobial agents

Again there is no evidence that the use of antimicrobial agents has influenced the incidence of the disease at a national level and even on the basis of official notifications the almost unrelenting increase in incidence has already been noted. Local evidence shows that only a minority of practitioners submit specimens from patients suffering from Sonne dysentery and one therefore assumes that the majority of practitioners prescribe antimicrobial agents without any reference to laboratory findings and their treatment with antimicrobial agents must therefore be of the 'crystal ball' variety which is nationally uneconomic, potentially dangerous and, at least on most occasions, unlikely to succeed.

In regard to the eradication of carriage of *Sh. sonnei* there is again no clear guidance from the numerous studies which have been published that antibiotics have any useful part to play nor is there evidence that the isolation of cases, either at home or in hospital, influences the spread of infection. The comparative incidence of Sonne dysentery in two Scottish cities shows that hospitalization of cases has no influence on the incidence of the disease in the community; the admission of cases of bacillary dysentery to an isolation hospital, other than for essentially social reasons, was discontinued in Edinburgh several years ago whereas in another Scottish city an isolation policy continued; yet over the years the relative incidence of the infection in the latter city has not been influenced. In summary, there would seem to be no place for the use of antibiotics in this, the most common gastro-intestinal infection in Britain.

THE ENTERIC FEVERS

There is no doubt from the wealth of publications (e.g. Marmion, 1952) that, in the case of true typhoid fever, treatment with chloramphenicol has quite spectacular effects and the same is probably true in cases of the paratyphoid fevers when these are truly systemic illnesses. Chloramphenicol does not, however, offer much in the eradication of the causal organisms from the small proportion of individuals who become chronic carriers of the enteric fever organisms although ampicillin is beneficial in this regard (Christie, 1968).

SALMONELLA FOOD POISONING

All of the evidence points unequivocally to the fact that specific therapy, even when guided by *in vitro* sensitivity tests, has no advantage in the treatment of gastro-enteritis caused by any of the members of the genus *Salmonella* and this statement encompasses such cases even when *S. paratyphi B* is the causal agent; as Christie (1969) states, 'The doctor may feel helpless, but this is no reason for using useless drugs'.

TOXIC FOOD POISONING

If one follows the rationale that antimicrobial treatment must not be instituted until one at least knows that the patient is suffering from infection, then in the case of toxic food poisoning such treatment would never be used since virtually every victim will have recovered before even the most competent laboratory could confirm the diagnosis. Another logical reason for withholding antimicrobial therapy in cases of toxic food poisoning is that the entire symptomatology is caused by preformed toxins and not by bacterial invasion but the logic of this argument is not acceptable to most patients and is apparently ignored by many clinicians. *Antibiotics have no place in the treatment of toxic food poisoning.*

CONCLUSIONS

In this brief communication I am aware that I am presenting a very anti-antibiotic attitude and would finally ask the question 'How can the bacteriologist help to ensure that patients suffering from gastro-intestinal infection are adequately treated?' Firstly, in a less benevolent society legislation might be invoked which denied the use of antibiotics (except in cases of real emergency) unless the prescription was accompanied by a certificate from a bacteriologist stating that on the basis of *in vitro* tests the agent was likely to be useful. More realistically, in Britain one wonders whether any good would come if bacteriologists stopped reporting the results of *in vitro* sensitivity tests to the clinician or alternatively reported the results of such tests with an accompanying statement reminding his clinical colleague of the futility of specific therapy in the majority of cases of gastro-intestinal infection.

REFERENCES

CHRISTIE, A. B. (1968). Acute infectious diseases. In *British Encyclopedia of Medical Practice.* Medical Progress, London.

CHRISTIE, A. B. (1969). *Infectious Diseases: Epidemiology and Clinical Practice.* E. and S. Livingstone, London.

GILLIES, R. R. (1968). Bacillary dysentery in Scotland: some epidemiological studies. *Archivum Immunologiae et Therapiae Experimentalis*, **16,** 410.

HUTCHINSON, R. I. (1956). Some observations on the method of spread of Sonne dysentery. *Monthly Bulletin of the Ministry of Health*, **15,** 110.

MARMION, D. E. (1952). A clinical study of 330 cases of enteric fever treated in Egypt. *Transactions of the Royal Society of Tropical Medicine and Hygiene*, **46,** 619.

17

TREATMENT OF GASTRO-INTESTINAL INFECTIONS: A CLINICIAN'S VIEWPOINT

A. B. CHRISTIE

INTESTINAL infection is a serious problem in this country. You do not have to go abroad to get infected. In 1965, for example, 22 people from England and Wales got typhoid fever while on holiday abroad, but 35 contracted the disease at home. In 1965 over 500 people in Blackpool were infected by drinking milk. They were thought to have paratyphoid fever, but the organism was, in fact, *Salmonella java*. In another recent year there were 160 cases of typhoid fever and 200 of paratyphoid in England and Wales: 50 of the typhoids were contracted at home, and 150 of the paratyphoids, 80 of them due to a waterborne infection in Yorkshire. Fortunately, typhoid is not a very infectious disease, and once the contaminated item of food or drink has been dealt with, there is very little risk of further spread of infection.

The same is not true of other intestinal infections. Sonne dysentery spreads very easily from person to person. I have never heard of typhoid spreading through a nursery school, but I have had painful experience of Sonne dysentery sweeping through and closing several. I need not dwell on the havoc caused in infant nurseries by outbreaks of *Escherichia coli* enteritis, nor need I describe the difficulties of eradicating salmonellae, once they have found lodgement in a farmstead, an abattoir, a poultry plant or a food factory.

Intestinal infections are still among the commonest infectious diseases in this country, and my task is to assess what place, if any, antibiotics have in their management. One might imagine that after 30 years that place would have been defined, but alas the practice of medicine is far from being an exact discipline, and I am tempted to quote from Hazlitt 'If we wish to know the force of human genius we should read Shakespeare. If we wish to see the insignificance of human learning we may study his commentators.' The essay is entitled 'On the ignorance of the learned.'

TYPHOID FEVER

Those of us who remember typhoid fever in the pre-antibiotic era must regard the effect of chloramphenicol in this disease as one of the most dramatic achievements of twentieth-century medicine. A long, low, muttering fever has been converted into a short, sharp, febrile illness. But the drug has not lowered the incidence of relapse in typhoid fever: indeed it may have increased it. It has not lowered the number of patients who become carriers after treatment of the infection and it is useless in the treatment of carriers. Both of these disappointing features are doubtless due to the fact that *Salmonella typhi* is an intracellular parasite, and that inside the cell it is in some way protected against the full action of the antibiotic. Tissue culture experiments have demonstrated that *S. typhi* outside cells is readily killed when an antibiotic is added to the culture, but that although organisms inside the cells stop multiplying they are not killed as long as the tissue culture cell remains alive. If the culture cells are destroyed, death of the *S. typhi* soon follows. In similar experiments, tissue culture cells have been infected with *S. typhi*, and then attempts made to 'cure' them with antibiotics. Some of the cultures appear to be 'cured', but in others *S. typhi* reappeared after the end of a 3-weeks course of treatment (Smadel, 1960; Hopps *et al.*, 1961; Showacre *et al.*, 1961).

Chloramphenicol

Do these experiments have any relevance to what occurs in the patient with typhoid fever? Does chloramphenicol simply stop the multiplication of extracellular *S. typhi*, enabling other defence mechanisms of the body to kill them off, while intracellular organisms are protected in some way and are able to emerge when the cell dies, and to multiply if the antibiotic is no longer present and in this way cause a clinical relapse? This seems theoretically reasonable, but it is not always easy to convert theory into practice. Can one prevent relapse in typhoid fever patients treated with chloramphenicol?

Various dosage schedules have been tried—a long course of 14 to 21 days, or two shorter courses separated by an interval, but none has given consistent results. The length of treatment and the total dose seem to be important. A 10-day course has always given better results than a 5-day course, and a total dose of 20 g has usually been followed by fewer relapses than total doses of 15 g and 10 g (Rowland, 1961; Christie, 1969). It is, however, salutary to note that in one series, of 122 patients not given the drug 13·9 per cent had a relapse, while of 200 given it 27·5 per cent relapsed (El Rami, 1950a,b). The date of that report is 1950 and the doses may have been too small to do other than temporarily interfere with the course of the disease, instead of allowing it to burn itself out. One is, however, tempted to wonder whether we get too worried about relapses as they are usually mild clinically and quickly respond to treatment. And one also wonders whether as clinicians we are expecting the impossible from chloramphenicol.

In recent trials in America (Hornick *et al.*, 1970) volunteers swallowed varying doses of live typhoid bacilli suspended in milk. When the dose was 10 million organisms, half of the volunteers became ill with typical typhoid fever and were treated with chloramphenicol while the other half remained well. In both groups however, *S. typhi* was excreted in the faeces for several weeks, and the authors stated that chloramphenicol 'did not shorten the period of multiplication or residence of typhoid bacilli in the gut', although it did cure the systemic illness in those who became ill.

Size of infecting dose of organisms

Although not completely relevant to antibiotic treatment, other findings from these volunteer studies are worth mentioning. The size of the infecting dose determined the clinical outcome. When the dose was 10^9 bacilli, 95 per cent of volunteers developed typhoid fever; at 10^7 50 per cent and at 10^5 28 per cent. When the dose was only 1000 bacilli however, none of the volunteers became ill. We cannot tell how closely these doses relate to infecting doses in nature, although a study of the incubation periods following varying doses suggested that in a water-borne outbreak such as in Zermatt the dose lay somewhere between 10^7 and 10^5 bacilli, with an illness rate therefore between 50 per cent and 28 per cent of those exposed.

Efficacy of vaccination

A second finding was that typhoid vaccination gave no protection at all when the dose administered was 10^7 or higher, but gave nearly 70 per cent protection against a dose of 10^5 bacilli. This is around the level of protection found in WHO field trials (Cvjetanović & Uemura, 1965), and the figures suggest that typhoid vaccines may be expected to give some protection against water-borne infections, but would fail against food-borne infections, where the dose is much higher. When typhoid fever did develop, the illness was equally severe in the vaccinated and the unvaccinated, and high antibody titre before challenge did not prevent infection and illness at the higher dosages. These, of course, are facts we know from studies of non-experimental typhoid fever, just as we know that relapses occur in typhoid fever when H and O antibodies are often at their highest in the patient's serum. It may well be that intestinal immunity is more important in preventing typhoid fever than are serum antibodies, and oral vaccination with attenuated streptomycin-dependent strains of *S. typhi* has apparently proved protective in volunteer experiments (Hornick *et al.*, 1970).

Typhoid carriers

In the experiments to which I have been referring 250 volunteers received antibiotic treatment for typhoid fever, but none became permanent typhoid carriers, a finding which we may find surprising and follow-up studies may not have been thorough enough. In my own series of 8 chronic typhoid carriers treated with ampicillin, I had only one failure who at one stage produced 196 consecutive negative faecal cultures, yet the 197th was positive! Table 1 shows the excretion pattern of the carriers during a 5-month observation period before treatment (the patients had been known carriers for between 7 and 27 years). Table 2 shows the treatment given, and Table 3 the results of treatment.

It has been stated (Smith, 1969) that the results of ampicillin treatment of typhoid carriers are 'to say the least equivocal'. I never understand the meaning of words like 'equivocal' or highly idiomatic phrases like 'to say the

TABLE 1

TYPHOID CARRIERS: BEFORE TREATMENT

Patient	*Years as carrier*	*Faeces positive before treatment*
A.I.	7	17/31
M.P.	13	41/44
E.F.	12	11/43
R.G.	12 (?53)	28/42
A.P.	27	40/41
E.L.	26	40/44
M.K.	?	31/31
M. Potts	11	43/44

least', but all I would say is that 500 negative faecal specimens after ampicillin therapy does suggest that ampicillin has altered a typhoid carrier's pattern of excretion! Other writers have reported on larger series with varying success (Merselis *et al.*, 1964; Jamieson *et al.*, 1968; Dinbar *et al.*, 1969). All are agreed that the state of the biliary tract is important. If it is normal, then treatment with ampicillin is often successful. If it is abnormal, ampicillin is still worth trying. If cholecystectomy is eventually decided on, ampicillin may improve the clearance rates. In some parts of the world, for example Hong Kong, the carrier state is associated with recurrent cholangitis rather than with cholecystitis (McFadzean & Ong, 1966). Cholecystectomy is very

TABLE 2

TYPHOID CARRIERS: TREATMENT

1st Week
- Ampicillin by mouth: 1 g every 6 hours
- Probenecid by mouth: 1 g twice daily
- Ampicillin injection: 500 mg every 6 hours

Weeks 2 to 12
- Ampicillin by mouth: 1 g every 8 hours
- Probenecid by mouth: 1 g twice daily

TABLE 3

TYPHOID CARRIERS: EFFECT OF TREATMENT WITH AMPICILLIN

	Years of observation after treatment	*Negative faecal specimens*	*Carrier state in* 1970
A.I.	7	500	Cured ?
M.P.	7	500	Cured ?
E.F.	5	300	Cured ? (Died 1968)
R.G.	7	500	Cured ?
A.P.	5	300	Cured ? (Died 1968)
E.L.	7	500	Cured ?
M.K.	9/12	31	Cured ??
M. Potts	7	196	Relapsed

unlikely to eradicate the intrahepatic carrier state. I do not know if prolonged ampicillin therapy has been tried in such cases.

Ampicillin

In the treatment of typhoid fever ampicillin has proved very inferior to chloramphenicol. It has been given along with chloramphenicol in the hope that chloramphenicol, which is bacteriostatic, would rapidly control the clinical illness while ampicillin, which is bactericidal, would prevent relapses and the carrier state. In my own very small experience this has not proved successful and I do not know of any large scale trials of the combination which might give a definate answer. When I have a typhoid patient, clinically well but persistently excreting the organism, I give them a 6-weeks course of ampicillin. So far this has proved successful, the patient passing fairly strict tests of cure including sterile duodenal bile specimens. Perhaps a short course of chloramphenicol followed by a long course of ampicillin is the surest way of avoiding the carrier state after typhoid fever, but my experience is limited and I do not know.

Co-trimoxazole

Co-trimoxazole has been used with success in the treatment of typhoid fever (Annotation, 1970). In Kamat's series (Kamat, 1970) of 220 patients, the 100 treated with co-trimoxazole did better in every way than the 120 treated with chloramphenicol. No report has yet been published, as far as I know, about follow-up. I understand there have been no permanent carriers, but Dr. Kamat is doubtful if his laboratory techniques and facilities have been adequate for such a study (Kamat, 1971). Farid and his colleagues also published a convincing paper on this form of treatment in typhoid fever (Farid *et al.*, 1970). As a clinician, I do not think it matters at all whether a patient's temperature comes down to normal in 4 instead of 4·3 days or in 4·7 instead of 5 days. All that matters is that treatment is effective and, at the same time, safe.

A more recent report from South Africa (Scragg & Rubidge, 1971) tells of alarming neutropenia in a few patients treated with co-trimoxazole, and the authors insist that, as with chloramphenicol, the blood picture must be monitored during co-trimoxazole treatment. They also reported that blood cultures remained positive in a few patients even in the second and third weeks of treatment and suggest that long-term bacteriological follow-up of patients is required. It must be emphasized that their patients were children, often undernourished, and that strains of *S. typhi* differ in virulence and perhaps in their response to drugs. The study by Dr. Geddes and his colleagues (Geddes *et al.*, 1971) is a model of caution. It confirms the efficacy of co-trimoxazole in the treatment of typhoid fever, but reports one or two failures, and concludes that 'in patients with severe enteric fever chloramphenicol may remain the drug of choice'. Those of us who have seen severe blood dyscrasia develop in a patient under treatment with chloramphenicol would certainly welcome a safer drug. The evidence that co-trimoxazole is such a drug is not completely convincing.

SALMONELLOSIS

In salmonella enteritis antibiotics are contra-indicated. They do not shorten the illness and they prolong the period of excretion. Why this is so is not clear. It may be that antibiotics inhibit the growth of some intestinal organisms which would otherwise help to maintain a pH range in the intestine unfavourable to the growth of salmonellae (Hornick *et al.*, 1970). In the volunteer experiments I mentioned earlier (Hornick *et al.*, 1970), when a dose of 1000 typhoid bacilli was fed in milk to 14 volunteers none of them became ill with typhoid fever, but when streptomycin was given to 4 volunteers before the dose of typhoid bacilli, one of the 4 did become ill. This seems to have given the experimenters some scientific satisfaction, but whether the volunteer was equally elated is not recorded! Similar results have, of course, been obtained by treating guinea-pigs with antibiotics before infecting them with an oral dose of salmonellae (Moore, 1957).

When salmonellae invade the bloodstream one must attempt, by treating the patient with antibiotics, to clear the bloodstream and prevent the salmonellae from invading other organs of the body. This sounds very rational, but I am uncertain whether this is achieved in practice. I have certainly not seen dramatic clinical responses such as one is accustomed to in typhoid fever. Many salmonellae are, of course, more resistant to antibiotics than is *S. typhi* to chloramphenicol, and much may depend on the type of salmonella and the minimum inhibitory concentration of the organism for the antibiotic. Most of my experience has been with *S. virchow* septicaemia. My patients have all recovered, but whether they would have done so equally quickly without antibiotics I do not know. In the series reported by Cherubin and colleagues (Cherubin *et al.*, 1969) the mortality from salmonella septicaemia was 33·6 per cent, higher than one would expect in typhoid fever.

DYSENTERY

For the mild type of dysentery seen in this country few of us would recommend routine antibiotic treatment. I have in the past treated such patients with various antibiotics, mainly ampicillin or streptomycin, and have felt that the treatment shortened the period of excretion, an important point when, as happens so often, the infected child has to be discharged to a residential institution. The present epidemic strains in Liverpool are, however, resistant to most of the common antibiotics, but sensitive to nalidixic acid. This drug has not shortened the period of excretion and we have stopped using it.

I have no experience of severe or fulminating shigellosis such as has been recently reported in Central America (Levine *et al.*, 1970; Reller, 1970) and do not know whether antibiotics would affect the clinical course of such illnesses although I would be inclined to try. The *Shigella dysenteriae* type 1 (Shiga bacillus) was certainly resistant to several antibiotics but sensitive to ampicillin, kanamycin and gentamicin. The pandemic was, according to Dupont and his colleagues (1971), the worst seen in the world for over 70 years. The effect of treating those patients with antibiotics might well be to widen the spectrum of antibiotic resistance, and accordingly most interest has since been focused on the feasibility of inducing mucosal immunity by the oral administration of live vaccines composed of artificially created mutants, recombinations or other bacterial variants (Formal *et al.*, 1966; Mel *et al.*, 1968; Dupont *et al.*, 1971; Edsall, 1971).

INFANTILE GASTROENTERITIS

From many infants with gastroenteritis no pathogens are ever grown from the faeces. It is irrational to treat such infants with antibiotics. But every clinician who treats infants knows that, even when an enteropathogenic *Escherichia coli* is isolated from the faeces, the infant recovers without antibiotics. When an infant with gastroenteritis is seriously ill it is dehydration which must be corrected and it is fluid not antibiotic which corrects dehydration. There is little if any evidence that enteropathogenic *Esch. coli* often invade the bloodstream of the infant, for in nearly every case when hydration is corrected the infants general condition rapidly improves.

I do not like to discharge from hospital infants who are still excreting enteropathogenic *Esch. coli*, though they are probably not very infectious once the diarrhoeal stage is past. On the other hand I do not like keeping an infant in hospital simply because there are some *Esch. coli* in its faeces, for there is always the danger of cross-infection by another serotype. When an infant has to return from hospital to a residential institution, you must be sure that it has stopped excreting *Esch. coli* and in such cases I usually prescribe an antibiotic to which the organism is sensitive, but am not convinced that this leads to more rapid disappearance of the *Esch. coli* from the faeces. I am very doubtful if the use of antibiotics does much to stop the spread of *Esch. coli* infection, for the surroundings of an infant with *Esch. coli* diarrhoea are rapidly and heavily contaminated with the organism, and an antibiotic can hardly act quickly enough to have a significant effect on this level of contamination. It is, of course, *logical* to give an antibiotic to cut down the weight of infection, and I know I would be defeated in any *argument* on this subject. But philosophers used to argue about how many angels could be balanced on the point of a needle and as far as I know they never reached an agreement. I do not think the facts at issue are so ethereal in the case of infantile gastroenteritis, but the last thing I would insist on in this connection is that 'experience teaches', for quite often it merely renders one intolerant. So I am open to correction on this matter.

TRAVELLERS' DIARRHOEA

The histories of expeditions, wars, pilgrimages and other mass migrations usually include accounts of diseases that broke out when 'the crowds left their normal haunts and met with the makeshifts and discomforts of travelling rough' (Christie, 1969). Package tours are the modern forms of mass migration but whether they can be described as 'travelling rough' is a matter of opinion. Disease or discomfort is certainly not unknown on the sunshine holidays, and the travellers often return to these shores less fit than when they left for their glamorous vacations (Christie, 1970–71).

You will be familiar with Kean's account of the outbreak of travellers' diarrhoea which occurred during the Eighth International Congress of Tropical Medicine and Malaria in Teheran in 1968 (Kean, 1969). The eminent patients gave many explanations for the affliction—change of diet, drinks, ices, the water, the sun, the voyage—explanations that might have been professed by less distinguished travellers! Only one or two thought a micro-organism might be to blame. Kean carried out no bacteriological tests, but did notice certain geographical factors in the aetiology.

He divided the countries of origin of the delegates into 'diarrhoeal' and 'non-diarrhoeal countries'. He had some difficulty with his classification. France, for example, he regarded as North European in general culture, but possibly Mediterranean in intestinal experience, and South African cities, though sub-tropical in climate, probably were North European with respect to diarrhoea. Making allowance for these difficulties, Kean found that of delegates from 'non-diarrhoeal' countries 41 per cent of 240 suffered from 'Turista', but only 8 per cent of 163 from 'diarrhoeal' countries. There were 48 delegates from Iran itself but only one was afflicted, so that it seemed that both culturally and microbiologically the Persians were very much at home in Teheran! The ninth congress was due to be held in Washington last year, but I have not heard whether 'Turista' again upset the proceedings, and, if so, whether the epidemiological findings were geographically reversed.

Other reports have suggested a microbiological cause for travellers' diarrhoea. Roantree (1969) pointed out that European travellers to India often suffered soon after arrival, but then became immune, until they moved to another station and presumably a new bacteriological environment. Neumann (1970) advised visitors to West Africa to drink water only out of hot-water taps as he had no difficulty in growing *Esch. coli* from water from the cold tap. You will, of course, all know the work of Rowe, Taylor and Bettelheim (1970) who isolated an unusual strain of *Esch. coli* from British troops suffering from diarrhoea in Aden, and later from a laboratory technician who went down with severe diarrhoea while working with the strain in Britain. All these reports seem to indicate that travellers' diarrhoea is microbiological in origin, and that intestinal immunity eventually develops after exposure. The many outbreaks one hears of among unfortunate holidaymakers have all the marks of an acute infectious disease. Have antibiotics any place to play in the prevention or the treatment of this increasingly common affliction? Roantree (1969) called for 'powerful remedies' and mentioned succinylsulphathiazole and ampicillin as being effective. Colistin cleared the organism from the faeces of the laboratory technician reported by Rowe and his colleagues (1970), or at least they disappeared after its use. I do not know if it shortened the diarrhoea. There are, of course, many so-called prophylactic agents on the market, some sponsored by travel agents or even recommended by doctors. Do any of them work? Do they bring the diarrhoea to an end? Or do they, as in salmonella enteritis, simply prolong the period of excretion? I have done much travel in many out of the way places, but usually in my motor caravan, with control over what I ate and, to some extent, over how it was cooked. I have recently sold the old van, and will, in future travels, be epidemiologically more insecure!

Travellers' diarrhoea is, I think, an urgent epidemiological problem in the twentieth-century world. It presents all the problems of the other intestinal infections I have touched on—causation, prevention and cure. After 30 years of antibiotics many of these are still unsolved.

REFERENCES

ANNOTATION (1970). Trimethoprim-sulphamethoxazole in typhoid. *British Medical Journal*, **3**, 297.

CHERUBIN, C. E., FODOR, T., DENMARK, L. L., MASTER, C. S., FUERST, H. T. & WINTER, J. W. (1969). Symptoms, septicaemia and death in salmonellosis. *American Journal of Epidemiology*, **90**, 285.

CHRISTIE, A. B. (1969). *Infectious Diseases: Epidemiology and Clinical Practice.* E. & S. Livingstone, Edinburgh.

CHRISTIE, A. B. (1970–71). In *Medical Progress* 1970–1971 (Ed., Richardson, Sir John). Butterworths, London.

CVJETANOVIĆ, B. & UEMURA, K. (1965). The present status of field and laboratory studies of typhoid and paratyphoid vaccines: with special reference to studies sponsored by the World Health Organization. *Bulletin of the World Health Organization*, **32**, 29.

DINBAR, A., ALTMANN, G. & TULCINSKY, D. B. (1969). The treatment of chronic biliary salmonella carriers. *American Journal of Medicine*, **47**, 236.

DU PONT, H. L., LEVINE, M. M., HORNICK, R. B., SNYDER, M. J., LIBONATI, J. B. & FORMAL, S. B. (1971). Oral attenuated vaccines in the control of shigellosis. In *Proceedings International Conference on the Application of Vaccines against Viral, Rickettsial and Bacterial Diseases of Man*, p. 364. Pan American Health Organization and World Health Organization, Washington D.C.

EDSALL, G. (1971). The evolution of bacterial vaccines. In *Proceedings International Conference on the Application of Vaccines against Viral, Rickettsial and Bacterial Diseases of Man*, p. 17. Pan American Health Organization and World Health Organization, Washington D.C.

EL RAMI, A. H. (1950a). Chloramphenicol in treatment of typhoid fever. *Lancet*, **i**, 618.

EL RAMI, A. H. (1950b). Chloramphenicol in treatment of enteric group of fevers. *Journal of the Egyptian Medical Association*, **33**, 40.

FARID, Z., HASSAN, A., WAHAB, M. F. A., SANBORN, W. R., KENT, D. C., YASSA, A. & HATHOUT, S. E. (1970). Trimethoprim-sulphamethoxazole in enteric fevers. *British Medical Journal*, **3**, 323.

FORMAL, S. B., KENT, T. H., MAY, H. C., PALMER, A., FALKOW, S. & LABREC, E. H. (1966). Protection of monkeys against experimental shigellosis with a living attenuated oral polyvalent dysentery vaccine. *Journal of Bacteriology*, **92**, 17.

GANGAROSA, E. J., PERERA, D. R., MATA, L. J., MENDIZABAL-MORRIS, C., GUZMAN, G. & RELLER, L. B. (1970). Epidemic Shiga bacillus dysentery in Central America II. Epidemiologic studies in 1969. *Journal of Infectious Diseases*, **122**, 181.

GEDDES, A. M., FOTHERGILL, R., GOODALL, J. A. D. & DORKEN, P. R. (1971). Evaluation of trimethoprim-sulphamethoxazole in treatment of salmonella infections. *British Medical Journal*, **3**, 451.

HOPPS, HOPE E., SMADEL, J. E., BERNHEIM, BARBARA C., DANAUSKAS, I. Y. & JACKSON, ELIZ. B. (1961). Effects of antibiotics on intracellular *Salmonella typhi*. II Elimination of infection by prolonged treatment. *Journal of Immunology*, **87**, 162.

HORNICK, R. B., GREISMAN, S. E., WOODWARD, T. E., DUPONT, H. L., DAWKINS, A. T. & SNYDER, M. J. (1970). Typhoid fever: pathogenesis and immunological control. *New England Journal of Medicine*, **283**, 686, 739.

JAMIESON, W. M., PROUDFOOT, MARY & SMALL, R. G. (1968). Paratyphoid carriers treated with ampicillin. *Health Bulletin*, **26**, 1.

KAMAT, S. A. (1970). Evaluation of therapeutic efficacy of trimethoprim-sulphamethoxazole and chloramphenicol in enteric fever. *British Medical Journal*, **3**, 320.

KAMAT, S. A. (1971). Personal communication.

KEAN, B. H. (1969). Turista in Teheran. *Lancet*, **ii**, 583.

LEVINE, M. M., DUPONT, H. L., FORMAL, S. B. & GANGAROSA, E. J. (1970). Epidemic Shiga dysentery in Central America. *Lancet*, **ii**, 607.

MATA, E. J., GANGAROSA, E. J., CÁCERES, A., PERERA, D. R. & MELICANOS, M. L. (1970). Epidemic Shiga bacillus dysentery in Central America I. Etiologic investigations in Guatemala. *Journal of Infectious Diseases*, **122**, 170.

MCFADZEAN, A. J. S. & ONG, G. B. (1966). The intrahepatic typhoid carrier. *British Medical Journal*, **i**, 1567.

MEL, D. M., ARSIĆ, B. L., NIKOLIĆ, B. D. & RADOVANOVIĆ, M. L. (1968). Studies on vaccination against bacillary dysentery. Oral immunization with live monotypic and combined vaccines. *Bulletin of the World Health Organization*, **39**, 375.

MERSELIS, J. G., KAYE, D., CONNOLLY, C. S. & HOOK, E. W. (1964). The typhoid carrier state: quantitative bacteriology and preliminary observations on therapy. *East African Medical Journal*, **41**, 219.

MOORE, B. (1957). Observations pointing to the conjunctiva as the portal of entry of salmonella infection of guinea pigs. *Journal of Hygiene* (*Cambridge*), **55**, 414.

NEUMANN, H. H. (1970). Travellers' diarrhoea. *Lancet*, **i**, 420.

RELLER, L. B. (1970). Epidemic Shiga dysentery in Central America. *Lancet*, **ii**, 661.

ROANTREE, W. B. (1969). Turista. *Lancet*, **ii**, 779.

ROWE, B., TAYLOR, J. & BETTELHEIM, K. A. (1970). An investigation of travellers' diarrhoea. *Lancet*, **i**, 7.

ROWLAND, H. A. R. (1961). The complications of typhoid fever. *Journal of Tropical Medicine and Hygiene*, **64**, 143.

SCRAGG, J. N. & RUBIDGE, C. J. (1971). Trimethoprim-sulphamethoxazole in typhoid fever in children. *British Medical Journal* **3**, 738.

SHOWACRE, JANE L., HOPPS, HOPE E. & SMADEL, J. E. (1961). Effects of antibiotics on intracellular *Salmonella typhi*. I. Demonstration by phase microscopy of prompt inhibition of intracellular multiplication. *Journal of Immunology*, **87**, 153.

SMADEL, J. E. (1960). Some aspects of intracellular infections. *Journal of Immunology*, **84**, 1.

SMITH, H. (1969). Chemotherapy in gastro-intestinal infections. *Medical Review*, April, 1969.

18

CHEMOTHERAPY OF VENEREAL DISEASE

R. R. Willcox

The three most important venereal diseases are syphilis, gonorrhoea and non-gonococcal urethritis. Today antibiotics are employed routinely in all three conditions.

SYPHILIS

Pre-penicillin treatment

Penicillin was first used in the treatment of syphilis by Mahoney *et al.* (1943) on four Norwegian sailors. No one doubted the statistical or other significance of this small series. Prior to this time the available therapy with arsenic and bismuth lasted for a whole year and the toxic effects were numerous and often severe. No wonder that only about one-quarter of patients completed the prescribed course (Chope & Malcolm, 1948) although for those that did so the results were good and because of the slow cure obtained reinfection was rare.

Penicillin therapy

Evolution of repository penicillins

With penicillins virtually all patients rapidly received a minimal curative dose with very few side-effects. The patients found the new treatment a mixed blessing as 60–80 or more 3–4-hourly round-the-clock injections were then required. Moreover, after a year or two, the results obtained with the early commercial penicillins deteriorated before it was found that manufacturers, in a striving for greater purity, had unconsciously included greater amounts of the relatively inactive K fraction (Willcox, 1947). This soon led to the purification of crystalline benzyl penicillin G and with the introduction at this time of penicillin in oil-beeswax (Romansky & Rittman, 1945), followed 3 years later by the more easily injected aqueous procaine penicillin G (Buckwalter & Dickison, 1948), injections only once daily now became possible.

With the suspension of procaine penicillin in arachis oil with aluminium monostearate (PAM), the subsequent minimum requirements for this preparation being established by the World Health Organization in 1952 (WHO, 1964), and the later introduction of benzathine penicillin providing even longer serum levels from each dose (Szabo *et al.*, 1951) the opportunity for spaced injections was now available, even successful therapy with a single injection.

Compared with many other diseases a low serum level of penicillin is required for the treatment of early syphilis (above 0·03 units/ml) but this has to be kept up continually for a minimum of 8 days as penicillin exerts its effect on the cell wall during multiplication and *Treponema pallidum* divides only every 30–33 hours (Magnuson *et al.*, 1948; Cumberland & Turner, 1949).

Results of treatment

It was soon shown that the results obtained with penicillin alone were clearly superior to those of arsenic and bismuth therapy (Shafer *et al.*, 1954) and that no gain resulted from adding arsenic and bismuth to penicillin, as data from St. Mary's shows in Table 1.

TABLE 1

SYPHILIS—RESULTS OBTAINED WITH PENICILLIN ALONE, PENICILLIN WITH BISMUTH AND PENICILLIN, ARSENIC AND BISMUTH
(St. Mary's—Willcox, 1962a; Jefferiss *et al.*, 1951)

Therapy	*Penicillin with arsenic and bismuth*	*Penicillin with bismuth*	*Penicillin alone*
Length of course (weeks)	11	11	6
No. treated	561	183	120
Followed one year or more			
No.	307	76	56
Per cent	54·5	41·5	46·7
Per cent failures of those followed one year or more	7·2	9·2	3·6

Better results are obtained in primary than in secondary syphilis and better still when the antibiotic is given in the incubation period. The treatment schedules for early syphilis are therefore based on those required for the secondary stage. If PAM is used it is recommended by WHO (WHO, 1960) that a minimum of 4·8 million units is given in 1–8 spaced injections. Single injections of 4·8 million units of PAM are superior to 2·4 million units but equally good results may be obtained with single doses of 2·5 mega units of benzathine penicillin (Smith *et al.*, 1956).

The schedules currently recommended by the United States Public Health Service for the treatment of primary and secondary syphilis are single injections of 2·4 million units of benzathine penicillin, 4·8 mega units of PAM (given as 2·4 mega units initially plus two injections of 1·2 million units 3 days apart) or eight daily injections of 600,000 units of aqueous procaine penicillin (USPHS, 1968).

These, of course, are minimum requirements and in many areas, including this country, more than these amounts are given although it has been shown that high doses (above 6 million units) do not give added advantage (Perdrup, 1960).

A recent WHO survey of 3749 patients with early syphilis treated with penicillin, according to established criteria, showed complete cure in sero-negative primary syphilis. In sero-positive primary syphilis and in secondary syphilis 93–100 per cent attained serological non-reactivity by reagin tests. No clinical or serological relapses were observed. In cases of unspecified 'early syphilis' retreatment rates varied around 8 per cent. Most retreated cases were considered to be reinfections (Guthe and Idsøe, 1968).

Although reagin sero-negativity is reached in nearly all cases following the treatment, TPI reactivity remains in about one-third of cases (Perdrup, 1960). What significance this has, if any, in relation to the persistence of treponemes in the lymph glands and other sites such as have been described in recent years particularly in late syphilis (Collart *et al.*, 1962)—the nature of which is not yet clear—has yet to be determined. No signs of *T. pallidum* developing resistance to penicillin have been observed but the inability to culture the organism *in vitro* would render its early detection difficult (Schamberg, 1963).

Overall effects of penicillin

Penicillin will rapidly abolish treponemes from the tissues of persons suffering from early infections with venereal and endemic syphilis, yaws and pinta, will heal the early lesions, cause sero-reversal to reagin tests and prevent later complications. It will also prevent the disease when given in the incubation period and will prevent the child of a syphilitic mother from becoming infected or will cure same *in utero*. It will effect a cure in asymptomatic neurosyphilis and prevent this condition from becoming symptomatic as also the occurrence of other late manifestations when given to latent cases. Its results in established late syphilis are less sure. Biological 'cure' may be obtained but clinical progression occurs from damaged tissues and from scarring.

Penicillin reactions

The reported incidence of penicillin reactions amongst 74,000 patients in the literature has been less than 1 per cent but such rates are usually associated with single injections. When multiple injections are used, as commonly in the treatment of syphilis, reaction rates as high as 6·6–10·2 per cent have been reported (Willcox, 1964a).

There is some evidence that the incidence of penicillin reactions has declined in recent years, partly no doubt from the taking of a more careful history of previous allergy, and using an alternative antibiotic when present, but also from the wider use of antibiotics other than penicillin for many conditions. In the venereal diseases clinics of the United States the incidence of allergic side-effects to penicillin declined from 9·71 per 1000 in 1959 to 7·57 in 1964 and 6·61 in 1969 (Rudolph, 1971) while at the London Hospital the rate of 8·9 per 1000 in 1967 fell to 6·8 in 1969 (Wilkinson, 1972).

Fatalities from penicillin are extremely rare. It is estimated from a collective survey of 858,024 patients with venereal diseases treated with penicillin that there was one death per 78,000 patients (Willcox, 1964a).

Alternative antibiotics

Penicillin is undoubtedly the best antibiotic for the treatment of syphilis and should be used in all cases in which possible allergy is not suspected. The tetracyclines, chloramphenicol, erythromycin and some other antibiotics —e.g. carbomycin—are also active. The cephalosporins (e.g. cephaloridine by injection) are considered by some to be a suitable substitute in cases of penicillin allergy but recent experience suggests the possibility of cross-sensitivity between penicillin and these drugs (Luger, 1968).

The schedules recommended by the United States Public Health Service consist of 20–30 g of demethylchlortetracycline, or 30–40 g of tetracycline, chlortetracycline, oxytetracycline or erythromycin, given orally in four daily doses over 10–15 days (USPHS, 1968). Trials have also been undertaken with intravenous injections of rolitetracycline (Luger, 1968).

GONORRHOEA

Pre-penicillin treatments

Prior to the introduction of the sulphonamides in 1937 the treatment of gonorrhoea was by means of daily urethral irrigations. The average duration of cure was 101 days and more than one-third of patients developed complications (Cokkinis and McElligott, 1938).

Even with the sulphonamides there were failures in 10 per cent or more of cases with the doses able to be given and the resistant organisms soon became predominant. By 1943, amongst the troops in Italy, the drugs had become effective in only 25 per cent of cases (Campbell, 1944) while in London 5 years later response was noted in but 14·1 per cent (Dunlop, 1949). Prior to the introduction of penicillin patients failing to sulphonamides had to return to urethral irrigations, cure being hastened in some instances by unpleasant pyretotherapy with intravenous TAB vaccine which required admission to hospital.

Penicillin therapy

Early experience with penicillin

Penicillin providentially arrived as the troops in Naples were standing in line for their urethral irrigations and prevented what otherwise would have been a major therapeutic set-back. Split doses of only 100,000–300,000 units of the then impure commercial penicillins were highly successful (Willcox, 1968). In one series the failure rate was only 2·5 per cent with 200,000 units (Hingson *et al.*, 1948).

Following the introduction of penicillin in oil-beeswax, aqueous procaine penicillin and PAM, single-injection treatments became general with highly satisfactory results. In Chicago in 1948, when over 33,000 cases had been treated with but 200,000 units, the failure rate was estimated not to exceed 2·8 per cent (Eisenberg & Easterly, 1948). Even a few years later at St. Mary's Hospital single injections of but 150,000 units of PAM were more than 90 per cent successful (Willcox, 1958).

Development of resistance to penicillin

With time, failure rates began slowly to increase particularly following single injections of long-acting preparations giving low serum levels (e.g. PAM and benzathine penicillin) although evidence of developing resistance was not immediately clearly forthcoming from laboratory testing. Correlation between strains less sensitive to penicillin and treatment failure, however, (Curtis & Wilkinson, 1958; Cradock-Watson *et al.*, 1958) brought realization of the problem and its significance.

Increasing proportions of circulating strains of gonococci less sensitive to penicillin have since been noted in most parts of the world. In many areas, e.g. the U.S.A. (Martin *et al.*, 1969) and in the United Kingdom (Wilkinson, 1972) the rise has been gradually progressive although the upper limit of resistance in London remains about the same as in 1957 (Wilkinson, 1972). The degree of resistance varies geographically and, as regards time, being more marked in the Far East—particularly in relation to the War zones and in Africa, while it is least marked in Northern Europe (Table 2).

The lessened sensitivity of the gonococcus to penicillin has been associated to some extent with a reduced sensitivity to other antibiotics (e.g. tetracycline, spiramycin, erythromycin) and is frequently accompanied by an absolute resistance to streptomycin.

TABLE 2

SENSITIVITY OF THE GONOCOCCUS TO PENICILLIN (PER CENT)

		Minimum inhibitory concentration (ug/ml)		
Area	*Authors*	*0·05 or less*	*0·06–0·12*	*>0·12*
EUROPE				
U.K. (London)	Lynn *et al.* (1970)	65·0	18·5	16·4
	Leigh *et al.* (1969)	63·0	18·0	19·0
Norway	Gundersen *et al.* (1969)	65·5	17·8	16·7
NORTH AMERICA				
Canada	Amies (1969)	34·9	19·0	46·1
U.S.A.	Fishnaller *et al.* (1968)	20·9	22·4	56·7
AUSTRALIA	Hatos (1970)	22·0	6·8	71·2
AFRICA				
Uganda	Arya & Phillips (1970)	19·1	7·5	73·4
FAR EAST				
Hawaii	Keys *et al.* (1969)	14·5	11·6	73·9
Japan				
Philippines				

The resistance observed has some relation to treatment practices and there is some evidence that it may improve when treatment becomes more effective (Lomholt & Berg, 1966; Nielsen, 1970; Lucas, 1971). Nevertheless a deteriorating situation is being observed in many areas and in some, very high doses of penicillin, even with probenecid, are now required if the disease can still be cured in a single injection.

The treatment for gonorrhoea currently recommended in the United States is by means of single sessions of 2·4 mega units of aqueous procaine penicillin for males and 4·8 mega units for females. In some parts of the Far East 4·8 mega units will fail in 30 per cent of male cases (WHO, 1969) but half of this amount can be made effective if probenecid is also given (Holmes *et al.*, 1967).

A single dose of 4·8 mega units of aqueous procaine penicillin plus 2·0 g of probenecid has been considered capable of overcoming the vast majority of circulating gonococcal strains in the U.S.A. Certainly the author has had no failures with this regime in patients previously repeatedly relapsing to lower doses of penicillin in London. Nevertheless the limit is reached with what can reasonably be injected with standard preparations of aqueous procaine penicillin and investigations are afoot with a more concentrated preparation (WHO, 1972).

Alternative antibiotics to penicillin

There is fortunately a number of alternative *injectable* antibiotics in addition to benzyl penicillin G and the various penicillin compounds, ampicillin, hetacillin and carbenecillin. These include the cephalosporins, the injectable tetracyclines including rolitetracycline, chloromycetin succinate, kanamycin and spectinomycin.

Those effective *orally* include the penicillins, penicillin V, phenethicillin, ampicillin, hetacillin, amoxycillin and pivampicillin; the cephalosporin, cephalexin; the tetracyclines, chlortetracycline, oxytetracycline, tetracycline hydrochloride and the phosphate complex, demethylchlortetracycline, lymecycline, methacycline, clomocycline, doxycycline and mixed tetracyclines; chloramphenicol and its analogue thiamphenicol; erythromycin; oleandomycin; spiramycin; pristinomycin; rifampicin; and co-trimoxazole.

It is virtually impossible for one physician to present personal experience with all of these but the results obtained with a number of them at St. Mary's Hospital, London W.2 and King Edward VII Hospital, Windsor, are presented.

Recent experiences with antibiotic treatment

Injectable antibiotics

Owing to the frequent mobility of patients with venereal diseases, and their overall poor record of attendance once symptoms have been ameliorated, 'one-shot', 'instant' or so-called 'one-minute' treatments have considerable epidemiological advantages. Moreover, when oral therapy is given, patients cannot by any means always be trusted to take their medication in the doses and at the times requested. The results described in this paper therefore concern only those obtained by means of single or at the most double dose therapy. Moreover, they concern male patients with urethral gonorrhoea only as these are more easy to assess and failing patients are more likely to return because of the presence of symptoms.

TABLE 3

GONORRHOEA—SINGLE DOSES OF 1·2 MEGA UNITS OF PROCAINE PENICILLIN
(St. Mary's)

Year	*Treated*	*Followed*	*Fail*	*Per cent fail of followed*
1961[a]	200	165	25	15·2
1963[b]	279	207	23	11·1
1966[c]	200	158	17	8·5
1968–69[d]	300	264	36	13·8
1970[e]	114	98	10	10·2
	1093	892	111	12·4

[a] Unpublished series.
[b] Willcox (1964b)
[c] Morrison *et al.* (1968).
[d] Cobbold *et al.* (1970).
[e] Willcox *et al.* (1971).

Penicillin is still more effective against the gonococcus in Great Britain than in many parts of the world. Indeed the failure rates obtained in males at St. Mary's Hospital with single doses of 1·2 million units or aqueous procaine penicillin have not materially changed during the past decade (Table 3).

It is possible to improve on these results either by increasing the dose or by using the same dose in conjunction with 1·0 g probenecid (Table 4).

Other antibiotics are required in cases of penicillin failure and for patients suspected of being allergic to penicillin. The results obtained at St. Mary's

TABLE 4

GONORRHOEA—SINGLE DOSES OF PROCAINE PENICILLIN WITH AND WITHOUT 1·0 g PROBENECID
(St. Mary's)

Dose (mega units)	*Treated*	*Followed*	*Fail*	*Per cent fail of followed*
2·4[a]	280	240	14	5·8
1·2 plus probenecid[b]	307	264	18	6·8

[a] Morrison *et al.* (1968).
[b] Cobbold *et al.* (1970).

and at Windsor in the treatment of 534 patients given one of six other antibiotics in single doses by injection are shown in Table 5.

TABLE 5

GONORRHOEA—SINGLE DOSES OF OTHER INJECTABLE ANTIBIOTICS
(St. Mary's)

Antibiotic	*Dose (g)*	*Treated*	*Followed*	*Fail*	*Per cent fail of followed*
Streptomycin[a]	1·0	130	104	33	31·7
Ampicillin[b]	0·25–0·5	106	83	23	27·7
Rolitetracycline plus tetracycline phosphate by mouth[c]	0·375 + 0·5	48	45	7	15·6
Tetracyclines[b]	0·5	46	37	5	13·5
Spectinomycin[d]	1·4–1·6	151	134	23	9·7
Chloromycetin succinate[e]	1·0	53	44	2	4·5
Total	0·25–1·0	534	447	93	20·8

[a] Spitzer & Willcox (1968).
[b] Willcox (1968)—note: ampicillin should not be given to patients suspected of being allergic to benzyl penicillin.
[c] Willcox (1970).
[d] Willcox (1962b).
[e] Willcox (1963).

Best results were obtained with the little used chloromycetin succinate, which is contra-indicated on account of toxicity, and with spectinomycin which is not yet on the general market in this country. Worst results were achieved with streptomycin. On the basis of exponentially increasing failure rates with this drug over consecutive 5-year periods it was forecast, from the 31·7 per cent failure rate obtained in 1966, that the antibiotic would fail in 85 per cent of cases by 1971. In a limited series of 8 patients treated in that year failure occurred in 5 out of 6 (83.3 per cent) of those followed (Willcox & Woodcock, 1971).

TABLE 6

GONORRHOEA—SINGLE DOSES OF OTHER INJECTABLE ANTIBIOTICS

Antibiotic	*Area*	*Dose (g)*	*Treated*	*Followed*	*Fail*	*Per cent fail of followed*
Cephaloridine	London[a]	2·0	40	35	6	17·1
	London[b]	2·0	46	34	3	8·9
	Bradford[c]	2·0–2·75	103	77	4	5·2
Kanamycin	London[d]	2·0	102	79	3	3·8
	London[e]	2·0	34	31	—	—
Total		2·0–2·75	325	256	16	6·3

[a] Csonka *et al.* (1967).
[b] Marshall & Curtis (1967).
[c] Oller (1967).
[d] Wilkinson *et al.* (1967).
[e] Csonka (1967).

Experience in other hospitals with two other injectable antibiotics—cephaloridine and kanamycin—are shown in Table 6. Better results were obtained with cephaloridine outside of rather than within London where excellent results were achieved with kanamycin.

Orally administered antibiotics

It is probably true that no antibiotic at present available gives as good results in single doses by mouth as can be obtained with single injections of adequate amounts of aqueous procaine penicillin. The experience at St. Mary's in 622 cases in which one of seven antibiotics was administered orally in a single dose is shown in Table 7. Best results were obtained with rifampicin, doxycycline and spiramycin.

TABLE 7

GONORRHOEA—SINGLE DOSES OF ORAL ANTIBIOTICS

Antibiotic	*Dose (g)*	*Treated*	*Followed*	*Fail*	*Per cent fail of followed*
Lymecycline[a]	0·816–1·22	75	66	13	19·7
Demethylchlortetracycline[b]	0·9–1·2	82	76	12	15·8
Ampicillin[c]	0·5–1·0	200	174	26	14·9
Amoxycillin[a]	0·5–2·0	76	67	10	14·9
Spiramycin[d]	2·0–3·4	54	47	6	12·8
Doxycycline[a]	0·9	32	25	3	12·0
Rifampicin[e]	0·9	103	89	10	11·2
Total	—	622	544	80	14·7

[a] Unpublished data.
[b] Willcox (1967).
[c] Willcox (1964b).
[d] Willcox (1956). There were no failures in 25 followed who were given 3·4 g.
[e] Cobbold *et al.* (1968).

The efficiency of treatment with the orally administered penicillins and cephalosporins can be improved with the simultaneous use of probenecid. The results obtained with cephalexin, ampicillin and the new amoxycillin, which is better absorbed than ampicillin when given orally (Acred *et al.*, 1971; Croydon & Sutherland, 1971; Geddes *et al.*, 1971), when used with probenecid are shown in Table 8.

With ampicillin the results proved markedly better in Swansea, where a collaborative series was conducted simultaneously using the same criteria, than at St. Mary's (Willcox *et al.*, 1971; Cobbold *et al.*, 1972). Amoxycillin, however, proved satisfactory in London.

Although venereal disease patients are unreliable in taking multiple doses of orally-administered drugs they can probably be trusted to take one additional dose 4–6 hours after receiving the first under supervision in the clinic. The results experienced in 488 patients given one of five antibiotics in this manner are shown in Table 9.

TABLE 8

GONORRHOEA—SINGLE ORAL DOSES OF SEMI-SYNTHETIC PENICILLINS WITH PROBENECID (1·0 g)

Antibiotic	*Area*	*Dose (g)*	*Treated*	*Followed*	*Fail*	*Per cent fail of followed*
Cephalexin	London[a]	3·0	87	66	11	16·7
Ampicillin	London[b]	2·0	114	94	10	10·6
	Swansea[c]	2·0	106	91	2	2·2
Amoxycillin	London[d]	1·0–2·0	70	62	5	6·3
Total		1·0–3·0	377	313	28	8·9

[a] Willcox & Woodcock (1970).
[b] Willcox *et al.*, (1971).
[c] Cobbold *et al.* (1972).
[d] Unpublished data.

TABLE 9

GONORRHOEA—DOUBLE DOSES OF ANTIBIOTICS GIVEN ORALLY (St. Mary's)

Antibiotic	*Dose (g)*	*Treated*	*Followed*	*Fail*	*Per cent fail of followed*
Cephalexin[a]	2·0 + 2·0	102	82	12	14·6
Ampicillin[b]	1·0 + 1·0	153	127	15	11·8
Triple tetracycline[c]	1·2 + 1·2	100	89	8	9·0
Amoxycillin[d]	0·5 + 0·5	26	19	1	5·3
Demethylchlortetracycline[e]	1·2 + 1·2	107	93	4	4·3
Total	1·0–4·0	488	410	40	9·8

[a] Willcox & Woodcock (1970).
[b] Willcox (1965).
[c] Willcox (1971).
[d] Unpublished data.
[e] Willcox (1969)

Failure rates in under 10 per cent of cases were noted with demethychlortetracycline, amoxycillin and a triple tetracycline mixture.

NON-GONOCOCCAL URETHRITIS

Earlier treatments

In recent years the numbers of cases of non-gonococcal urethritis in males have exceeded those of gonorrhoea. As with gonorrhoea the treatment of this condition, prior to the introduction of the sulphonamides, was by means of urethral irrigations. Sulphonamides were then used but the results were less impressive than for gonorrhoea. The advent of penicillin represented no new advance for non-gonococcal urethritis and the sulphonamides remained the drugs of choice. When streptomycin was introduced, improved results were obtained with single doses of this antibiotic when combined with a 5-day course of sulphonamides, and this became the staple treatment in the clinics and remained so for many years on account of its relative cheapness, even after a number of more effective but more expensive broad-spectrum antibiotics had been discovered.

Modern treatments

The results of treating 2184 male patients with non-gonococcal urethritis at St. Mary's or at Windsor with one of twenty-five different methods are shown in Table 10.

TABLE 10

RESULTS OF TREATMENT OF 2184 CASES OF NON-GONOCOCCAL URETHRITIS USING TWENTY-FIVE DIFFERENT TREATMENT METHODS

Drug	*Usual dosage (g)*	*Treated*	*Followed*	*Retreated*	*Per cent retreated*
Tetracycline and oleandomycin	6	106	82	12	14·6
Oxytetracycline	5–6	85	82	13	15·9
Lymecycline	4·9	101	65	11	16·9
Triple tetracycline	7·2	71	57	10	17·5
Tetracycline hydrochloride	6	124	108	20	18·5
Chlortetracycline	5–6	115	108	20	18·5
Spiramycin	10–20	134	123	25	20·3
Triacetyloleandomycin	6	100	85	19	22·4
Streptomycin + sulphonamides	1·0[b] 8–12	150	113	31	27·4
Erythromycin	6	207	177	49	27·7
Tetracycline phosphate[a]	4	150	130	36	27·7
A.B.O.B.	2·4	58	54	20	37·0
Sulphonamides	8–28	215	195	73	37·4
Penicillin	1–3.6 mega units	70	65	26	40·0
Chloramphenicol	5–6	39	37	16	40·5
Spectinomycin + sulphonamides	1·6[b] 10	42	34	15	44·1
Streptomycin b	1–4	164	141	65	46·1
Metronidazole	4·2	70	58	28	48·3
Aminitrozole	1·8–2·1	49	45	22	48·9
Spectinomycin	1·6	30	26	14	53·8
Compound 17025	2	13	13	7	53·8
Novobiocin	6–12	40	36	20	55·6
Nalidixic acid	28	10	8	5	62.5
Ampicillin	6	12	12	8	66·7
Placebo	—	29	22	15	68·2
Total	—	2184	1876	580	30·9

[a] With and without 4 mg methyl prednisolone.
[b] With and without phenylbutazone.

The most effective antibiotics are the tetracyclines, alone or with oleandomycin, providing cure rates in excess of 80 per cent. In most cases treatment with these drugs was spread over 6 days. When given for less than this time (e.g. with tetracycline phosphate over 4 days) the results were less striking. That this condition responds to tetracyclines gives added support to the view that *Chlamydia* may be responsible for many of the cases encountered. If this is so it is not unlikely that a 6-day course may be too short always to eradicate the organism. Indeed it has been shown that improved results may be obtained by extending the treatment period to up to 21 days (John, 1971).

Close behind the tetracyclines with 20·3–27·7 per cent of failures are the macrolide antibiotics spiramycin, triacetyl-oleandomycin and erythromycin, the results achieved with the latter being similar to those obtained by streptomycin and the sulphonamides.

The sulphonamides alone, and penicillin and chloramphenicol, provided 37·0–40·5 per cent of failures while little or no activity was noted with streptomycin alone, metronidazole, spectinomycin, novobiocin, nalidixic acid or ampicillin. Ampicillin proved the least effective and yet this drug is commonly prescribed for urethritis by private practitioners.

SUMMARY AND CONCLUSIONS

Data are presented of the results of treating 6749 patients with venereal disease (864 of syphilis, 3701 of gonorrhoea and 2184 of non-gonococcal urethritis) attending St. Mary's Hospital, London, W.2. or King Edward VII Hospital, Windsor, in recent years and the results are compared with some of the published findings at other centres.

Penicillin remains the drug of choice for the treatment of syphilis and is still first choice for the treatment of gonorrhoea although, owing to the development of resistance, large doses are now required with or without probenecid if the disease is still to be cured by a single injection. The limits of what can be achieved by treatment in this way, however, have now been reached in some areas. Continued research is therefore required to discover new effective products to keep pace with a deteriorating situation.

The tetracyclines continue to give the best results in non-gonococcal urethritis.

Although the impact that antibiotics have made on the treatment of venereal diseases is truly vast it is a sobering thought that, apart from syphilis, they have not succeeded in reducing their incidence, indeed the opposite.

In some ways antibiotics have contributed to the present adverse situation. Reinfection is now possible with both syphilis and gonorrhoea much more frequently than formerly. Fear of these diseases, at one time one of the brakes on promiscuity, has been removed with the new easy treatments and there is some suggestion that under antibiotic impact both syphilis and gonorrhoea are becoming milder diseases and therefore more difficult to diagnose.

The mind boggles however, when the present runaway rise in incidence of gonorrhoea and non-gonococcal urethritis is considered—as to what the present situation would be without them.

REFERENCES

ACRED, P., HUNTER, P. A. & MIZEN, L. (1971). Chemotherapy and pharmacology of alpha-amino-*p*-hydroxybenzylpenicillin (BRL 2333) a new broad spectrum semi-synthetic penicillin. Paper presented at VIIth International Congress of Chemotherapy, Prague.

AMIES, C. R. (1969). Sensitivity of *Neisseria gonorrhoeae* to penicillins and other antibiotics. Studies carried out in Toronto during the period 1961 to 1968. *British Journal of Venereal Diseases*, **45**, 216.

ARYA, O. P. & PHILLIPS, I. (1970). Antibiotic sensitivity of gonococci and treatment of gonorrhoea in Uganda. *British Journal of Venereal Diseases*, **46**, 149.

BUCKWALTER, F. H. & DICKISON, H. L. (1948). New absorption delaying vehicle for penicillins. *Journal of the American Pharmaceutical Association*, **37**, 472.

CAMPBELL, D. J. (1944). Gonorrhoea in North Africa and Central Mediterranean. *British Medical Journal*, **2**, 44.

CHOPE, H. D. & MALCOLM, J. C. (1948). Administrative advantages of rapid syphilotherapy on out-patient basis. *Journal of Venereal Disease Information*, **29**, 173.

COBBOLD, R. J. C., MORRISON, G. D. & WILLCOX, R. R. (1968). Treatment of gonorrhoea with single oral doses of rifampicin. *British Medical Journal*, **4**, 681.

COBBOLD, R. J. C., SPITZER, R. J., MORRISON, G. D. & WILLCOX, R. R. (1970). One-session treatment of gonorrhoea in males with procaine penicillins plus probenecid. *Postgraguate Medical Journal*, **46**, 142.

COBBOLD, R. J. C., REES, G. D. & PARKER, R. B. (1972). In press.

COKKINIS, A. J. & MCELLIGOTT, G. L. M. (1938). Sulphanilamide in gonorrhoea; analysis of 633 cases. *Lancet*, **2**, 355.

COLLART, P., BOREL, L. J. & DUREL, P. (1962). Study of the effect of penicillins in late syphilis. Persistance of *Treponema pallidum* following treatment 1. Late syphilis—experimental. *Annals Institute Pasteur (Paris)*, **102**, 596.

CRADOCK-WATSON, J. E., SHOOTER, R. A. & NICOL, C. S. (1958). Sensitivity of strains of gonococci to penicillin, sulphathiazole and streptomycin. *British Medical Journal*, **1**, 1091.

CROYDON, E. A. P. & SUTHERLAND, R. (1971). Microbiology and human pharmacology of a new penicillin—alpha-amino-*p*-hydroxybenzylpenicillin (BRL 2333). Paper presented at VIIth International Congress of Chemotherapy, Prague.

CSONKA, G. W. (1967). Kanamycin in non-gonococcal urethritis. *Postgraduate Medical Journal, May supplement*, p. 63.

CSONKA, G. W. & MURRAY, M. (1967). Cephaloridine in the treatment of non-gonococcal urethritis. *Postgraduate Medical Journal, August Supplement*, **43**, 123.

CUMBERLAND, M. C. & TURNER, T. B. (1949). Rate of multiplication of *Treponema pallidum* in normal and immune rabbits. *American Journal of Syphilis*, **33**, 201.

CURTIS, F. R. & WILKINSON, A. E. (1958). A comparison of the *in vitro* sensitivity of gonococci to penicillins with the results of treatment. *British Journal of Venereal Diseases*, **34**, 70.

DUNLOP, E. M. C. (1949). Gonorrhoea and sulphonamides. *British Journal of Venereal Diseases*, **25**, 81.

EISENBERG, H. & EASTERLY, M. E. (1948). Efficiency of penicillins in gonorrhoea, analysed by sampling method. *Journal of Venereal Disease Information*, **29**, 269.

FISCHNALLER, J. E., PEDERSEN, H. B., RONALD, A. R., BONIN, P. & TRONCA, E. L. (1968). Kanamycin sulphate in the treatment of acute gonorrhoeal urethritis in men. *Journal of American Medical Association*, **203**, 909.

GEDDES, A. M., WILLIAMS, J. D., KOSMIDIS, J., GOODALL, J. A. D. & ANDREWS, J. (1971). Clinical pharmocological studies with a new semi-synthetic penicillin—alpha-amino-*p*-hydroxybenzylpenicillin. Paper presented at VIIth International Congress of Chemotherapy, Prague.

GUNDERSEN, T., ODEGAARD, E. & GJESSING, H. C. (1969). Treatment of gonorrhoea by one oral dose of ampicillin and probenecid combined. *British Journal of Venereal Diseases*, **43**, 235.

GUTHE, T. & IDSØE, I. (1968). Antibiotic treatment of venereal diseases. In *Current Problems in Dermatology*, Vol. 2, p. 2. Karger, Basel and New York.

HATOS, G. (1970). Treatment of gonorrhoea by penicillin and a renal blocking agent (probenecid). *Medical Journal of Australia*, **1**, 1096.

HINGSON, R. A., EASLEY, E. J., GRAY, A. L., TUCKER, C. B., KIESSELBACH, M. R., PARKHURST, G. E., USHER, G. S. & DAVIDSON, H. H. (1948). Hypospray administration of penicillin in treatment of gonorrhoea. *Journal of Venereal Disease Information*, **29**, 61.

HOLMES, K. K., JOHNSON, D. W. & FLOYD, T. M. (1967). Studies of venereal disease. 1. Probenecid-procaine penicillin G combination and tetracycline hydrochloride in the treatment of 'penicillin-resistant' gonorrhoea in men. *Journal of American Medical Association*, **202**, 461.

JEFFERISS, F. J. G., WILLCOX, R. R. & MCELLIGOTT, G. L. M. (1951). Treatment of early syphilis with penicillin, neoarsphenamine and bismuth, and with penicillin and bismuth alone. *Lancet*, **1**, 83.

JOHN, J. (1971). Efficacy of prolonged regimes of oxytetracycline in the treatment of non-gonococcal urethritis. *British Journal of Venereology*, **47**, 266.

KEYS, T. F., HALVERSON, C. W. & CLARK, E. J. (1969). Single-dose treatment of gonorrhoea with selected antibiotic agents. *Journal of American Medical Association*, **210**, 857.

LEIGH, D. A., LE FRANC, J. & TURNBULL, A. R. (1969). Sensitivity to penicillin of *Neisseria gonorrhoea*. Relationship to the results of treatment. *British Journal of Venereal Diseases*, **45**, 151.

LOMHOLT, G. & BERG, I. (1966). Gonorrhoea situation in South Greenland in the summer of 1964. *British Journal of Venereal Diseases*, **42**, 1.

LUCAS, J. B. (1971). Paper presented at National Venereal Disease Conference, Atlanta, Georgia.

LUGER, A., (1968). Antibiotic therapy of venereal diseases. In *Current Problems in Dermatology*, Vol. 2, p. 58. Karger, Basel and New York.

LYNN, R., NICOL, C. S., RIDLEY, M., RIMMER, D., SYMONDS, M. A. E. & WARREN, C. (1970). Further studies of penicillin resistant gonococci. *British Journal of Venereal Diseases*, **46**, 404.

MAGNUSON, H. J., EAGLE, H. & FLEISCHMAN, R. (1948). Minimal infectious inoculum of *Spirochaeta pallida* (Nichols strain) and consideration of its rate of multiplication *in vivo*. *American Journal of Syphilis*, **32**, 1.

MAHONEY, J. F., ARNOLD, R. C. & HARRIS, A. (1943). Penicillin treatment of early syphilis; preliminary report. *American Journal of Public Health*, **33**, 1387.

MARSHALL, M. J. & CURTIS, F. R. (1967). Single doses of cephaloridine in the treatment of gonococcal urethritis in males. *Postgraduate Medical Journal, August Supplement*, **43**, 121.

MARTIN, J. E., LESTER, A., KELLOGG, D. S. & THAYER, J. D. (1969). *In vitro* susceptibility of *Neisseria gonorrhoeae* to nine antimicrobial agents. *Applied Microbiology*, **18**, 21.

MORRISON, G. D., COBBOLD, R. J. C., BOR, S., SPITZER, R. J., FOSTER, D. N. & WILLCOX, R. R. (1968). Treatment of gonococcal urethritis with single injections of 2–4 mega units of aqueous procaine penicillin. *British Journal of Venereal Diseases*, **44**, 319.

NIELSON, R. (1970). Sensitivity of gonococci to antibiotics in strains isolated from 'prostitutes' in Copenhagen. *British Journal of Venereal Diseases*, **46**, 153.

OLLER, L. Z. (1967). Further experience with cephaloridine in gonorrhoea. *Postgraduate Medical Journal, August Supplement*, **43**, 124.

PERDRUP, A. (1960). Penicillin treatment of early syphilis. A follow-up study of 213 patients observed for one to eleven years. Comparison between the effect of six and twelve million units. *Acta Dermato-Venereologica* (*Stockholm*), **40**, 340.

ROMANSKY, M. J. & RITTMAN, G. E. (1945). Penicillin blood levels for 24 hours following single intramuscular injection of calcium penicillin in beeswax and peanut oil. *New England Journal of Medicine*, **233**, 577.

RUDOLPH, A. H. (1971). Paper presented at National Venereal Disease Conference, Atlanta, Georgia.

SCHAMBERG, I. L. (1963). Syphilis and Sisyphus. *British Journal of Venereal Diseases*, **39**, 87.

SHAFER, J. K., USILTON, L. J. & PRICE, E. V. (1954). Long-term studies of results of penicillin therapy in early syphilis. *Bulletin of World Heath Organisation*, **10, 563.**

SMITH, C. A., KAMP, M., OLANSKY, S. & PRICE, E. V. (1956). Benzathine penicillin G in the treatment of syphilis. *Bulletin of World Health Organisation*, **15**, 1087.

SPITZER, R. J. & WILLCOX, R. R. (1968). Streptomycin in the treatment of gonorrhoea in London in 1966. *Acta Dermato-Venereologica, Stockholm*, **48**, 537.

SZABO, J. L., EDWARDS, C. D. & BRUCE, W. F. (1951). *N,N*-dibenzylethylenediamine penicillin: preparation and properties. *Antibiotic and Chemotherapy, New York*, **1**, 499.

UNITED STATES PUBLIC HEALTH SERVICE (1968). *Syphilis a Synopsis.* United States Public Health Service Publication, Number 1660, Washington.

WILKINSON, A. E. (1972). Problems in the treatment of venereal disease: Bacterial resistance: Allergy. *Journal of Royal College of Physicians of London*, **6**, 175.

WILKINSON, A. E., RACE, J. W. & CURTIS, F. R. (1967). Kanamycin in the treatment of gonorrhoea in males. *Postgraduate Medical Journal, May Supplement*, p. 65.

WILLCOX, R. R. (1947). Commercial penicillins and treatment of syphilis; some recent American developments. *British Journal of Venereal Diseases*, **23**, 11.

WILLCOX, R. R. (1956). Treatment of gonorrhoea with spiramycin. *British Journal of Venereal Diseases*, **32**, 117.

WILLCOX, R. R. (1958). *Bulletin of the World Health Organisation*, **19**, 503.

WILLCOX, R. R. (1962a). Treatment of early venereal syphilis with antibiotics. *British Journal of Venereal Diseases*, **38**, 109.

WILLCOX, R. R. (1962b). Trobicin (actinospectacin), a new injectable antibiotic in the treatment of gonorrhoea. *British Journal of Venereal Diseases*, **38**, 150.

WILLCOX, R. R. (1963). Treatment of acute gonorrhoea with single injections of chloromycetin succinate. *British Journal of Venereal Diseases*, **39**, 160.

WILLCOX, R. R. (1964a). Influence of penicillin allergic reactions on venereal disease control programmes. *British Journal of Venereal Diseases*, **40,** 200.

WILLCOX, R. R. (1964b). The newer penicillins in the treatment of gonorrhoea. *Postgraduate Medical Journal, May Supplement*, **40,** 202.

WILLCOX, R. R. (1965). Ampicillin divided doses in the treatment of gonorrhoea. *British Journal of Clinical Practice*, **19,** 689.

WILLCOX R. R. (1967). Demethylchlortetracycline in the treatmeat of gonorrhoea. *British Journal of Venereal Diseases*, **43,** 157.

WILLCOX, R. R. (1968). Antibiotic therapy of venereal diseases. In *Current Problems in Dermatology*, Vol. 2, p. 58. Karger, New York.

WILLCOX, R. R. (1969). Treatment of gonorrhoea with double doses of demethylchlortetracycline. *Acta Dermato-Venereologica* (*Stockholm*), **49,** 103.

WILLCOX, R. R. (1970). Recent developments in the treatment of gonorrhoea. *British Journal of Venereal Diseases*, **46,** 141.

WILLCOX, R. R. (1971). Treatment of gonorrhoea with two oral doses of antibiotics. Trials of cephalexin and of triple Tetracycline (Deteclo). *British Journal of Venereal Diseases*, **47,** 31.

WILLCOX, R. R. & WOODCOCK, K. S. (1970). Cephalexin in the oral treatment of gonorrhoea by a double-dose method. *Postgraduate Medical Journal, October Supplement*, **46,** 103.

WILLCOX, R. R. & WOODCOCK, K. S. (1971). Unpublished data.

WILLCOX, R. R., WOODCOCK, K. S. & LATTO, D. (1971). Ampicillin and probenecid in the treatment of gonorrhoea. Paper presented at VIIth International Congress of Chemotherapy, Prague.

WORLD HEALTH ORGANISATION (1960). *World Health Organisation Expert Committee on Venereal Infections and Treponematoses. Fifth report.* World Health Organisation Technical Report Service, number 190, Geneva.

WORLD HEALTH ORGANISATION (1964). *World Health Organisation Expert Committee on Biological Standardisation. Sixteenth report.* World Health Technical Report Service, number 274, Geneva.

WORLD HEALTH ORGANISATION (1969). *Report on the Second Regional Seminar on Venereal Disease Control.* World Health Organisation Regional Office for the Western Pacific Region, Manila.

WORLD HEALTH ORGANISATION (1972). *Report of World Health Organisation and I.U.V.D.T. Travelling Seminar to the United States of America.* In press.

19

THE SELECTION OF ANTIBIOTICS IN GENERAL PRACTICE

J. C. GOULD

GREAT emphasis is given to the resistance of pathogenic bacteria to antibiotics and antibacterial agents, and an observer might be forgiven for gaining the impression that the treatment of infection is now a very difficult thing for the clinician, fraught with numerous hazards and often with an unfavourable outcome for the patient.

My remit, however, is to discuss the choice of antibiotic in general practice, and I wish to say from the outset that as far as my own geographical area is concerned the majority of pathogenic bacteria isolated from patients remain antibiotic sensitive, and although a proportion of strains show some *in vitro* resistance to some of the commonly used antibacterial agents there does not appear to be any particular problem in treatment that can be related to this resistance.

PREDICTABLE SENSITIVITY PATTERNS

Not all bacteria are sensitive to each and every antibiotic, nor have they ever been. Each group of organisms, whether it be described as a 'species' or 'genus' has its characteristic pattern of sensitivity to a range of antibiotics, and this may be referred to as the 'antibiogram'. This tends to be 'fixed' with many of the common pathogens, e.g. streptococci and Pasteurella and Haemophilus species and allows the use of the 'predictable sensitivity pattern' (Table 1). With other organisms such as staphylococci and *Escherichia coli* the pattern of antibiotic sensitivity is more variable and it may be less certain to predict sensitivity or resistance for individual strains. Within each of these groups of organisms however, it is possible to describe the reaction of the majority of strains to antibiotics with sufficient accuracy for the treatment of infections. Thus, since so many strains of *Staphylococcus pyogenes* are resistant to penicillin because of penicillinase production, it is reasonable to regard all such strains as resistant to penicillin; on the other hand so many strains are sensitive to cloxacillin and flucloxacillin, lincomycin, fucidic acid and chloramphenicol, that these drugs may be accepted as active unless there is some special reason to question the sensitivity in an individual case, e.g. because the patient is not responding to treatment. This is not to say that the patient will fail to respond to treatment with an antibiotic which appears to be inactive *in vitro* against the infecting bacterium; many patients do respond favourably in such a situation and just as many fail to respond when it appears that the strain of bacterium is fully sensitive to the chemotherapeutic agent being used.

TABLE 1

PREDICTABLE SENSITIVITIES

	Sensitive to:	*Resistant to:*
Pneumococcus	P, E, L, C, Cep	S, K, G
Strept. pyogenes	P, E, L, C, Cep. Less sensitive to other penicillins	S, K, G. In some cases to T
Strept. faecalis, Other streptococci	A, E, L, Cep	
H. influenzae and other Haemophilus species	A, T, Co, C. Less sensitive to Cep	E, L
Staph. pyogenes when 'Penicillin-sensitive'	P, T, E, L, Fuc, G. Penicillinase-resistant penicillins	
'Penicillinase-producer but antibiotic sensitive'	Usually sensitive to all above antibiotics except P	
'Antibiotic-resistant'		Often resistant to T and E. More rarely resistant to one or more of the other antibiotics
Esch. coli		
(a) antibiotic sensitive	Usually to A, C, T, Su, Na, Co, S, K, G, N	
(b) antibiotic resistant		May be resistant to one or more of these drugs: S, T
Ps. aeruginosa	Poly, G, Car, C, K. Moderately sensitive to a combination of A+Clox. T+Su or Co	
P. mirabilis	A, K, G, Co, Su, C, Na, N	Cy, Poly
Other Proteus sp.		May be resistant to one or more of above agents

Abbreviations: A, Ampicillin; C, Clindamycin; Car, Carbenicillin; Cep, Cephalosporins; Clox, Cloxacillin and other penicillinase resistant penicillins; Co, Co-trimoxazole; Cy, Cycloserine; E, Erythromycin; Fuc, Fucidic acid; G, Gentamicin; K, Kanamycin; L, Lincomycin; N, Nitrofurantoin; Na, Nalidixic acid; P, Penicillin; Poly, Polymyxins; S, Streptomycin; Su, Sulphonamides; T, Tetracycline.

Thus resistance is relative, but one of the great difficulties is to define to what criterion it is relative. It is logical to relate our *in vitro* laboratory results to a level which approximates to the amount of antibiotic likely to be circulating in the blood during normal dosage of the antibiotic, but it must always be remembered that the laboratory models used are poor representations of the complex conditions pertaining in the host's tissues during the infection. The ultimate measurement, and often the only one of real value, is the clinical response of the patient—does he respond to the treatment or not. In this context the overall outstanding success of chemotherapy in the past 30 years both in and out of hospital must not be forgotten or looked at in false perspective. In general practice one of the results of chemotherapy has been a reduction in the number of patients requiring admission to hospital because of infection.

Thus most of the infection occurring in hospital is incidental to the primary condition of the patient which necessitated admission, or is secondary to procedures carried out on the patient while he is in hospital.

INFECTIONS IN DOMICILIARY PRACTICE

It should be remembered that most of the episodes of infection in the community occur among the general population outside hospital. Most of these infections are self limiting and resolve spontaneously. The more severe are seen by the general practitioner to be treated or more likely referred to hospital. In spite of this large number of infections in general practice only a small proportion of the bacteriological diagnostic work comes from general practitioners. In the Edinburgh area the amount is less than 20 per cent of the laboratory work in microbiology, and this is one very good reason why there is a bias in the information which is obtained from studies carried out in chemotherapy and reported to Societies and in the Journals. Further, it must be true that a great deal of treatment of infection is being carried out without specific laboratory diagnosis and without antibiotic sensitivity tests to direct chemotherapy. In the main however, such treatment appears to be successful.

SELECTION OF ANTIBIOTIC IN DOMICILIARY PRACTICE

The choice of antibiotic is based on the basic principles that,
(1) a diagnosis is established,
(2) the causative organisms are isolated, and
(3) specific antibiotic sensitivity tests are carried out on the isolated organism.

In practice it is difficult to follow these procedures and the general practitioner is faced with making,
(1) a rapid diagnosis,
(2) a decision whether or not to treat with antibiotic,
(3) having decided to use an antibiotic, he must choose a drug, and
(4) the drug to be used must be convenient to the patient and to a certain extent to himself.

The choice of antibiotic is therefore most often an empirical one and depends upon decisions about,
(a) the probable diagnosis,
(b) the probable nature of the infecting organism, and
(c) its predictable sensitivity.

A disadvantage of this policy is the possible masking of the true nature of infection, using the wrong antibiotic, encouraging the development of resistance in the infecting strains, altering unnecessarily the microflora of the patient and the development of immunological hypersensitivity, and it cannot be denied that frequently no definitive diagnosis is possible after antibiotics have been given in this empirical way. However, the speedy recovery of the patient whether the antibiotic is prescribed for a specific reason or not is sufficient to justify this procedure in most practitioners minds. In a few patients treatment is unsuccessful but it is doubtful if this frequency is any higher than when prescription of the antibiotic is on the basis of laboratory tests.

The general practitioner must approach the problem of chemotherapy as he does most others, on the basis of his experience, and in this he should be supported by the experience of the microbiologist. A great deal of the success of co-operation between the general practitioner and the microbiologist depends upon encouraging the practitioner to make greater use of the laboratory and the key to this is better communication. Specimen containers must be improved and made readily available; the samples to be examined must be collected rapidly and taken to the laboratory where rapid reports can be prepared and communicated to the practitioner.

Where possible general practitioners should be encouraged to participate in the laboratory work either by coming to the laboratory or by carrying out the initial stages of bacteriological examination such as the plating of urines in their own side rooms, and having the diagnosis completed within the laboratory.

Finally the microbiologist must act in his capacity as a consultant and provide an adequate commentary not only on specific results, but upon epidemiological trends which include the predictable sensitivity of pathogenic bacteria. Table 1 shows some of the predictable sensitivities for the main pathogenic bacteria and this is intended to be a guide to the practitioner. It is subject to revision at any time depending upon the results of local bacteriology as determined by the microbiologist.

The choice of antibiotics in respiratory infection

In acute upper respiratory tract infection including pharyngitis, tonsillitis, tracheitis, otitis and stomatitis, pathogenic bacteria are frequently important though not always as the primary infective agents. The majority of those of consequence are penicillin-sensitive, e.g. *Streptococcus pyogenes*, Pneumococcus, Vincent's organisms and Corynebacteria, so that benzylpenicillin is the drug of choice. Where necessary erythromycin or lincomycin are second choice. The prescription of these antibiotics will not affect the clinical course of viral infections but may shorten the course of those which involve secondary bacterial invasion and will abort most primary bacterial infections. The main exception to this is in infections due to Haemophilus species which are quite common as a cause of recurrent tonsillitis and pharyngitis. Small epidemics of *Haemophilus parainfluenzae* infection may occur and epidemiological information from the microbiologist can be of great value to the general practitioner when this occurs. Ampicillin or tetracycline are indicated as the drugs of choice for such infections and the only important contra-indication is infectious mononucleosis for which ampicillin should not be used.

When bacteria are involved in acute bronchitis and tracheitis they are usually haemophilus species with or without pneumococcus or *Strept. pyogenes*; large doses of penicillin are often helpful in these patients but probably ampicillin and tetracycline are more generally effective. Tetracycline is particularly useful if mycoplasma is involved as the infecting agent.

Pneumonia and bronchopneumonia are most often due to pneumococcus; more rarely species such as klebsiella, *Haemophilus influenzae* and *Staph. pyogenes* may be the cause but such patients are largely candidates for bacterial investigation and the individual estimation of the antibiotic sensitivity of the infecting organism. Failure to respond to therapy may be due to unresolved or atypical pneumonia and detailed investigations including serology will be required to establish a diagnosis and carry out management of the patient.

Acute exacerbations in chronic bronchitis are invariably associated with pneumococcal and *H. influenzae* infection. The exacerbation may be treated with any of the antibiotics or combinations of antibacterial agents effective against these bacteria—tetracycline, ampicillin, cotrimoxazole, chloramphenicol, and penicillin + streptomycin. The clinical response is similar irrespective of which drug is used providing adequate dosage and time of treatment is given. Cephalosporins and lincomycin are somewhat less active because of the variable sensitivity found *in vitro* with many strains of haemophilus. Pneumococcal infections are highly sensitive to both of these antibiotics.

The choice of antibiotic in intestinal infection

Bacterial infections with or without flux are very common in general practice. In the United Kingdom most are due to *Shigella sonnei* or *Shigella flexneri*; an indefinite number are due to 'type specific' *Esch. coli*, especially in younger children, and salmonella infection is much less common. The toxic forms of food poisoning with gastro-enteritis are also very common, but as there is no true infection in these patients chemotherapy is not indicated.

The general consensus of current opinion is against the use of chemotherapy in most cases of shigella and salmonella infection; it is unlikely that antibiotics significantly shorten the clinical course of infection and there is some evidence that they frequently make it worse and increase both the rate of relapse and the period of carriage of the organism. In hospital the administration of antibiotic does appear to increase the chances of antibiotic resistant Gram negative bacilli colonizing the intestinal tract and this may have important epidemiological consequences. In general practice this appears, but it is true that many strains of shigella are now resistant to several antibiotics such as the sulphonamides, streptomycin, neomycin and tetracycline which have been much used in the past for the treatment of diarrhoea. Thus the continued use of these, and other antibiotics may result in further spread of resistant strains. It is not suggested that this resistance is a factor in the failure to cure these patients with antibiotic, but it would be wiser to restrict the use of antibiotics to prevent spread of resistant organisms within the community.

The choice of antibiotic in urinary tract infection

In general practice the majority of uncomplicated (primary) infections are due to *Esch. coli*, and 90 per cent of the strains when examined are sensitive to the usually used antibacterial agents namely, ampicillin, cotrimoxazole, cephalosporins, the amino sugars, tetracycline, chloramphenicol, cycloserine, sulphonamide, nalidixic acid and the furazones. Most of the remainder are due to *Streptococcus faecalis* and *Proteus mirabilis* which are always sensitive to ampicillin, the cephalosporins and cotrimoxazole. The treatment of patients with a significant bacteriuria, with or without a pyuria, therefore presents no immediate problem and the choice of antibiotic is a clinical one. The response to the first course of treatment of 5–10 days seems to be much the same whichever drug is used, and approximates to 75 per cent, and if the second course does not eradicate the organisms from the urine, further investigation of the urinary tract is strongly indicated.

Secondary infection of the urinary tract that has resulted from instrumentation, operation, or failure of previous treatment, may be found to be due to *Esch. coli*, *Strept. faecalis*, proteus, pseudomonas and klebsiella species and a number of other organisms either occurring singly or in a mixed infection, and more frequently these strains are resistant to one or more of the antibacterial agents quoted above, and often this is paralleled by a refractory response to treatment. In such cases individual assessment of antibiotic sensitivity of the infecting microbes should be carried out.

Chronic pyelonephritis and other chronic renal infections may involve organisms which are intermittently present on urine examination and they may be difficult or impossible to eradicate. Individual sensitivity tests may indicate a suitable antibiotic but management of the patient may be best effected by the use of combinations of antibacterial agents. When treatment has to continue for an extended period, sometimes indefinitely, the choice must be from oral preparations and the mixture can be altered each month or 6 weeks to reduce the chance of selecting resistant flora.

CONCLUSION

The greater amount of infection in the community is seen by the general practitioner and every encouragement should be given to increase the amount of laboratory diagnosis. However, it must be recognized that much treatment with antibiotics will continue to be empirical and under these conditions the use of predictable sensitivity is of value in the management of the patient. The microbiologist can help in this by maintaining a commentary on the antibiotic sensitivity of the main pathogenic bacteria isolated in his region; this experience coupled with the clinical experience of the practitioners should ensure successful treatment in most patients. In those whose infection is more serious or refractory it will be necessary to carry out detailed laboratory examinations to isolate the causative organism and determine its specific antibiotic sensitivity.

In hospital, selective pressures which led to the emergence and spread of antibiotic resistant strains will continue and make the treatment of some infections contracted in hospital more difficult. The same basic mechanisms are present in the general community but the pressure is less so that there is less disturbance of the ecological balance of antibiotic sensitive bacteria.

DISCUSSION

Tests for antibiotic synergy

Question. Can Dr. Gould describe the methods used for examination of sensitivities to combinations of antibiotics, particularly as these are sometimes of value in bowel preparation for surgery, and it is often difficult to persuade a bacteriologist to test antibiotic combinations for synergy.

Dr. J. C. Gould. In the simplest situation the one that we most frequently use is the development of the primary sensitivity tests where material from the patient, be it urine, sputum or faeces, is spread out in a uniform lawn on a culture plate or a combination of culture plates. Discs impregnated with the antibiotics are then either placed one on top of the other or are placed at arbitrary distances from one another, the centres of the two discs being approximately 20 mm apart.

This is not the method that we would use if we were asked for a combination for the treatment of endocarditis. In this condition we would perform more sophisticated tests such as combined serial dilution tests, or perhaps a modified abbreviated Chabbert test initially, before carrying out more complicated tube dilution tests.

I might trail my coat a little bit further as you have asked this question. I was going to mention it in the text. For the treatment of chronic urinary tract infection I don't think that sensitivity tests are of much value. If we have a patient in the far north of Scotland who is many days train, canoe and pony time from the nearest centres she sends in dip-slide cultures from time to time but we only see her once every 6 months. We say to the local practitioner—you have a list of antibiotics which includes the usual antibacterial agents and it's rather like a pool form, you can permute two of any of this group and change them each month. It seems to work, that is, the patients continue to be suppressed.

The general practitioner

Dr. J. S. Stevenson. Although I very much admired what Dr. Gould said about the combination of general practice and laboratories, I feel that I must disagree with him regarding general practitioners working either in a laboratory or with infective material. After 20 years of encouraging practitioners to come to my laboratory I don't think I would allow the average general practitioner to work with sonné, typhimurium, etc., anymore than I would allow the average venereologist to remove my appendix!

Professor R. E. O. Williams. Is anybody going to attack Dr. Gould on any of the heretical statements that he made? I must say I wonder whether if one trained general practitioners they wouldn't be just as safe in handling sonné bacteria as we are!

General Practitioner. As a much maligned general practitioner, I might perhaps have a say. The thing about general practice, especially the busy urban practice, is that infections are seen every day and it would be quite impossible to use the laboratory as one would perhaps like to, by sending sputum specimens from all chest infections and so forth. I find that what you must do it to make a careful clinical diagnosis and choose an antibiotic. One's choice is right in 99 per cent of cases. In the other 1 per cent you need the help of the laboratory but these cases often require admission to hospital anyway

Dr. J. C. Gould. I would agree. This is essentially what I was saying.

20

ANTIVIRAL AGENTS

D. J. BAUER

INTRODUCTION

COMPARED with the successes of antibacterial chemotherapy, the discovery of drugs acting specifically on virus infections has made relatively little progress so far. This is partly due to the fact that the first antibacterial drugs were brought into use 30 years ago, providing the stimulus for the intensive development which has taken place since then, whereas antiviral drugs were used in man for the first time barely 10 years ago. A further reason is that the problem of antiviral chemotherapy is intrinsically much more difficult. Bacteria possess metabolic systems which differ from those of the host, and which can therefore be selectively attacked, whereas viruses are largely dependent on the synthetic machinery of the host cell, which offers no opportunity for selective attack. The pace of antiviral research has also been slowed by a general attitude of pessimism, which holds that virus diseases cannot be treated since their onset is too acute and their duration too limited. Nevertheless, definite progress has been made, and at the present time there are three specific antiviral drugs which are in use in human medicine.

At the same time the realization has gradually dawned that the main place of antiviral drugs is in prophylaxis, since they confer immediate protection during the incubation period, whereas the protection conferred by vaccination develops too late under these particular circumstances.

POINTS OF ATTACK BY ANTIVIRAL AGENTS

There are three situations in which a virus could be attacked by an antiviral drug. After it gains access to the body the virus particle is at first in an extracellular position, in the blood stream or tissue fluid. In this position it is not doing harm, in distinction to a bacterium, which will be multiplying and producing toxins. Although the virus would appear to be vulnerable this is in fact not the case. The most potent agent for inactivating extracellular virus is specific neutralizing antibody, but this is nearly always ineffective in practice, with the sole exceptions of gamma-globulin in the prophylaxis of infective hepatitis and the treatment of infective complications of smallpox vaccination. There is little likelihood of finding a chemical compound with specificity as high as that of antibody, and an attack on the virus in the extracullular position seems unlikely to succeed.

From the tissue space the virus particle becomes attached to the surface of a cell. In certain cases this takes place by means of specific receptors, and any compound which can block these receptors should prevent the attachment of the virus and its entry into the cell. This has been achieved with amantadine hydrochloride, which will prevent the attachment of influenza virus, but the method is unlikely to succeed with viruses which enter cells by other means.

After entry into the cell the virus particle separates into its individual components. It may contain enzymes for replicating its own nucleic acids, or it may induce the host cells to do this by means of their own mechanism of transcription and translation. Although host cell systems are used, the products are specific for the virus, and the degree of difference between host and parasite which is required as a point of chemotherapeutic attack is thus present. Methisazone and idoxuridine act in this kind of way.

VIRUS INFECTIONS SUSCEPTIBLE TO CHEMOTHERAPY

In describing the use of drugs in the chemotherapy of virus infections reference will be made only to those drugs which are available commercially and are in regular use in clinical practice.

Vaccinia

Smallpox vaccination consists of an artificial infection of the skin with vaccinia virus. This usually proceeds within tolerable limits, but occasionally there may be a very severe local and general reaction. Also, vaccination may be necessary but contraindicated for various reasons, such as age, certain diseases of the skin and concomitant disease of other systems. In such cases the course of the vaccinial infection can be moderated by treatment with methisazone (Marboran), a compound which specifically inhibits the multiplication of vaccinia virus. In a series reported by Jaroszyńska-Weinberger and Mészáros (1966), 55 children aged 2½–9 years with various contraindications to primary vaccination were vaccinated and divided into 2 groups; 26 were treated with methisazone and 29 were given antivaccinial gamma-globulin. No untreated control group was used, on account of the danger of vaccinating without cover in such cases. Treatment was begun on the 4th day after vaccination and methisazone was given by mouth in an initial dose of 100 mg/kg followed by 50 mg/kg daily for 3–6 days. The severity of the local lesion was significantly reduced in comparison with the gamma-globulin group and the total duration from vaccination to detachment of the scab was also reduced.

Ectopic primary vaccinia may occur in dangerous sites such as the orbit, nose and mouth. Jaroszyńska-Weinberger (1970) used methisazone in 16 such cases, and compared the results with a control group of 23 patients, 5 of whom were treated with gamma-globulin. Methisazone was given by mouth in a dose of 150 mg/kg for up to 8 days. Healing occurred more rapidly in the methisazone group.

If smallpox vaccination is carried out in eczematous persons, whether the disease is active or not, *eczema vaccinatum* may develop. This is a serious condition, resembling smallpox in many features, which carries a high mortality. The course is very variable, and assessment of response to treatment can only be based on clinical impressions, but good results have been obtained with methisazone given in a loading dose of 200 mg/kg, followed by 50 mg/kg every 6 hours for 48 hours (Bauer, 1965).

If the immune response is defective, as in hypogammaglobulinaemia, or treatment with immunosuppressive drugs, the vaccinial lesion may spread indefinitely without any tendency to heal, and metastatic lesions may appear anywhere in the body. This condition is called *vaccinia gangrenosa*, and is invariably fatal in the absence of treatment. Recovery can sometimes be obtained with antivaccinial gamma-globulin, but cases which fail to respond can be cured with methisazone in the same dosage as used for eczema vaccinatum (Bauer, 1965). Virological cure can usually be obtained in 50 per cent of cases, but the patient is still left with the underlying condition which may itself be fatal.

Introduction of smallpox vaccine into the eye may give rise to vaccinial keratitis. This is a serious condition which may leave corneal opacities or give rise to perforation of the cornea. It responds very well to idoxuridine. This is instilled into the eye in the form of a 0·5 per cent solution, and should be given every 2 hours around the clock until the lesions have healed. Simultaneous lesions on the palpebral conjunctiva and eyelids can be treated with oral methisazone.

Smallpox and alastrim

Persons who have been in contact with smallpox are always vaccinated, but the immunity produced by vaccination usually develops too slowly to prevent the onset of the disease, although it may give rise to a milder course. Methisazone will give immediate protection, and 2 doses of 3 g in an adult will usually eradicate the infection. In a trial carried out in Madras in 1963 there were 18 cases of smallpox among 2610 contacts treated with methisazone, and 113 among 2710 contacts who were not treated. There was thus a 6-fold reduction in case incidence (Bauer *et al.*, 1969).

Methisazone is also effective in the prophylaxis of alastrim, a milder form of smallpox which occurs in South America. In a trial reported by Ribeiro do Valle *et al.* (1965), 8 cases of alastrim occurred among 215 contacts given 3 or 6 g of methisazone, and 49 among 306 who were untreated, or refused treatment. There was a 4·3-fold reduction in case-incidence.

Herpes simplex infections

Infection with herpes virus (herpes simplex) can cause keratitis, vesicular eruptions of the skin, mouth and genital area, and encephalitis. The standard treatment is with idoxuridine. Herpetic keratitis will respond to idoxuridine drops given in the same dosage régime as for vaccinial keratitis. Resistant strains of herpes virus may develop during repeated courses of treatment, and the drug has little effect if there is deep stromal involvement.

The course of cutaneous herpes can be considerably shortened by local treatment with a 5 per cent solution of idoxuridine in dimethylsulphoxide, and there is some evidence that the treatment prevents recurrences in the same area (MacCallum & Juel-Jensen, 1966). Primary herpes infection of the skin occurs fairly frequently in hospital staff, and may take the form of herpetic whitlow. This is a painful condition which may take 3–4 weeks to heal. It responds very rapidly to 40 per cent idoxuridine in dimethylsulphoxide. The lesion should be covered with lint which is kept constantly moistened with the solution. Severe generalized primary herpes responds well to cytarabine, given intravenously in doses up to 2 mg/kg daily (Juel-Jensen, 1970). The treatment of herpetic encephalitis is less satisfactory. Idoxuridine has been given intravenously or into the carotid artery by slow infusion in total doses of up to 1000 mg/kg over a period of 5 days. Some survivals have been obtained, but the disease is not invariably fatal and there has been residual mental and neurological defect in every case. The low solubility and rapid inactivation of the drug render it unsatisfactory for use in this condition.

Herpes zoster

There is one report of the successful treatment of zoster keratitis with idoxuridine. The drug was given as 0·5 per cent eye drops administered 2-hourly for 5 days. The lesion began to regress on the second day of treatment. The use of idoxuridine in cutaneous zoster has been investigated by Juel-Jensen *et al.* (1970) in a controlled trial against a placebo. The best results were obtained with a 40 per cent solution in dimethylsulphoxide applied locally on gauze which was kept continuously moist with the solution. In comparison with the placebo group the treatment caused rapid disappearance of pain and drying of the lesion. Waltuch and Sachs (1968) obtained a rapid cure with intravenous idoxuridine in a total dose of 25 g over 5 days in a case of severe generalized zoster with underlying Hodgkin's disease. Intravenous idoxuridine has been used with some beneficial effect in an infant suffering from congenital cytomegalovirus infection (Conchie *et al.*, 1968).

Influenza

The prophylaxis and treatment of influenza is on a less satisfactory footing than that of the other virus infections. The only drug available as yet is amantadine hydrochloride, and its degree of activity leaves much to be desired. A number of trials have given negative results, and only those in which a significant effect was obtained will be mentioned here. The best report is that given by Galbraith *et al.* (1969). The drug was given prophylactically to family contacts of patients suffering from A2 influenza in 1967–68 in a dose of 100 mg orally every 12 hours. Treatment was continued for 10 days, and a placebo was used. No case of influenza occurred during the treatment period among 48 contacts given the drug, whereas there were 10 cases during the same period among 69 contacts given placebo. The difference was highly significant. No effect was observed in a similar trial carried out during an outbreak caused by the Hong Kong variant in 1969. Some therapeutic effect in A2 influenza has been claimed by Hornick *et al.* (1969), in a trial carried out during an epidemic in a prison in 1968. The chemotherapy of influenza is thus still in an unsatisfactory state, and derivatives of amantadine with higher activity are needed, or more active compounds of a different chemical class.

Adenovirus infections

A start has been made on the chemotherapy of adenovirus infections. Little *et al.* (1968) carried out a trial of oral methisazone and trifluorothymidine eye drops against placebos in 160 volunteers with experimentally induced adenovirus 3 conjunctivitis. Trifluorothymidine was inactive, but after the code had been broken the observers considered that the disease might have been milder in the group given methisazone. There is clearly a need for a compound effective in the prophylaxis and treatment of adenovirus infections in view of their prevalence during the winter months.

CONCLUSION

In conclusion, it is evident that antiviral chemotherapy is an established fact, but suffers at present from the disadvantage that the diseases which are susceptible to treatment or prevention are not of widespread occurrence, but the drugs which are available, which may be life-saving in certain circumstances, nevertheless constitute a notable advance in therapeutics.

REFERENCES

BAUER, D. J. (1965). Clinical experience with the antiviral drug Marboran (1 methylisatin 3-thiosemicarbazone). *Annals of the New York Academy of Sciences*, **130**, Art. 1, 110.

BAUER, D. J., VINCENT, L. S., KEMPE, C. H., YOUNG, P. A. & DOWNIE, A. W. (1969). Prophylaxis of smallpox with methisazone. *American Journal of Epidemiology*, **90**, 130.

CONCHIE, A. F., BARTON, B. W. & TOBIN, J. O'H. (1968). Congenital cytomegalovirus infection treated with idoxuridine. *British Medical Journal*, **4**, 162.

GALBRAITH, A. W., OXFORD, J. S., SCHILD, G. C. & WATSON, G. I. (1969). Protective effect of 1-adamantanamine hydrochloride on influenza A2 infections in the family environment. *Lancet*, **ii**, 1026.

HORNICK, R. B., TOGO, Y., MAHLER, S. & IEZZONI, D. (1969). Evaluation of amantadine hydrochloride in the treatment of A2 influenzal disease. *Bulletin of the World Health Organization*, **41**, 671.

JAROSZYŃSKA-WEINBERGER, B. (1970). Treatment with methisazone of complications following smallpox vaccination. *Archives of Diseases of Childhood*, **45**, 573.

JAROSZYŃSKA-WEINBERGER, B. & MÉSZÁROS, J. (1966). A comparison of the protective effect of methisazone and a hyperimmune antivaccinial gamma-globulin in primary smallpox vaccination carried out in the presence of contraindications. *Lancet*, **i**, 948.

JUEL-JENSEN, B. E. (1970). Severe generalized primary herpes treated with cytarabine. *British Medical Journal*, **2**, 154.

JUEL-JENSEN, B. E., MACCALLUM, F. O., MACKENZIE, A. M. R. & PIKE, M. C. (1970). Treatment of zoster with idoxuridine in dimethylsulphoxide. Results of two double-blind controlled trials. *British Medical Journal*, **4**, 776.

LITTLE, J. M., LORENZETTI, D. W. C., BROWN, D. C., SCHWEEN, H. H., JONES, B. R. & KAUFMAN, H. E. (1968). Studies of adenovirus type III infection treated with methisazone and trifluorothymidine. *Proceedings of the Society for Experimental Biology and Medicine*, **127**, 1028.

MACCALLUM, F. O. & JUEL-JENSEN, B. E. (1966). Herpes simplex virus skin infection in man treated with idoxuridine in dimethylsulphoxide. *British Medical Journal*, **2**, 805.

RIBEIRO DO VALLE, L. A., DE MELO, P. R., DE SALLES GOMES, L. F. & PROENÇA, L. M. (1965). Methisazone in prevention of variola minor among contacts. *Lancet*, **ii**, 976.

WALTUCH, G. & SACHS, F. (1968). Herpes zoster in a patient with Hodgkin's disease. Treatment with idoxuridine. *Archives of Internal Medicine*, **121**, 458.

21

ANTIFUNGAL AGENTS

H. I. Winner

DERMATOPHYTE INFECTIONS

Infections of the ringworm type, such as athlete's foot and favus, are among the most common infectious diseases in the world, rivalling in frequency the common cold, malaria, bilharzia and other mass diseases. There are vast reservoirs in both the human and the animal population. For years the traditional treatment of these has been by means of keratolytic and fungicidal applications of various kinds which is not relevant to the present symposium. However, it was long evident that even in economically advanced communities there were a small number of persistent local infections which were not amenable to local treatment or even to surgery. Such were the affections of the finger-nails and toe-nails due to *Trichophyton rubrum*.

Another common and distressing disease was ringworm of the scalp, which frequently occurred as an epidemic in children and which was often treated by the brutal method of complete depilation. Children would have all their hair shaved off and after this operation, disfiguring both physically and mentally, it took the child many months to get back to normal.

In 1939 Oxford, Raistrick and Simonart discovered a substance produced by *Penicillium griseofulvum* which prevented the growth of certain fungi which were plant parasites. It was named griseofulvin and became much used in plant pathology. In 1958 Gentles in Glasgow found that griseofulvin given systemically could cure *Microsporon canis* infection in guinea pigs. He and his colleagues (1959) also showed that the antibiotic given systemically got into the hair of treated animals from which it could be extracted only with methanol. It was soon applied to human cases of dermatophyte infections with striking results. Patients who had deformed finger-nails and toe-nails became cured within months by taking these tablets by mouth. It was a miraculous effect for many of these people and completely altered their lives. Moreover, children with tinea capitis are now treated by oral griseofulvin.

Griseofulvin is virtually harmless. Although there are occasional refractory infections and the drug has to be taken for a long time, it has completely altered the outlook in dermatophyte diseases. People who were seriously afflicted and deformed can now live normal lives.

SUPERFICIAL CANDIDA INFECTIONS

Candida albicans causes superficial infections which may be trivial but can be serious. Oral and vaginal thrush and candidosis of the skin are all common and usually trivial, though often persistent. Occasionally superficial candida infections are serious and widespread, causing disseminated eruptions or profound disorders such as granuloma. Also, rarely, candida may cause serious systemic disease.

In the past, superficial infections were traditionally treated by the local application of disfiguring, depressing, and dirty dyes, such as gentian violet. Today the best form of treatment is the application of an antifungal antibiotic of which there are several.

Nystatin

The best known is nystatin, first described by Hazen and Brown in 1950. It is active against fungi but not against bacteria. In particular, it is active against candidas and other yeast-like organisms. The pure substance has the form of white crystal needles, with the chemical formula $C_{46}H_{77}NO_{19}$; they are only slightly soluble in water. It is a polyene, that is, it contains numerous double bonds of the CH=CH type. It is stable as a dry powder but the solution is unstable to heat, acid and alkali; solutions have to be kept refrigerated if they are to keep more than a few days.

Nystatin is much used for surface application in cases of superficial candidosis such as infections of the mucous membranes and the skin. About 90 per cent of cases clear up at the first application. Because it is so toxic and unstable the drug cannot be given intravenously. It can however be given by mouth and also it is sometimes given by inhalation in cases of pulmonary candidosis and by urethral instillation in candidosis of the bladder.

Amphotericin B

The second antibiotic used widely is amphotericin B. This was derived from *Streptomyces venuzuelae* and was first described in 1955 by Gold and by Vandeputte and their colleagues. Pure amphotericin B consists of deep yellow prismatic crystals which are amphoteric. The dry powder is stable for long periods. It is not very soluble. Like nystatin, it is a polyene. The growth of cultures of *C. albicans* is suppressed by amphotericin B which is now widely used for superficial application as a second line of attack after nystatin. Used in this way, it is harmless.

Candicidin

A third polyene used for local application is candicidin, about as active as nystatin (Waksman *et al.*, 1965). There are various others which are not much used in this country.

Locally applied, these drugs are quite safe and usually effective. They are not absorbed from the skin or mucous membranes. They are clean and pleasant, unlike the dyes which they have supplanted. No natural resistance to them has been encountered.

SYSTEMIC INFECTIONS

Systemic fungus infections are serious diseases. Systemic candidosis, and other opportunistic infections such as Histoplasmosis, Cryptococcosis and Coccidioidomycosis all occur in economically advanced communities but they are rare in this country. There are also several infections which occur in economically backward communities, such as South American Blastomycosis, Sporotrichosis, Chromoblastomycosis, Rhinosporidiosis, Mucormycosis, Phycomycosis and Mycetoma—incidentally the only one of these which responds to penicillin.

The problems of treating these conditions may be formidable. The patient's defence mechanisms may have been depressed by some such cause as systemic disease, irradiation, immunosuppressive therapy or malnutrition. Or the patient may be a poor man in a poor country, with a multiple infection of which the fungus infection is only one. In such cases the disease may start as a trivial affliction and be slow and chronic, progressing for many years during which disability and deformity appear and become crippling. We do not know how frequent these infections are in economically backward countries, or even how they are transmitted. They appear to be common and they are usually multiple. Moreover, these infections occur as rarities in this country, brought in by immigrants and travellers.

The associated conditions of course should be treated if possible. But it is often not possible to treat the cause of a general reduction in immunity mechanisms, or the economic conditions, which may be important factors in the disease. There is also the fundamental problem of attacking a sophisticated complicated fungus which is much more complicated than a bacterium or virus, and often multicellular. It is difficult to find substances which are able to kill such organisms in human tissues without damaging the human host.

Amphotericin B

However, there are some antibiotics which can be used systemically of which the best is amphotericin B. This is toxic; patients are liable to develop febrile reactions, some become nauseated, some vomit, and about two-thirds, after a few days, show a rise in the blood urea-nitrogen which may be accompanied by renal damage. Patients should never be put on systemic amphotericin B unless they are under hospital surveillance. On the other hand, of course, patients are very ill with a systemic infection before they need to be put on a systemic antifungal at all, and the cases are often so desperately serious that a calculated risk in therapy is justified.

Newer agents

Another drug, also developed in the U.S.A., is 5-fluorocytosine, which is similar in its mode of action and toxicity to amphotericin B (Tassel & Madoff, 1968; Utz *et al.*, 1969). Hamycin is a third line of attack; this was discovered, investigated and developed in India (Anjaneyulu *et al.*, 1961; Maniar & Mavdikar, 1966). It is similar in its usage and toxicity to amphotericin B. The latest of these drugs is clotrimazole which has been developed and marketed within the last few years (Plempel *et al.*, 1969; Oberste-Lehn *et al.*, 1969). It is still too early to assess its place in therapeutics.

There are various other systemic antifungals, not much used in this country, where systemic fungus infections are uncommon. Trichomycin is a polyene which has been developed in Japan. It appears to be effective in various types of candidosis. Pimaricin is a polyene from South Africa on which much work has been done in the Netherlands. I have no personal experience with either of these substances.

No natural resistance to these drugs by any of the fungi I have mentioned has been found. Systemic fungus infections can now be satisfactorily treated by antibiotics and treatment saves many lives.

THE DEVELOPMENT OF ANTIBIOTIC RESISTANCE IN VITRO

By numerous transfers to gradually increasing concentrations of antibiotic it is possible to obtain isolates of candida resistant to nystatin and amphotericin B (Athar & Winner, 1971). These organisms are less pathogenic than the isolates from which they are derived, and show other features such as smaller colonies and reduced development of mycelium. The mode of action of amphotericin B is of general interest. It makes holes in the lipid membrane surrounding the cell, and this action is inhibited by ergosterol. The mechanism of this is intriguing and has important implications in cytology.

It appears that the chances of candida becoming resistant to antibiotics under natural conditions are very small. The reason is that such organisms would be likely to lose their pathogenicity. Normally the organism is not very pathogenic at the worst of times so that if it became less pathogenic it probably would not cause disease even in people with impaired immunity mechanisms. This is probably the reason why resistant candidas have not been found in clinical isolates.

THE PRESENT SITUATION IN THERAPY

With improved diagnostic facilities the number of known cases of systemic fungus infections is increasing though it is doubtful whether this is a real increase.

My first choice of antibiotic is amphotericin B, followed by 5-fluorocytosine or hamycin. The position of clotrimazole in therapy is still doubtful.

There is a real need for less toxic systemic antifungal antibiotics, for a drug as non-toxic as penicillin or some of the later antibacterials. The difficulties both theoretical and practical of developing such substances are formidable, but it seems likely that they will be overcome within a much shorter time than the next 30 years.

REFERENCES

ANJANEYULU, R., APTE, P. P. & PADHYE, A. A. (1961). *Journal of Obstetrics and Gynaecology of India*, **11.**

ATHAR, M. A. & WINNER, H. I. (1971). The development of resistance by candida species to polyene antibiotics *in vitro*. *Journal of Medical Microbiology*, **4,** 505.

GENTLES, J. C. (1958). Experimental ringworm in guinea pigs: oral treatment with griseofulvin. *Nature* (*London*), **182,** 476.

GENTLES, J. C., BARNES, M. J. & FANTES, K. H. (1959). Presence of griseofulvin in hair of guinea pigs after oral administration. *Nature* (*London*), **183,** 256.

GOLD, W., STOUT, H. A., PAGANO, J. F. & DONOVICK, R. (1956). Amphotericins A and B, antifungal antibiotics produced by a streptomycele. I. *In vitro* studies. *Antibiotics Annual*, 1955–56, p. 579.

HAZEN, E. L. & BROWN, R. (1950). Two antifungal agents produced by a soil actinomycete. *Science*, **112,** 432.

MANIAR, A. C. & MAVDIKAR, S. (1966). Biological activities of Hamycin. *Canadian Journal of Microbiology*. **12,** 377.

OBERSTE-LEHN, H., BAGGESEN, I. & PLEMPEL, M. (1969). Erste klinische Erfahrungen bei System-Mykosen mit einem neuen oralen Antimykotikum. *Deutsche Medizinische Wochenschrift*, **94,** 1365.

OXFORD, A. E., RAISTRICK, H. & SIMONART, P. (1939). Studies in the biochemistry of microorganisms. Griseofulvin, $C_{17}H_{17}O_6Cl$, a metabolic product of *Penicillin Griseofulvum Dierckx*. *Biochemical Journal*, **33,** 240.

PLEMPEL, M., BARTMANN, K., BUCHEL, K. H. & REGEL, E. (1969). Experimentelle Befunde uber ein neues, oral wirksames Antimykotikum mit breiten Wirkungs-spektrum. *Deutsche Medizinische Wochenschrift*, **94,** 1356.

TASSEL, D. & MADOFF, M. A. (1968). Treatment of Candida sepsis and cryptococcus meningitis with 5-fluorocytocine. A new antifungal agent. *Journal of the American Medical Association*, **206,** 830.

UTZ., J. P., SHADOMY, S., MCGEHEE, R. F. & TYNES, B. S. (1969). 5-Fluorocytocine: experience in patients with pulmonary and other forms of cryptococcosis. *American Review of Respiratory Diseases*, **99,** 975.

VANDEPUTTE, J., WACHTEL, J. L. & STILLER, E. T. (1956). Amphotericins A and B, antifungal antibiotics produced by a streptomycete. II. The isolation and properties of the crystalline amphotericins. *Antibiotics Annual*, 1955–56, p. 587.

WAKSMAN, S. A., LECHEVALIER, H. A. & SCHAFFNER, C. P. (1965). Candicidin and other polyenic antifungal antibiotics. *Bulletin of the World Health Organisation*, **33,** 219.

DISCUSSION

Candida infections of the urinary tract

Mr. R. L. Lamming. Candida is being cultured much more frequently from the urine of patients who have received many antibiotics, particularly in ill people in intensive care units. When candida is present in the urine in large quantities how do you establish whether this is a local infection or one which has infected the kidneys, and how do you set about investigation and treatment of this problem?

Professor H. I. Winner. I would agree with your observation on the increased frequancy of candida in urinary infection. If the infection is localized to the bladder then give nystatin by instillation through a catheter. If you are quite satisfied that it is a renal infection, a systemic drug is necessary, and you would have to give amphotericin B if it persisted. I must say that I've seen one or two cases in which there has been a transient candida infection and I feel that irrigation with large volumes of fluid clears up some of these. In my experience the patient is often not very ill. It's a serious thing to put a patient on amphotericin B and it is worth changing the pH of the urine and giving alkali and large quantities of fluid for a week or so before starting amphotericin B.

22

UNTOWARD REACTIONS DURING ANTIBIOTIC THERAPY

A. M. GEDDES

All antibiotics are potentially toxic. They act therapeutically by killing or inhibiting the growth of bacteria and it is not surprising that they occasionally have similar actions on human cells. Some seldom cause side-effects but when they do the result can be disastrous. The use of chloramphenicol is rarely associated with untoward side-effects but very occasionally it can cause a fatal aplastic anaemia. On the other hand, although as many as as 15 per cent of patients treated with lincomycin develop diarrhoea, serious toxicity has not been reported with this antibiotic.

The side-effects of an antibiotic can frequently be *prevented or minimized* by understanding the mechanism of their production which may be related to one or more of the following factors:

1. The dose of antibiotic.
2. Increased patient susceptibility which may be either innate or acquired.
3. Interaction with other drugs.
4. Microbiological effects of the antibiotic.

THE DOSE OF ANTIBIOTIC

This may be excessive due either to error in administration or failure to consider the age and weight of the patient when calculating the dose. Apart from the neo-natal period, children metabolize and excrete drugs remarkably well. Elderly patients, on the other hand, may require a reduction in the recommended adult dose of an antibiotic whose toxicity is dose-related.

The amount of antibiotic which is safe when administered by one route can be lethal if given by another. Penicillin is remarkably non-toxic even in large doses by intramuscular injection whereas intrathecal administration of more than 20,000 units can cause the death of the patient. I have seen two examples of this tragic error. There are also certain rare hazards associated with the intravenous injection of excessively high doses of benzylpenicillin. The first is haemolytic anaemia (Petz & Fudenberg, 1966) while a second is the danger of cardiac arrhythmias induced by the potassium salt of penicillin. Sixteen megaunits of benzylpenicillin contain 25 milli-equivalents of potassium cation (Stewart, 1968). Finally, encephalopathy has been reported in patients being given 25 million or more units of penicillin per day by I.V. injection (Bloomer *et al.*, 1967).

The neurotoxicity of certain other antibiotics is also dose-related. Isoniazid in the high dose of 600 milligrams (mg) which is normally given to treat tuberculous meningitis can cause confusion, convulsions and neuropathy by competitive inhibition of pyridoxine. These can be prevented by the simultaneous administration of 10 mg of Vitamin B6. If the serum level of cycloserine exceeds 20 micrograms (μg) per millilitre (ml) neurotoxicity results (Gray *et al.*, 1967). The polymixins can cause neurological side-effects and also respiratory arrest if given in excessive doses (Pohlmann, 1966). We have seen acute hydrocephalus in two small babies given relatively large doses of nalidixic acid. This complication, which has also been reported with tetracycline (Fields, 1961), is probably related to a critical dose of nalidixic acid (Boreus & Sundstrom, 1967).

The ototoxicity of the streptomycin (amino-hexose) group of antibiotics, is well known. Damage to the auditory and vestibular portions of the eighth cranial nerve results from excessively high serum levels of these antibiotics and can be prevented by restricting the dose. Ototoxicity was not observed in a series of 228 patients treated by us with kanamycin, none of whom were given more than 1 gram (g) of the antibiotic daily (Murdoch *et al.*, 1966).

Cephaloridine in a daily dose of more than 6 g can cause renal tubular damage leading to renal failure (Foord, 1969) and the nephrotoxicity of amphotericin B is similarly dose-related (Butler *et al.*, 1964).

We have seen children's teeth which have been discoloured by the administration of tetracycline. This finding, which was first reported by Schwachman and his colleagues in 1959, is normally related to the total dose of tetracycline administered (Wallman & Hilton, 1962; Bevelander & Nakahara, 1966). The tetracyclines stain and can cause hypoplasia of both primary and secondary dentition and because of this should not be given to children under the age of ten. If it is *essential* to prescribe tetracycline in this age group, oxytetracycline, which has the least effect on teeth, should be given (*Lancet*, 1968).

Bone marrow toxicity due to chloramphenicol, particularly reversible marrow depression, is commoner following high doses of the antibiotic (McCurdy, 1963) although fatal aplastic anaemia can occur after even small doses. The 'grey syndrome' of circulatory collapse, reported in neonates given chloramphenicol, occurred when the babies were given the antibiotic in doses in excess of 100 mg per kilogram (kg) per day (Weiss *et al.*, 1960). Because of the serious toxicity associated with its use, chloramphenicol should be reserved for the treatment of typhoid fever and severe *Haemophilus influenzae* infections.

Kahn and his colleagues in 1968 reported blood dyscrasias in elderly patients given large doses of trimethoprim, a component of co-trimoxazole and an inhibitor of folic acid metabolism. There have been reports of granulopenia in patients with typhoid fever being treated with co-trimoxazole (Scragg & Rubidge, 1971; Stamps & Wicks, 1972). Granulocytes have the fastest turnover of the marrow cells and might be expected to be the first to show folate deficiency (Fowle, 1970). We have treated a number of patients suffering from typhoid fever with co-trimoxazole in a relatively high dose of 640 mg of trimethoprim and 3·2 g of sulphamethoxazole daily and have seen an instance of neutropenia (100 neutrophils per cubic millimetre). Two of the other patients in this study became anaemic, one with macrocytosis, during or after treatment with co-trimoxazole (Geddes *et al.*, 1971).

Rifampicin competes with bilirubin for excretion by the liver and large doses may thus lead to jaundice (Aquinas *et al.*, 1972). The ocular toxicity (retrobulbar neuritis) of ethambutol is dose dependent (Leibold, 1966).

INCREASED PATIENT SUSCEPTIBILITY

Innate

Certain patients have an increased susceptibility from birth to side effects of certain antibiotics. This may be related to hypersensitivity or allergic mechanisms, or is occasionally genetically determined.

The penicillins

The best known example of hypersensitivity to antibiotics is penicillin allergy. The major antigenic determinant in penicillin allergy is the penicilloyl group derived from the penicillanic acid 'nucleus', the basis of all the penicillins, and a patient allergic to one penicillin is thus allergic to them all. The proportion of the population who are truly allergic to the penicillins is unknown as there is no satisfactory test for penicillin allergy. Skin testing with penicillin or penicilloyl-polylysine, which is derived from penicillin G, is not a completely reliable method of testing for allergy although a recent report suggests that it may be of some value in detecting susceptible patients and reducing the incidence of reactions to the penicillins (Adkinson *et al.*, 1971).

The frequency of allergic reactions to penicillin vary in different reports from 1 to 10 per cent with anaphylaxis occurring in 0·015–0·004 per cent and a mortality of all those treated of 0·0015–0·002 per cent (Idsoe *et al.*, 1968). In our experience the incidence of allergic reactions to benzylpenicillin agrees with the figure of 1 per cent quoted by Van Arsdell (1968). The incidence of skin rash in patients treated with ampicillin is, however, considerably higher. In 1968 we reported that of a group of patients treated with ampicillin, 24 per cent suffering from enteric fever and 11 per cent with pyelonephritis developed skin rashes (Geddes *et al.*, 1968). Reports from other centres have quoted lower figures which are still in excess of the rash incidence with benzylpenicillin (Knudsen, 1969).

Ampicillin is a semi-synthetic antibiotic which is manufactured by a biological process employing Gram-negative bacilli and it has been postulated that the maculo-papular ampicillin skin rash may be caused by protein and polypeptide impurities derived from these fermentation reactions (Knudsen *et al.*, 1970). Certainly, these protein impurities can cause maculo-papular eruptions when injected into baboons (Knudsen *et al.*, 1970). Because of the known cross-allergenicity between the penicillins, the majority of patients developing a rash with ampicillin will be labelled as penicillin-allergic and thus denied any penicillin in the future. In view of the extensive use of ampicillin the number of patients developing skin rashes must be considerable and it is extremely important to determine whether these eruptions are related to true penicillin allergy mediated by the 6-amino-penicillanic acid (6-APA) nucleus or caused by another mechanism.

We have recently completed a prospective study in Edinburgh, Leeds and Birmingham in which we have investigated the incidence of the ampicillin skin rash. Nine hundred and thirty-three patients were treated with ampicillin and 68 (7·3 per cent) developed a rash. Sixty-one of the 68 skin rashes in our study were macular or maculo-papular but only two were exclusively urticarial, the type of rash normally associated with penicillin allergy (*Lencet*, 1969) and none of the patients developed anaphylaxis. Skin rashes caused by other drugs such as the barbiturates are normally macular or maculo-papular and are not associated with anaphylactic reactions. It would, therefore, seem that the maculo-papular, measles-like rash associated with the administration of ampicillin, is not related to true penicillin allergy but is probably caused by impurities which may be proteins, polypeptides or polymers. Further studies are in progress to investigate the cellular immunological aspects of the eruptions.

The cephalosporins

The cephalosporins may occasionally cause allergic reactions, the incidence being quoted as 1·7 per cent of those treated (Petz, 1971). It is probable that they can be given safely to patients allergic to penicillin although reactions to the cephalosporins occur in 8·2 per cent of patients who are also allergic to the penicillins (Petz, 1971). Although this could be related to cross-allergenicity it is probably only a manifestation of multiple hypersensitivity in a particularly allergic patient. We have recently seen a woman who has developed severe allergic reactions to penicillin, cephalexin, tetracycline and sulphonamides.

Sulphonamides

Hypersensitivity to the sulphonamides is well recognized and can take several forms (Murdoch, 1965). Beveridge and his colleagues in 1964 reported an association between the use of long-acting sulphonamides and the Stevens-Johnson syndrome. We have recently seen 12 cases of this syndrome of whom only 6 had received antimicrobial chemotherapy prior to the onset of the skin and mucous membrane lesions, 4 being given penicillin and 2 erythromycin. The only feature common to all patients was an antecedent respiratory tract infection and it is tempting to speculate that the Stevens-Johnson syndrome is a manifestation of hypersensitivity to a micro-organism, the relationship with antibiotic therapy given to treat the 'triggering' infection being coincidental. We have recently studied the use of co-trimoxazole in patients suffering from salmonella infection and have noted a skin rash incidence of 8 per cent which is probably related to the sulphonamide component of this compound (Geddes *et al.*, 1971).

Other compounds

Antibiotic hypersensitivity may be manifested in organs other than the skin, nitrofurantoin for example causing pulmonary eosinophilia (Nicklaus & Snyder, 1968) while erythromycin estolate given for more than 14 days can occasionally be associated with cholestatic jaundice associated with eosinophilia (Robinson, 1961). The usually fatal aplastic anaemia which occurs in approximately one in 50,000 patients given chloramphenicol may be related to hypersensitivity reaction in the bone marrow, especially when the dose of antibiotic is not excessive. We have seen thrombocytopenia develop in a patient receiving only three tablets of co-trimoxazole daily, less than the recommended dose, suggesting a possible hypersensitivity mechanism.

Innate susceptibility to antibiotic toxicity can be related to mechanisms other than hypersensitivity. Certain people are slow acetylators of isoniazid, this factor probably being genetically controlled (Garrod & O'Grady, 1971). Slow acetylators of isoniazid are more likely to develop side effects during treatment with the drug (Devadatta, 1965). Glucose-6-phosphate dehydrogenase deficiency is associated with increased sensitivity to the sulphonamides, nitrofurantoin and nalidixic acid. Finally, sex may predispose to toxicity to antibiotics. In a study in Belfast, Hurwitz (1969) found that women were more likely to develop side-effects to drugs in general than men. Our ampicillin rash study showed a similar female predominance and nitrofurantoin toxicity also is commoner in women (Koch-Wesser *et al.*, 1971).

Acquired

Increased susceptibility to antibiotic toxicity may be acquired. Renal disease can be exacerbated by tetracyclines (Stott *et al.*, 1971) and renal failure will lead to cumulation in the blood of potentially toxic antibiotics normally excreted by healthy kidneys such as the amino-hexoses, polymyxins and nitrofurantoin. We have seen a child with renal failure develop an irreversible peripheral neuropathy as a result of long-term nitrofurantoin administration.

Similarly, drugs excreted by the liver, like the tetracyclines and erythromycin, should be avoided in patients with hepatic disease because of possible increased toxicity. Neomycin given orally over a prolonged period to patients with liver failure may be absorbed from the small bowel with resultant ototoxicity (Berk & Chalmers, 1970). It is probably better to avoid the use of neomycin for reducing gut flora in liver failure and to prescribe colistin instead.

Ampicillin given to patients suffering from glandular fever almost invariably causes a skin rash (Pullen *et al.*, 1967). A similar high incidence of rash with ampicillin occurs in cytomegalovirus mononucleosis (Klemola, 1970) and lymphatic leukaemia (Cameron & Richmond, 1971). Folic acid deficiency may develop in elderly, malnourished and seriously ill patients who might therefore become more liable to blood dyscrasias during treatment with co-trimoxazole.

Antibiotics which are safe in the non-pregnant woman are contra-indicated when she becomes pregnant. The effect of tetracyclines on foetal teeth (and possibly developing bone) have already been mentioned. Tetracycline should not be given intravenously during pregnancy because of reports of fatal liver failure associated with this route of administration in pregnant women (Kunelis *et al.*, 1965). Sulphonamides may precipitate or exacerbate kernicterus by competing with bilirubin for plasma protein binding sites (Harris *et al.*, 1958) and should be avoided if possible in the last trimester of pregnancy as should nalidixic acid which, as already mentioned, can be neurotoxic in small children.

DRUG INTERACTION

Antibiotics may interact with other drugs with resultant toxicity. Cephaloridine administered along with frusemide can lead to renal failure (Foord, 1969; Dodds & Foord, 1970) while a combination of ethacrynic acid and an aminoglycoside may be ototoxic (Kabins, 1972). Neomycin given intraperitoneally to anaesthetized patients receiving muscle relaxants may cause respiratory arrest (Craig *et al.*, 1966). Sulphonamides, including the sulphonamide containing co-trimoxazole, may potentiate the hypoglycaemic action of the sulphonylureas while broad spectrum antibiotics can increase the activity of anticoagulants by reducing the absorption of Vitamin K from the small bowel (Coon & Willis, 1970). Sulphonamides such as sulphamethoxypyridazine, which are highly protein-bound, may displace warfarin from serum carrier sites and enhance its anticoagulant action while griseofulvin may reduce this effect by stimulation of hepatic enzymes which control the metabolism of warfarin (Kabins, 1972). Tetracycline absorption from the gut may be prevented by binding with oral iron with possible increase in gastro-intestinal side-effects (Neuvonen *et al.*, 1970).

MICROBIOLOGICAL SIDE-EFFECTS

Broad spectrum antibiotics administered orally can alter the gut flora and lead to super-infection with pathogenic organisms. The tetracyclines and ampicillin may cause overgrowth with *Candida albicans*, and staphylococcal entero-colitis can complicate oral tetracycline or neomycin therapy. The administration of cephalexin is reported as being associated with an increase in pseudomonas species in the faeces (Gaya *et al.*, 1970). Although the clinical significance of this finding has been disputed we have seen a child suffering from measles, who was treated with tetracycline followed by cephaloridine for suspected pneumonia, who developed a fatal pseudomonas septicaemia.

CONCLUSION

Most toxic reactions to antibiotics are preventable if the following principles are observed:

1. Care should be taken with the amount of antibiotic given when side-effects are known to be dose-related, especially in the elderly.
2. Known hypersensitivity to an antibiotic is a contra-indication to its use.
3. Babies should not be given nalidixic acid or tetracycline and chloramphenicol and sulphonamides are best avoided in the neonatal period.
4. Tetracyclines must not be prescribed for children under the age of ten.
5. Pregnancy is a contra-indication to tetracycline administration, and sulphonamides (including co-trimoxazole) and also nalidixic acid should not be given during the last trimester.
6. Tetracyclines should be avoided in patients with renal disease and tetracyclines, erythromycin and neomycin in liver disease. The frequency of administration of the amino-hexoses and polymyxins must be reduced in renal failure in which nitrofurantoin and amphotericin B are contra-indicated.
7. Ampicillin should not be given to patients suffering from glandular fever, cytomegalovirus infections or lymphatic leukaemia.
8. Chloramphenicol should be reserved for the treatment of typhoid fever and severe haemophilus infections.
9. Antibiotics and drugs with which they are known to interact should not be administered simultaneously.

REFERENCES

ADKINSON, N. F., THOMPSON, W. L., MADDREY, W. C. & LICHTENSTEIN, L. M. (1971). Routine use of penicillin skin testing on an inpatient service. *New England Journal of Medicine*, **285,** 22.

AQUINAS, M., ALLAN, W. G. L., HORSFALL., P. A. L., JENKINS, P. K., KUNG-YAN, W., GIRLING, D., TALL, R. & FOX, W. (1972). Adverse reactions to daily and intermittent rifampicin regimes for pulmonary tuberculosis in Hong Kong. *British Medical Journal*, **1,** 765.

BERK, D. P. & CHALMERS, T. (1970). Deafness complicating antibiotic therapy of hepatic encephalopathy. *Annals of Internal Medicine*, **73,** 393.

BEVELANDER, G. & NAKAHARA, H. J. (1966). The effect of diverse amounts of tetracycline on fluorescence and coloration of teeth. *Journal of Pediatrics*, **68,** 114.

BEVERIDGE J., HARRIS, M., WISE, G. & STEVENS, L. (1964). Long-acting sulphonamides associated with Stevens Johnson syndrome. *Lancet*, **2,** 593.

BLOOMER, H. A., BARTON, L. J. & MADDOCK, R. K. (1967). Penicillin-induced encephalopathy in uremic patients. *Journal of American Medical Association*, **200,** 121.

BOREUS, L. O. & SUNDSTROM, B. (1967). Intracranial hypertension in a child during treatment with nalidixic acid. *British Medical Journal*, **2,** 744.

BUTLER, W. T., BENNETT, J. E., ALLING, D. W., WERTLAKE, P. T., UTZ, J. P. & HILL, G. J. (1964). Nephrotoxicity of amphotericin B—Early and late effects of 81 patients. *Annals of Internal Medicine*, **61,** 175.

CAMERON, S. J. & RICHMOND, J. (1971). Ampicillin hypersensitivity in lymphatic leukaemia. *Scottish Medical Journal*, **16,** 425.

COON, W. W. & WILLIS, P. W. (1970). Some aspects of the pharmacology of oral anticoagulants. *Clinical Pharmacology & Therapeutics*, **11,** 312.

CRAIG, H. V., GUILLET, G. G., WALKER, J. A. & ARTZ, C. P. (1966). Respiratory depression related to intraperitoneal neomycins. Experimental study and review of recent literature. *American Surgery*, **32,** 27.

DODDS, M. G. & FOORD, R. D. (1970). Enhancement of potent diuretics of renal tubular necrosis induced by cephaloridine. *British Journal of Pharmacology*, **40,** 227.

DEVADATTA, S. (1965). Isoniazid-induced encephalopathy. *Lancet*, **2,** 440.

FIELDS, J. P. (1961). Bulging fontanelle: a complication of tetracycline therapy in infants. *Journal of Pediatrics*, **58,** 74.

FOORD, R. D. (1969). Cephaloridine and the kidney. *Progress in Antimicrobial & Anticancer Chemotherapy*, **1,** 597.

FOWLE, A. S. E. (1970). National use of trimethoprim and sulphamethoxazole for one year—problems and solutions. *Supplement to South African Medical Journal*, 15th August, 1970.

GARROD, L. P. & O'GRADY, F. (1971). Tuberculosis. In *Antibiotic and Chemotherapy*, 3rd ed., p. 403. E. & S. Livingstone, Edinburgh and London.

GAYA, H., ADNITT, P. I. & TURNER, P. (1970). Changes in gut flora after cephalexin treatment. *British Medical Journal*, **3,** 624.

GEDDES, A. M., MURDOCH, J. MCC., WRIGHT, N. W., ORMONDE, N. W. H. & WALLACE, E. T. (1968). Clinical and laboratory experience with ampicillin. *Proceedings of Symposium on Semi-synthetic Penicillins & New Antibiotics*, p. 252. Sao Paulo, Brasil.

GEDDES, A. M., FOTHERGILL, R., GOODALL, J. A. D. & DORKEN, P. R. (1971). Evaluation of trimethoprim-sulphamethoxazole compound in treatment of salmonella infections. *British Medical Journal*, **3,** 451.

GRAY, J. A., GEDDES, A. M., WALLACE, E. T. & MURDOCH, J. MCC. (1967). The long-term management of urinary infections with cycloserine. In *Symposium on Pyelonephritis*, p. 34. E. & S. Livingstone, Edinburgh and London.

HARRIS, R. C., LUCEY, J. F. & MACLEAN, J. R. (1958). Kernicterus in premature infants associated with low concentrations of bilirubin in the plasma. *Pediatrics*, **21,** 875.

HURWITZ, N. (1969). Predisposing factors in adverse reactions to drugs. *British Medical Journal*, **1,** 536.

IDSOE, I., GUTHE, T., WILLCOX, R. R. & DE WECK, A. L. (1968). Nature and extent of penicillin side-reactions, with particular reference to fatalities from anaphylactoid shock. *Bulletin of World Health Organization*, **38,** 159.

KABINS, S. A. (1972). Interactions among antibiotics and other drugs. *Journal of the American Medical Association*, **219,** 206.

KAHN, S. B., FEIN, S. A. & BRODSKY, I., (1968). Effects of trimethoprim on folate metabolism in man. *Clinical Pharmacology & Therapeutics*, **9,** 550.

KLEMOLA, E. (1970). Hypersensitivity reactions to ampicillin in cytomegalovirus mononucleosis. *Scandinavian Journal of Infectious Diseases*, **2,** 29.

KNUDSEN, E. T. (1969). Ampicillin and urticaria. *British Medical Journal*, **1,** 846.

KNUDSEN, E. T., DEWDNEY, J. M. & TRAFFORD, J. A. P. (1970). Reduction in incidence of ampicillin rash by purification of ampicillin. *British Medical Journal*, **1,** 469.

KOCH-WESER, J., SIDEL, V. W., DEXTER, M., PARISH, P., FINER, D. C. & KANAREK, P. (1971). Adverse reactions to sulfisoxazole, sulfamethoxazole and nitrofurantoin. *Archives of Internal Medicine*, **128,** 399.

KUNELIS, C. T., PETERS, J. L. & EDMONDSON, H. A. (1965). Fatty liver of pregnancy and its relationship to tetracycline therapy. *American Journal of Medicine*, **38,** 359.

Lancet (1968). Tetracyclines and teeth. Leading article, **1,** 1360.

Lancet (1969). Ampicillin rashes. Leading article, **2,** 993.

LEIBOLD, J. E. (1966). The ocular toxicity of ethambutol and its relationship to dose. *Annals of the New York Academy of Sciences*, **135,** 904.

MCCURDY, P. R. (1963). Plasma concentration of Chloramphenicol and bone marrow suppression. *Blood*, **21,** 363.

MURDOCH, J. MCC. (1965). Toxicity of the sulphonamides. *Practitioner*, **194,** 26.

MURDOCH, J. MCC., GRAY, J. A., GEDDES, A. M. & WALLACE, E. T. (1966). Clinical experiences with kanamycin in septicaemia caused by gram-negative organisms. *Annals of New York Academy of Sciences*, **132,** 842.

NEUVONEN, P. J., GOTHONI, G., HACKMAN, R. & AF. BJÖRKSTEN, K. (1970). Interference of iron with the absorption of tetracyclines in man. *British Medical Journal*, **4,** 532.

NICKLAUS, T. M. & SNYDER, A. B. (1968). Nitrofurantoin pulmonary reaction—a unique syndrome. *Archives of Internal Medicine*, **121,** 151.

PETZ, L. D. & FUDENBERG, H. H. (1966). Coombs-positive haemolytic anaemia caused by penicillin administration. *New England Journal of Medicine*, **274,** 171.

PETZ, L. D. (1971). Immunologic reactions of humans to cephalosporins. *Postgraduate Medical Journal*, **47,** February supplement, p. 64.

POHLMANN, G. (1966). Respiratory arrest associated with intravenous administration of polymyxin B sulphate. *Journal of the American Medical Association*, **196,** 181.

PULLEN, H., WRIGHT, N. & MURDOCH, J. MCC. (1967). Hypersensitivity reactions to antibacterial drugs in infectious mononucleosis. *Lancet*, **2,** 1176.

ROBINSON, M. M. (1961). Antibiotics increase incidence of hepatitis. *Journal of the American Medical Association*, **178,** 89.

SCHWACHMAN, H., FEKETE, E., KULCZYCKI, L. L. & FOLEY, G. E. (1958–59). The effect of long-term antibiotic therapy in patients with cystic fibrosis of the pancreas. *Antibiotics Annual*, p. 692.

STOTT, R. B., CAMERON, J. S., OGG, C. S. & TOSELAND, P. (1971). Tetracyclines and impaired renal function. *Lancet*, **2,** 1378.

SCRAGG, J. N. & RUBIDGE, C. J. (1971). Trimethoprim and sulphamethoxazole in typhoid fever in children. *British Medical Journal*, **3,** 738.

STAMPS, T. J. & WICKS, A. C. B. (1972). Trimethoprim-sulphamethoxazole in typhoid fever. *British Medical Journal*, **1,** 176.

STEWART, G. T. (1967). Allergenic residues in penicillins. *Lancet*, **1,** 1173.

STEWART, G. T. (1968). Clinical and epidemiologic impact of penicillins old and new. *Pediatric Clinics of North America*, **15,** 23.

VAN ARSDELL, P. P. (1968). The risk of penicillin reactions. *Annals of Internal Medicine*, **69,** 1071.

WALLMAN, I. S. & HILTON, H. B. (1962). Teeth pigmented by tetracycline. *Lancet*, **1,** 827.

WEISS, C. F., GLAZKO, A. J. & WESTON, J. K. (1960). Chloramphenicol in the newborn infant. A physiologic explanation of its toxicity when given in excessive doses. *New England Journal of Medicine*, **262,** 787.

23

ANTIBIOTICS IN PROSPECTIVE

Round Table Discussion

Chairman: F. W. O'GRADY

IMMEDIATE PROBLEMS

Professor F. W. O'Grady

Dr. Lambert and I left antimicrobial therapy in a fairly satisfactory state at the end of the morning. Professor Brumfitt and his colleagues on resistance this afternoon left a very sad state as far as I can see. Can I start by asking the physicians around the table to what extent they feel that resistance amongst organisms is at the present time, and as far as they see in the immediate foreseeable future, seriously interfering with their clinical practice?

Professor O. L. Wade

A great change has occurred in the pattern of bacterial infection in our hospitals during the last 15 years. There is a much higher prevalence of infections with gram-negative organisms causing serious trouble and this does worry me greatly because there is good evidence that much of it is preventable. One of the major factors which seems to influence it is the unnecessary use of antibiotics especially for prophylaxis.

Dr. H. P. Lambert

You could say that we are only just ahead. It may be fairly infrequently that resistance alone is the dominant limitation of treatment, but if one adds to the problem of resistance other limitations such as the many unwanted effects of drugs and especially drug hypersensitivity you can finish up with a very serious situation.

Dr. J. F. Munro

I couldn't understand at first why a general physician without any real interest in infection was invited here, but having listened today, I am aware that for many years I have been prescribing antibiotics too often, in too high a dose, with too broad a spectrum and for too long. The only sin that I have not been guilty of is using them excessively prophylactically. One gets the impression that the pharmaceutical industry is geared to increasingly broad-spectrum drugs. This is the way which antibiotics are being advertised and I have a lot of sympathy with general practitioners who misuse drugs like ampicillin. I hope that in the future emphasis will go back to much narrower spectrum antibiotics, even possibly antibiotics specific to certain conditions.

For example, in chronic bronchitis and emphysema it would be useful to have an antibiotic which was active against pneumococci and *Haemophilus influenzae* without producing a radical alteration in other flora. I should like to see antibiotics which were organism specific, for example, specifically against *Pseudomonas spp.* It strikes me as paradoxical that when one is treating an opportunist which has crept in because other antibiotics have been exhibited or because there is a breakdown in the patient's immunological mechanism we have to rely on a very wide spectrum antibiotic.

Professor F. W. O'Grady

Several people have said in the course of the afternoon that they think that the prophylactic use of antibiotics makes a tremendous impact on the emergence of resistance. It is hard to see just how the germs know the difference between whether the drug is being given prophylactically or therapeutically. Is this really an important factor?

Professor W. Brumfitt

We use chemotherapeutic agents very badly as you indicated earlier. Either we don't give enough when there is a severe infection, or we give them arbitrarily when there is no indication. In this latter circumstance the smaller dose, which is inadequate in relation to the MIC, may play a part in selection for resistance and I wonder whether this may not be one answer to Professor O'Grady's question. In any event, the arbitrary administration is bound to lead to unnecessary, inefficient and greater use of antibiotics which is especially undesirable in hospital. We all know that if you decrease the use of a particular chemotherapeutic agent given to patients in hospital then you reduce the number of bacteria resistant to that drug. This has been shown over and over again. It is a great pity that so many hospitals have no antibiotic policy. There is too much arbitrary prescribing according to fashion and if clinicians and bacteriologists got closer together then I think we could rationalize therapy. If only we could think of some method of getting the infectious disease physician closely involved with the laboratory, we should have more rational chemotherapy.

Finally, bacteriologists should remember that a great deal could be done by more rapid diagnosis. A paper appeared in the *Lancet* suggesting that patients with leukaemia (and of course these are a high risk group and have to be treated) should receive five antibiotics simultaneously for up to 5 days. To me this is an unhappy suggestion and I cannot imagine why there was a delay of 5 days before the bacteriological diagnosis was made. In patients suddenly developing fever and suspected of having bacteraemia why not look at the buffy coat? Knowledge of the bacterial ecology in the hospital would also be important and if the organism was suspected of being a *Pseudomonas spp.* then gentamicin should be given and so on. In the same report we were told that the aspergillus was a problem and therefore it was necessary to add other toxic substances such as amphotericin B.

Dr. S. Eykyn

Professor Brumfitt speaks out against multiple therapy in acute leukaemia and I agree with him, but what would he do in the situation described?

Professor W. Brumfitt

I think it is very dangerous indeed to exhibit chemotherapeutic agents in a rash way. A patient with leukaemia is often transfused repeatedly and is therefore a candidate for hepatitis. In the pre-icteric phase of hepatitis it would be unwise and of no value to give antibiotics. Patients with leukaemia are also often receiving immunosuppressive drugs and are therefore candidates for opportunistic infections. Thus they may get aspergillus in the lung and candida in the bronchial tree and the alimentary canal and so on. I feel that in this high risk group and others such as transplant patients, we must put in a great deal of bacteriological effort. The patients must be kept under surveillance by regular culture of throat swabs, faeces, urine and blood cultures. Often a pseudomonas is found in the throat, then the faeces, and then in the urine and subsequently in the kidneys and finally in the blood. Thus there is plenty of time to isolate the pathogens and do sensitivities. Often the patient can be treated with gentamicin alone. The patient's blood level can be monitored to give a safe level of antibiotic thus avoiding side effects.

Dr. J. F. Munro

I accept what you are saying and often you can and should have monitored the patient but some patients are admitted with bacteraemia and as a straight answer to Dr. Eykyn's question I would say gentamicin. I would qualify it by saying that whenever possible you should try, where appropriate, to narrow your spectrum as soon as you have bacteriological evidence.

Professor O. L. Wade

It is becoming much more important for physicians to collaborate closely with bacteriologists. The idea of the broad-spectrum antibiotic was good. It saved a lot of trouble because it saved us from the need to make a precise diagnosis. The clinician would say, 'this man has a fever', and would give him a broad spectrum antibiotic. We now understand the disadvantages such a policy carries, but if we want to tailor antibiotic therapy for the individual infection, we have to work closely with the bacteriologists.

The main difficulty in introducing antibiotic policies into hospitals is the doctors! The trouble with medical education is that we turn out our students as independently minded doctors who want to direct their own lives, their own patients and their own therapy. Then we turn round and say we want them all to collaborate on an agreed policy. With Professor Elmes I have fought this battle over the years and it is a very very difficult one.

Dr. S. Campbell

I should like to ask Professor Wade about the influence of the hospital consultant on general practitioner prescribing and the responsibility that rests with the consultant to influence this prescribing?

Professor O. L. Wade

I haven't looked at this closely in the field of antibiotics, but I have with other drugs and there is no doubt that the family doctor is very much influenced by the advice which is given by consultants. One of the difficulties is that most of us who are consultant physicians have not worked as general practitioners and therefore don't always appreciate what the results of our advice are going to be.

Professor M. H. Richmond

Could I say one thing in connection with broad-spectrum and narrow-spectrum antibiotics? I agree that if you can get an antibiotic to hit one situation only, that's fine; but there is one real worry about narrow-spectrum compounds and that is that aiming at a specific organism doesn't stop the antibiotic coming into contact with many other organisms which may require higher inhibitory concentrations. Unless you can get a range of really specific agents, I think there are risks in partially specific therapy. For example, a particular penicillin which is very useful for staphylococcal infection, may well inadvertently come into contact with enteric bacteria and, unless it is highly organism-selective, this could have unwanted effects. A case arises in Dr. Lowbury's Burns Unit where it looks as though ampicillin and other penicillins allowed an R-factor (which undermines carbenicillin therapy when it gets into the pseudomonas) to persist in the enteric bacteria. The antibiotic that is keeping the R-factor in the enterobacteria in the Burns Unit may not be carbenicillin but ampicillin.

Professor G. R. F. Hilson

I should just like to comment on two aspects. The first is that Professor Richmond was producing a tremendous logical fallacy when he criticized narrow-spectrum antibiotics because they would half-act on other organisms, since wide-spectrum antibiotics will half-act on a much wider spectrum of organisms! The second point that nobody mentioned—although Professor Richmond introduced the idea—is that before antibiotics were thought of organisms existed in a certain state. If we stopped all treatment by antibiotics, if that were ethically possible, then in 30 years all organisms would have reverted to their original state because that was the optimum one for evolutionary advantage.

Professor M. H. Richmond

Of course the bacterial population will have shifted enormously in 30 years but I think you can't guarantee that the situation would go back to where it was before.

Professor F. W. O'Grady

We now come to another point which Professor Richmond made: that we are only keeping one step ahead by courtesy of the drug companies. Mr. Acred, to what extent do you think that we are dependent on the production of new compounds?

Mr. P. Acred

Do you mean completely novel ones as opposed to modifications to existing ones? We obviously are always searching for new compounds, either completely new or modifications of existing agents. The comments on the question of specific or broad-spectrum attack are important to us as this is one of our problems. We have basically been looking for an antibiotic which will be a panacea of all ills. However, our thinking has changed in the last two or three years, certainly to more specific antibiotics able to attack a single bacterial species. On the other hand, the general practitioner may feel that he would rather have the panacea of all ills than the problem of diagnosis which we spoke about earlier in the day.

Dr. E. A. P. Croydon

We cannot think of modern England as a closed community and must spare a thought for the developing world. It's possible to improve the bacteriological services of this country, but in countries like Africa, which are now only hours away by air, this is irrelevant. With the problems there the broad-spectrum antibiotics are absolutely essential and I don't think that we can formulate a policy that doesn't take into consideration what is happening beyond these shores.

FUTURE PROBLEMS

Professor F. W. O'Grady

Time is getting on; perhaps I could just ask the panel in turn the specific question—'Where do we go from here'?

Dr. J. F. Munro

There are two things I would mention very briefly. The drug interactions that we know about are many, but we must pay much more attention to the drug interactions that we do not know about. How do the drugs which we are prescribing along with antibiotics in the general medical wards influence their action? The other point which has been mentioned is the need for antimicrobial therapy in patients who are immunologically impotent. But what we don't know much about is the effect of antibiotics on the immunological mechanisms. These are the questions I would like to see answered in the future.

Mr. P. Acred

From our point of view we will look for more antibiotics and more specific therapy. It is important that we should look for antibiotics which hopefully will have the non-toxicity of penicillin but which will improve on the pharmacological characteristics. If we could have a penicillin in which the half-life was considerably prolonged this I feel would be an advantage to the clinician.

Professor W. Brumfitt

It is 61 years since Ehrlich said that we must search for a substance effective against pathogens and not against human cells. Hitchings succeeded when he produced a compound (trimethoprim) which has 10,000 to 100,000 times the toxicity for a bacterial enzyme (dihydrofolate reductase) that it has for the corresponding human enzyme. This was a major step forward and points the way to future research. We must not forget that there is a great deal of room for pharmacological development such as improved absorption. We now have penicillins which can be taken by mouth and give high blood levels, for example, the indanylester of carbenicillin, amoxycillin and pivampicillin. Finally we need a rational antibiotic policy to stop the indiscriminate and unnecessary use of antibiotics. I feel that such a policy would improve the efficiency and results of chemotherapy.

Professor F. W. O'Grady

Antibiotic policy in hospital or antibiotic policy outside hospital?

Professor W. Brumfitt

Antibiotic policy in hospital is based to some extent upon the knowledge of the bacterial ecology. Since most bacteria outside hospitals will be sensitive to a wide range of drugs it is merely a matter of educating the general practitioners so that he knows which drug to use for a particular infection, e.g. urinary infections outside hospital are nearly always due to *Esch. coli* and are sensitive to a wide range of antibiotics.

Dr. H. P. Lambert

I would pass up new drugs for a year or so if we could get better diagnosis and better applied clinical pharmacology of existing agents. We have been a bit exotic discussing leukaemia and bacteraemia, but I keep thinking about more fundamental problems such as Professor Richmond's sewage outfall in Bristol and how difficult it is for a general practitioner to limit his use of antibiotics. This phrase 'indiscriminate use of antibiotics' is really an insult which always seems to be aimed at somebody other than oneself! The things which really determine what we call indiscriminate antibiotic usage are not only carelessness but also matters which are never talked about in symposia. They can't easily be written down but they underlie day to day action. How ill do you think this patient is? How ill do you think he is going to be in

12 hours time? Can you go back and see him? It is upon the answers to this kind of question that the decision to use antibiotics depends. If we could improve early diagnosis we would be able to improve our antibiotic policies.

Professor O. L. Wade

I am impressed at how clever these bacteria are and am a bit doubtful as to whether the chemists are going to keep level. We have got to think more about reducing cross-infection. I took the message from Dr. Ayliffe that cross-infection is one of the major factors rather than just straight mutation in the presence of antibacterials. It is the ecology of the hospital as a whole that determines which R-factors are around and which antibiotic-resistances one has to deal with. This means a difference in the way we design hospitals. Many people get into hospital now who don't need to be in there; they could be investigated just as well outside. Perhaps patients could be put up in local hotels! I am all in favour of keeping patients out of hospital, and, to quote Miss Nightingale, 'the least a hospital can do is no harm to its patients'. There is one other area of work which may impact on clinical practice with antibiotics and that is the work on the pharmacology of cytotoxic drugs. As this work develops, there may be cross-fertilization in that the mechanisms which are effective against malignant cells may throw some light on what is useful in viral and bacterial disease.

Professor M. H. Richmond

I think that the search for new antibiotics is still important and the pharmaceutical industry have an uphill struggle at present. They would admit themselves that it is getting more and more expensive to produce therapeutically effective agents. This must be one of the pressures for using broad-spectrum drugs because the cost of development of a drug is so high that if you want to produce 10 specific agents it is going to cost quite a bit more than one broad spectrum agent. Some of the cost factors are not operating perhaps to the best effect, but I don't think we can escape that. The other big area that no one has touched on in discussion is the use of antibiotics for treatment of conditions other than infections in man. Do we treat animals or do we destroy them? There is also the big area of the use of antibiotics for food production as opposed to therapy where much could be done which would help the situation.

Professor F. W. O'Grady

Unfortunately time is short and we have only been able to touch on the answers to several important questions. There is one that we have not even asked. If we are to have new agents—especially ones with very specific and limited uses—who is going to pay for them? Regrettably we must wait to debate that important question on another occasion.

INDEX